EVOLVING KNOWLEDGE BASES

Frontiers in Artificial Intelligence and Applications

Volume 81

Published in the subseries

Dissertations in Artificial Intelligence

Under the Editorship of the ECCAI Dissertation Board
Proposing Board Member: Luís Moniz Pereira

Recently published in this series:

Vol. 80, T. Welzer et al. (Eds.), Knowledge-based Software Engineering
Vol. 79, H. Motoda (Ed.), Active Mining
Vol. 78, T. Vidal and P. Liberatore (Eds.), STAIRS 2002
Vol. 77, F. van Harmelen (Ed.), ECAI 2002
Vol. 76, P. Sinčák et al. (Eds.), Intelligent Technologies – Theory and Applications
Vol. 75, I.F. Cruz et al. (Eds), The Emerging Semantic Web
Vol. 74, M. Blay-Fornarino et al. (Eds.), Cooperative Systems Design
Vol. 73, H. Kangassalo et al. (Eds.), Information Modelling and Knowledge Bases XIII
Vol. 72, A. Namatame et al. (Eds.), Agent-Based Approaches in Economic and Social Complex Systems
Vol. 71, J.M. Abe and J.I. da Silva Filho (Eds.), Logic, Artificial Intelligence and Robotics
Vol. 70, B. Verheij et al. (Eds.), Legal Knowledge and Information Systems
Vol. 69, N. Baba et al. (Eds.), Knowledge-Based Intelligent Information Engineering Systems & Allied Technologies
Vol. 68, J.D. Moore et al. (Eds.), Artificial Intelligence in Education
Vol. 67, H. Jaakkola et al. (Eds.), Information Modelling and Knowledge Bases XII
Vol. 66, H.H. Lund et al. (Eds.), Seventh Scandinavian Conference on Artificial Intelligence
Vol. 65, In production
Vol. 64, J. Breuker et al. (Eds.), Legal Knowledge and Information Systems
Vol. 63, I. Gent et al. (Eds.), SAT2000
Vol. 62, T. Hruška and M. Hashimoto (Eds.), Knowledge-Based Software Engineering
Vol. 61, E. Kawaguchi et al. (Eds.), Information Modelling and Knowledge Bases XI
Vol. 60, P. Hoffman and D. Lemke (Eds.), Teaching and Learning in a Network World
Vol. 59, M. Mohammadian (Ed.), Advances in Intelligent Systems: Theory and Applications
Vol. 58, R. Dieng et al. (Eds.), Designing Cooperative Systems
Vol. 57, M. Mohammadian (Ed.), New Frontiers in Computational Intelligence and its Applications
Vol. 56, M.I. Torres and A. Sanfeliu (Eds.), Pattern Recognition and Applications
Vol. 55, G. Cumming et al. (Eds.), Advanced Research in Computers and Communications in Education
Vol. 54, W. Horn (Ed.), ECAI 2000
Vol. 53, E. Motta, Reusable Components for Knowledge Modelling
Vol. 52, In production
Vol. 51, H. Jaakkola et al. (Eds.), Information Modelling and Knowledge Bases X
Vol. 50, S.P. Lajoie and M. Vivet (Eds.), Artificial Intelligence in Education
Vol. 49, P. McNamara and H. Prakken (Eds.), Norms, Logics and Information Systems
Vol. 48, P. Návrat and H. Ueno (Eds.), Knowledge-Based Software Engineering
Vol. 47, M.T. Escrig and F. Toledo, Qualitative Spatial Reasoning: Theory and Practice
Vol. 46, N. Guarino (Ed.), Formal Ontology in Information Systems
Vol. 45, P.-J. Charrel et al. (Eds.), Information Modelling and Knowledge Bases IX
Vol. 44, K. de Koning, Model-Based Reasoning about Learner Behaviour

ISSN: 0922-6389

Evolving Knowledge Bases

Specification and Semantics

João Alexandre Leite

Centro de Inteligência Artificial (CENTRIA), Departamento de Informática, Faculdade de Ciências e Tecnologia, Universidade Nova de Lisboa, Caparica, Portugal

IOS Press

Ohmsha

Amsterdam • Berlin • Oxford • Tokyo • Washington, DC

ISBN 1 58603 278 X (IOS Press)
ISBN 4 274 90571 3 C3055 (Ohmsha)
Library of Congress Control Number: 2002116113

Publisher
IOS Press
Nieuwe Hemweg 6B
1013 BG Amsterdam
The Netherlands
fax: +31 20 620 3419
e-mail: order@iospress.nl

Distributor in the UK and Ireland
IOS Press/Lavis Marketing
73 Lime Walk
Headington
Oxford OX3 7AD
England
fax: +44 1865 75 0079

Distributor in the USA and Canada
IOS Press, Inc.
5795-G Burke Centre Parkway
Burke, VA 22015
USA
fax: +1 703 323 3668
e-mail: iosbooks@iospress.com

Distributor in Germany, Austria and Switzerland
IOS Press/LSL.de
Gerichtsweg 28
D-04103 Leipzig
Germany
fax: +49 341 995 4255

Distributor in Japan
Ohmsha, Ltd.
3-1 Kanda Nishiki-cho
Chiyoda-ku, Tokyo 101-8460
Japan
fax: +81 3 3233 2426

PRINTED IN THE NETHERLANDS

Acknowledgements

I must start by thanking Ana for *being* with me and everything else..., and my parents, as ever, for being the best parents in the world.

On the academic side, I would like to start by thanking my supervisor, Prof. Dr. Luís Moniz Pereira, for everything he has provided me with, during these unforgettable years. His almost full devotion to the academic and scientific causes constitutes an example filled with fruitful lessons to be learnt. His leadership has played the fundamental role in bringing our research group to where it stands now. Thank you for everything you taught me.

A special acknowledgment must go to Prof. Dr. José Júlio Alferes for his collaboration and joint work. His presence, support, and insightful comments, were always of crucial importance.

I would also like to thank both Prof. Dr. Luís Moniz Pereira and Prof. Dr. José Júlio Alferes for sharply proofreading a draft of this work.

For valuable discussions and joint work throughout these years, I would also like to thank Prof. Dr. Antonio Brogi, Dr. Pierangelo Dell'Acqua, Prof. Dr. Teodor Przymusinski and Prof. Dr. Halina Przymusinska.

I would also like to acknowledge the comments and suggestions made by Prof. Dr. Carlos Damásio, Prof. Dr. Thomas Eiter which helped the improvement of the submitted version of this Thesis into this published version.

Thanks are also due to Dr. Miguel Calejo and Prof. Dr. Paulo Quaresma for their comments and suggestions.

The warmest of thanks goes to Carolina Sobral, Dina Luís, Francisco Pereira, Joana Lima, Joana Sobral, Leonor Barata, Luís Trindade, Miguel Ferrand and Vitor Nogueira, for being the best of friends.

A thank you also goes to the guys at FBA, in particular to Alexandre Matos, Cristina Alves, Conceição Miranda and João Bicker.

For always turning scientific conferences into very pleasant experiences, I would like to thank Daniela Carbogim, David Pearce and Paolo Torroni.

Quebra-Costas in Coimbra, and Tertúlia Bar in Lisbon, have always been my places of choice for relaxing from work (although Tertúlia has often served as an alternative working place), for which I thank them.

I would like to acknowledge the Departamento de Informática, and the Centro de Inteligência Artificial, for the working conditions provided. A special word of appreciation goes to Prof. Dr. Pedro Barahona for all his effort in making it possible to write this Thesis in English.

A special word of gratitude goes to the Secretarial staff for being so friendly and efficient.

This work was partially supported by PRAXIS XXI scholarship no. BD/13514/97, and conceived out within the MENTAL project PRAXIS XXI 2/2.1/TIT/1593/95, directed by my supervisor.

Abstract

Most of the work conducted so far in the field of logic programming has focused on representing static knowledge, i.e., knowledge that does not evolve with time. This is a serious drawback when dealing with dynamic knowledge bases in which not only the extensional part (the set of facts) changes dynamically but so does the intensional part (the set of rules).

In this thesis we investigate updates of knowledge bases represented by logic programs, where the updates are far more expressive than a mere insertion and deletion of facts since they can be specified by means of arbitrary program rules and thus they themselves are logic programs. Based on the notion of logic program updates, we define the notion of *Dynamic Logic Programming* (*DLP*) which characterizes knowledge given by a sequence of logic programs, each representing a state of the world. This notion is further extended to the case where such modules can be organized according to an acyclic digraph, introducing *Multi-dimensional Dynamic Logic Programming* (*MDLP*), thus allowing the concurrent representation of several dimensions of a knowledge system (e.g. time, hierarchy, etc.).

We then investigate the concept of *Evolving Knowledge Bases* (*EKB*). An *EKB* is a knowledge base which can not only be externally updated, but is capable of self evolution by means of its internally specified behaviour. To accomplish a uniform specification of such self and external updates, we extend the language of updates *LUPS*, otherwise only capable of specifying external updates, to be able to specify both the external updates as well as the internal behaviour and its updates.

The so defined *Evolving Knowledge Bases*, with an *MDLP* based knowledge representation, allow: the combination of knowledge from different sources; the specification of external updates to the knowledge of each individual source; the specification of relations between the sources of knowledge according to elaborate precedence relations; the update of such precedence relations; the specification and update of the evolution of such precedence relations; the specification and update of the knowledge base's internal behaviour; the access to and reasoning about external observations; the specification of multiple entities (sub-agents), within an *Evolving Knowledge Base*, each independently carrying out part of the internal behaviour; the specification and update of precedence relations among such sub-agents.

Throughout this thesis, we incrementally specify, semantically characterize, and illustrate with examples, the concepts and tools necessary to the development of *Evolving Knowledge Bases*.

Contents

List of Figures

Preface

This work started out with a *belief* and a *desire*. The *belief* that symbolic based representation and logic reasoning are (still) powerful and useful approaches to the study of *Artificial Intelligence* (*AI*), and that to follow such a stance *Logic Programming and Non-monotonic Reasoning* (*LP&NMR*) are probably the best available vehicles. The *desire* to prove *LP&NMR* to be a useful framework within the context of the latest *AI* trend: *intelligent agents*.

When facing with the fact that very little had been done in what concerns the use of *Logic Programming* to represent and reason about dynamic knowledge, i.e. knowledge that evolves with time, we soon realized that this job was going to be more of a ground breaking bottom-up task instead of a goal oriented top-down one. And this is how things went.

This rather long volume introduces several completely novel approaches, such as the framework of *Dynamic Logic Programming* to represent knowledge base updates, with no distinction between the extensional and intensional part of a knowledge base, and the introduction of the concept of an *Evolving Knowledge Base* - a knowledge base which also incorporates a specification of its dynamic behaviour and where both the knowledge and the behaviour can be updated. But most importantly, this volume should be regarded as an intermediate step of a long journey. Even though several solid and stable results are presented throughout, bringing closure to some problems, many other issues are addressed for which a fully satisfactory solution is not achieved, thus opening many doors. Some people may argue that such unpolished results should not be reported in a PhD Thesis. We argue the contrary: this is *just* a PhD Thesis - the beginning, not the end.

This Thesis, as well as the authors' M.Sc. Dissertation[?] where some preliminary results on the subject of Logic Program Updates first appeared, grew within the context of our *MENTAL* agents project[1], led by the authors' supervisor Prof. Dr. Luís Moniz Pereira, at the Centro de Inteligência Artificial, and Departamento de Informática, Universidade Nova de Lisboa. The aim of the *MENTAL* project was that of establishing, on a sound theoretical basis, the design of an overall architecture for mental agents based on, and building upon the strengths of logic programming. The *MENTAL* project will be followed by the *FLUX* project[2], led by Prof. Dr. José Júlio Alferes, within which we will carry on our research efforts in these directions.

Parts of this work are based on the following publications[3]:

- J. A. Leite, J. J. Alferes and L. M. Pereira, *MINERVA - A Dynamic Logic Programming Agent Architecture*, In J. J. Meyer and M. Tambe (eds.), Intelligent Agents VIII, pages 141-157, Springer, LNAI 2333, 2002.

[1]Portuguese research funding programme *PRAXIS XXI*, project *MENTAL* (2/2.1/TIT/1593/95).
[2]Portuguese research funding programme *POSI*, project *FLUX* (POSI/SRI/40958/2001).
[3]These publications are available at `http://centria.di.fct.unl.pt/~jleite/`

- J. A. Leite, J. J. Alferes, L. M. Pereira, H. Przymusinska, and T. C. Przymusinski. *A Language for Multi-dimensional Updates*, In J. Dix, J. A. Leite, and K. Satoh (eds.), Proceedings of the 3rd International Workshop Computational Logic in Multi-Agent Systems (CLIMA'02), number 93 in Datalogiske Skrifter (Writings on Computer Science), pages 19–34, Roskilde University, Denmark, 2002. Appeared also in the Electronic Notes on Theoretical Computer Science 70(5), 2002.

- J. J. Alferes, A. Brogi, J. A. Leite and L. M. Pereira, *Computing Environment-Aware Agent Behaviours with Logic Program Updates*, In A. Pettorossi (ed), Proceedings of the Eleventh International Workshop on Logic-based Program Synthesis and Transformation (LOPSTR'01), Selected Papers, pages 216-232, Springer, LNCS 2372, 2002.

- J. A. Leite, J. J. Alferes and L. M. Pereira, *Multi-dimensional Dynamic Knowledge Representation*, In T. Eiter, W. Faber and M. Truszczynski, Procs. of the Sixth International Conference on Logic Programming and Nonmonotonic Reasoning (LPNMR'01), pages 365-378, Springer, LNAI 2173, 2001.

- J. J. Alferes, P. Dell'Acqua, E. Lamma, J. A. Leite, L. M. Pereira and F. Riguzzi, *A Logic Based Approach to Multi-Agent Systems*, Invited paper in The Association for Logic Programming Newsletter, 14(3): 13 pages, August 2001.

- J. A. Leite, *A Modified Semantics for LUPS*, In P. Brazdil and A. Jorge (eds.), Progress in Artificial Intelligence, 10th Portuguese International Conference on Artificial Intelligence (EPIA'01), pages 261-275, Springer, LNAI 2258, December 2001.

- J. A. Leite, J. J. Alferes and L. M. Pereira, *On the Use of Multi-dimensional Dynamic Logic Programming to Represent Societal Agents' Viewpoints*, In P. Brazdil and A. Jorge (eds.), Progress in Artificial Intelligence, 10th Portuguese International Conference on Artificial Intelligence (EPIA'01), pages 276-289, Springer, LNAI 2258, December 2001.

- P. Dell'Acqua, J. A. Leite and L. M. Pereira, *Evolving Multi-Agent Viewpoints - an architecture*, In P. Brazdil and A. Jorge (eds.), Progress in Artificial Intelligence, 10th Portuguese International Conference on Artificial Intelligence (EPIA'01), pages 169-182, Springer, LNAI 2258, December 2001.

- J. A. Leite, J. J. Alferes and L. M. Pereira, *Combining Societal Agents' Knowledge.* In L. M. Pereira and P. Quaresma (eds.), Procs. of the APPIA-GULP-PRODE'01 Joint Conference on Declarative Programming (AGP'01), pages 313-327, Évora, Portugal, September 2001.

- J. J. Alferes, J. A. Leite, L. M. Pereira, H. Przymusinska and T. C. Przymusinski, *Dynamic Updates of Non-Monotonic Knowledge Bases*, The Journal of Logic Programming 45(1-3): 43-70, September/October 2000.

- J. A. Leite, J. J. Alferes and L. M. Pereira, *Dynamic Logic Programming with Multiple Dimensions*, In L. Garcia and M. Chiara Meo (eds.), Procs. of the APPIA-GULP-PRODE'00 Joint Conference on Declarative Programming (AGP'00), La Habana, Cuba, December 2000.

- J. A. Leite, J. J. Alferes and L. M. Pereira, *Multi-dimensional Dynamic Logic Programming*, In F. Sadri and K. Satoh (eds.), Procs. of the CL-2000 Workshop on Computational Logic in Multi-Agent Systems (CLIMA'00), pages 17-26, London, England, July 2000.

- J. A. Leite, F. C. Pereira, A. Cardoso and L. M. Pereira, *Metaphorical Mapping consistency via Dynamic Logic Programming*, In G. Wiggins (ed.), Procs. of the AISB Symposium on Creative and Cultural Aspects and Applications of AI and Cognitive Science (AISB'00), pages 41-50, AISB, Birmingham, England, April 2000.

- J. J. Alferes, J. A. Leite, L. M. Pereira, P. Quaresma, *Planning as Abductive Updating*, In D. Kitchin (ed.), Procs. of the AISB Symposium on AI Planning and Intelligent Agents (AISB'00), pages 1-8, AISB, Birmingham, England, April 2000.

- J. A. Leite and L. M. Pereira, *Generalizing updates: from models to programs*, In J.Dix, L.M. Pereira and T.C.Przymusinski (eds), Logic Programming and Knowledge Representation, Selected Extended Papers from LPKR'97, pages 224-246, Springer-Verlag, LNAI 1471, 1998.

- J. A. Leite and L. M. Pereira, *Iterated Logic Program Updates*, In J. Jaffar (ed.), Procs. of the 1998 Joint International Conference and Symposium on Logic Programming (JICSLP'98), Manchester, England, pages 265-278, MIT Press, June 1998.

- J. J. Alferes, J. A. Leite , L. M. Pereira, H. Przymusinska and T. C. Przymusinski, *Dynamic Logic Programming*, In A. Cohn, L. Schubert and S. Shapiro (eds.), Procs. of the Sixth International Conference on Principles of Knowledge Representation and Reasoning (KR'98), Trento, Italy, pages 98-109, Morgan Kaufmann, June 1998.

- J. J. Alferes, J. A. Leite , L. M. Pereira, H. Przymusinska and T. C. Przymusinski, *Updates of Logic Programs by Logic Programs*, In M. Klopotek, M. Michalewicz, Z. Ras (eds), Procs. of Intelligent Information Systems VII (IIS'98), Malbork, Poland, pages 160-177, Wydawnictwo IPI PAN, June 1998.

- J. J. Alferes, J. A. Leite , L. M. Pereira, H. Przymusinska and T. C. Przymusinski, *Dynamic Logic Programming*, In J. L. Freire, M. Falaschi and M. Vialres-Ferro (eds.), Procs. of the 1998 Joint Conference on Declarative Programming (AGP'98), La Coruña, Spain, pages 393-408, July 1998.

- J. A. Leite, *Logic Program Updates*, M.Sc. Dissertation, Departamento de Informática, Faculdade de Ciências e Tecnologia, Universidade Nova de Lisboa, November 1997.

- J. A. Leite and L. M. Pereira, *Generalizing updates: from models to programs*, In J.Dix, L.M. Pereira and T.C.Przymusinski (eds), Procs. of the ILPS'97 workshop on Logic Programming and Knowledge Representation (LPKR'97), Port Jefferson, Long Island, NY, USA, pages 1-24, October 1997.

The order of authors, where alphabetical, is not intended to indicate the extent of the individual contributions. Part of the results presented throughout this work have been obtained in collaboration with the co-authors, and for it I thank them profusely. At the beginning of each Chapter, there is mention to the publications where the results have partially appeared. This work was partially supported by PRAXIS XXI scholarship no. BD/13514/97. The author's home page is located at `http://centria.di.fct.unl.pt/~jleite/`, and he can be reached at `jleite@di.fct.unl.pt`.

Lisbon, 28th of August, 2002

João Alexandre Leite

Chapter 1

Introduction

In this introductory Chapter we briefly outline the directions taken throughout the remainder of the work, with special emphasis on the motivation which constitutes the starting point of our explorations. It aims only at providing a birds-eye view of this thesis. Rather more detailed motivation is to be found throughout, as each step is taken.

1.1 Starting Point

The development of machines that exhibit an intelligent behaviour has always been at the very core of *Artificial Intelligence (AI)*. Representing and reasoning about knowledge is one of the most fundamental and challenging tasks of AI. Since the mid-fifties there has been a strong desire to use logic-based languages to deal with such issues. The advantages of the approach were expressed by John McCarthy [161, 164] as follows:

> Expressing information in declarative sentences is far more modular than expressing it in segments of computer programs or in tables. Sentences can be true in a much wider context than programs can be used. The supplier of a fact does not have to understand much about how the receiver functions or how or whether the receiver will use it. The same fact can be used for many purposes, because the logical consequences of collections of facts can be available.

This stance originated a wide and lasting research effort, initially leading to two main independent streams: *Non-Monotonic Reasoning (NMR)*, and *Logic Programming (LP)*.

Non-Monotonic Reasoning, diverging from the use of classical logic and its closed and monotonic domains, aims at establishing formal reasoning methods that allow an adequate representation of common-sense reasoning, inherently non-monotonic: we are constantly forced to withdraw conclusions in face of new information, something that is not possible to represent with the intrinsically monotonic classical logic.

Logic Programming (LP) combines logic as a representation language, with the theory of automated deduction. LP introduced in Computer Science the important concept of declarative, as opposed to procedural programming. A procedural language can be seen as one to specify "*how*", whereas a declarative language is one to specify "*what*". According to this declarative view, summarized by Robert Kowalski [120] as *Algorithm=Logic+Control*, a programmer should only be concerned with the declarative meaning of the program, while the procedural aspects of its execution should be handled automatically.

The declarative nature of logic programming together with its amenability to implementation made it an important candidate for knowledge representation and non-monotonic reasoning, based on the so called "logical approach to knowledge representation". The cross-fertilization with Non-Monotonic Reasoning gave rise to the field of Logic Programming for Non-monotonic Reasoning, this being the area of research of this work.

Most of the work conducted so far in the field of Logic Programming has focused on representing *static* knowledge, i.e., knowledge that does not evolve with time. If we are to move to a more open and dynamic environment, typical of these web and agent days, we need to consider ways of representing knowledge which may evolve in time. If we are to accept the Logic Programming based approach to knowledge representation and reasoning, it must prove to be an appropriate framework capable of representing not only static knowledge, i.e. knowledge that does not evolve with time, but also dynamic knowledge, i.e. knowledge that does.

When dealing with modifications to a knowledge base represented by a propositional theory, two kinds of abstract frameworks have been distinguished both by Keller and Winslett [117] and by Katsuno and Mendelzon [116]. One, theory revision, deals with incorporating new knowledge about a static world whose previous representation was incomplete or incorrect. The other deals with changing worlds, and is known as theory update. Theory revision has been extensively studied in the context of Logic Programming (cf. [3, 10, 11, 33, 87, 88, 184, 202, 229, 230]), but in this work, we are concerned with representing and reasoning about worlds that change, i.e. we will investigate the problem of theory update.

Several authors have addressed the issue of updates of logic programs and deductive databases (see e.g. [12, 56, 102, 103, 157, 194, 197]), most of them following the so called *"interpretation update"* approach, originally proposed in [116, 228].

This approach is based on the idea of reducing the problem of finding an update of a knowledge base DB by another knowledge base U to the problem of finding updates of its individual interpretations (models[1]). More precisely, a knowledge base DB' is considered to be the update of a knowledge base DB by U if the set of models of DB'coincides with the set of updated models of DB, i.e., "the set of models of DB'" = "the set of updated models of DB". The update of models is governed by the update rules specified in U, and also by inertia applied to those literals of the models not directly affected by the update program. Thus, according to the interpretation update approach, the problem of finding an update of a *deductive* database DB is reduced to the problem of finding individual updates of all of its *relational instantiations* (models) M. Unfortunately, such an approach suffers, in general, from several important drawbacks:

- In order to obtain the update DB' of a knowledge base DB one has to first compute all the models M of DB (typically, a daunting task) and then individually compute their (possibly multiple) updates M_U by U. An update M_U of a given

[1]The notion of a model depends on the type of considered knowledge bases and on their semantics. Here, we are considering (generalized) logic programs under the stable model semantics.

interpretation M is obtained by changing the status of only those literals in M that are *"forced"* to change by the update U, while keeping all the other literals intact by *inertia* (see e.g. [157, 194, 197]).

- The updated knowledge base DB' is not defined directly but, instead, it is indirectly characterized as a knowledge base whose models coincide with the set of all updated models M_U of DB. In general, there is therefore no natural way of computing DB', which may even not exist at all, because the only straightforward candidate for DB' is the typically intractably large knowledge base DB'' consisting of all clauses that are entailed by all the updated models M_U of DB.

- Most importantly, while the *semantics* of the resulting knowledge base DB' indeed represents the *intended* meaning when just the *extensional* part of the knowledge base DB (the set of facts) is being updated, it leads to strongly *counter-intuitive* results when also the *intensional* part of the database (the set of rules) undergoes change, as the following example shows.

Example 1 *Consider the logic program P consisting of the following rules:*

$$\begin{aligned} sleep &\leftarrow not\, tv\_on \\ tv\_on &\leftarrow \\ watch\_tv &\leftarrow tv\_on. \end{aligned}$$

Clearly $M = \{tv\_on, watch\_tv\}$ is its only stable model. Suppose now that the update U states that there is a power failure, and if there is a power failure then the TV is no longer on, as represented by the logic program U:

$$\begin{aligned} not\, tv\_on &\leftarrow power\_failure \\ power\_failure &\leftarrow \end{aligned}$$

According to the above mentioned interpretation approach to updating, we would obtain $M_U = \{power\_failure, watch\_tv\}$ as the only update of M by U. This is because $power\_failure$ needs to be added to the model and its addition forces us to make tv_on false. As a result, even though there is a power failure, we are still watching TV. However, by inspecting the initial program and the updating rules, we are likely to conclude that since "watch_tv" was true only because "tv_on" was true, the removal of "tv_on" should make "watch_tv" false by default. Moreover, one would expect "sleep" to become true as well. Consequently, the intended model of the update of P by U is the model $M_U' = \{power\_failure, sleep\}$.

Let us look at another example:

Example 2 *Consider the logic program:*

$$\begin{aligned} free &\leftarrow not\, jail \\ jail &\leftarrow jail\_for\_eutanasia \\ jail\_for\_eutanasia &\leftarrow eutanasia \end{aligned}$$

whose only stable model is $M = \{free\}$. Suppose now that the update U states that "eutanasia becomes true, i.e. $U = \{eutanasia \leftarrow\}$. According to the interpretation approach to updating, we would obtain $\{free, eutanasia\}$ as the only update of M by U.

However, by inspecting the initial program and the update, we are likely to conclude that, since "free" was true because "jail" could be assumed false, which was the case because "eutanasia" was false, now that "eutanasia" became true "jail_for_eutanasia" and "jail" should also have become true, and "free" should be removed from the conclusions.

These two examples, we believe, are sufficient evidence to support the claim that existing methods, based on the notion of interpretation updates, are not adequate when we also wish to update the intensional part of a knowledge base. This constitutes the starting point to this work, its goal being to investigate the problem of updating knowledge bases represented by (generalized) logic programs.

1.2 The Roadmap

Why are we obtaining these somewhat unintuitive results when performing updates using the interpretation based approach? To answer this question we must first consider the role of inertia in updates.

Newton's first law, also known as the law of inertia, states that: *"every body remains at rest or moves with constant velocity in a straight line, unless it is compelled to change that state by an unbalanced force acting upon it"* (adapted from [174]). Commonsense often tends to interpret this law as things keeping as they are unless some kind of force is applied to them. This is true but it doesn't exhaust the meaning of the law. It is the result of all applied forces that governs the outcome. Take a body to which several forces are applied, and which is in a state of equilibrium due to those forces cancelling out. Later one of those forces is removed and the body starts to move.

The same kind of behaviour presents itself when updating programs. Before obtaining the truth value, by inertia, of those elements not directly affected by the update program, one should verify whether the truth of such elements is not indirectly affected by the updating of other elements.

These examples illustrates that, when updating knowledge bases, it is not sufficient to just consider the truth values of literals figuring in the heads of its rules because the truth value of their rule bodies may also be affected by the updates of other literals. In other words, it suggests that the *principle of inertia* should be applied not just to the individual literals in an interpretation but rather to *entire rules of the knowledge base.*

The first part of this work will be devoted to the problem of updating knowledge bases represented by generalized logic programs, where we propose a new solution that attempts to eliminate the drawbacks of the previously proposed approaches. Specifically, given one generalized logic program P (the initial program) and another logic program U (the updating program) we characterize the result of updating P with U, denoted by $P \oplus U$. Due to the application of the inertia principle not just to literals but to entire program rules, the semantics of our updated program $P \oplus U$ avoids the drawbacks of interpretation updates and seems to properly represent the intended semantics. Nevertheless, while our notion of program update significantly differs from the notion of interpretation update, it coincides with the latter (as originally introduced in [157] under the name of *revision program* and later reformulated in the language of logic programs in [194, 197]) when the initial program P is purely *extensional*, i.e., when the initial program is just a set of facts.

Subsequently, we introduce the paradigm of *Dynamic Logic Programming (DLP)*. The idea behind this paradigm is simple and quite fundamental. Suppose that we are given a set of program modules P_s, indexed by a sequence of states s, each representing a time period. Each program P_s contains some knowledge that is supposed to be true at the state s. Consequently, the individual program modules may contain mutually contradictory as well as overlapping information. The role of dynamic logic programming is to use the mutual relationships existing between different states (and specified in the form of the ordering relation) to precisely determine, at any given state s, the *declarative* as well as the *procedural* semantics of the combined program, composed of all modules, denoted by $P_1 \oplus ... \oplus P_s$. The introduction of *Dynamic Logic Programming* extends Logic Programming, making possible for a logic program to undergo a sequence of modifications, opening up the possibility of incremental design and evolution of logic programs, therefore significantly facilitating *modularization* of logic programming and, thus, modularization of non-monotonic reasoning as a whole.

Whereas *Dynamic Logic Programming* provides a meaning to sequences of logic programs, it says nothing about how to obtain them. Each logic program can represent newly incoming information, totally independent from the previous states, but can also depend on the previous state of affairs. To allow the specification of such logic programs whose construction can depend on the previous state, Alferes et al. introduced the language of updates LUPS [15]. The language LUPS is based on a notion of update commands that allow the specification (construction) of logic programs. Each command in LUPS, which can be issued in parallel with other such commands, specifies an update action which, in its basic form, encodes the assertion or retraction of a logic program rule. A collection of such commands, whose execution can be made dependent on the semantics of the current sequence of logic programs, specifies the next logic program to be added to such sequence. An example of one such commands is:

$$\textbf{assert } L \leftarrow L_1, \ldots, L_k \textbf{ when } L_{k+1}, \ldots, L_m$$

This command, when issued at some state s, means that if $L_{k+1}, \ldots, L_m$ holds at state $s-1$, then the rule $L \leftarrow L_1, \ldots, L_k$ should belong to the logic program at state s. Besides such basic commands that specify the next logic program in the sequence, LUPS also allows for so called persistent commands. These, when issued, will not only contribute to the specification of the next logic program, but they will contribute as well to the specification of every future logic program, until cancelled.

This notion of allowing commands to specify more than one state transition leads us to introduce the concept of *Evolving Knowledge Bases*, i.e. transform an otherwise static knowledge base which is only capable of responding to outside stimuli into a dynamic one where update commands are made part of the knowledge base, making its evolution viable according to its own behaviour specification, possibly without any external updates.

An *Evolving Knowledge Base* is a knowledge base which can change due to external update commands, but which also contains an internal specification encoding its behaviour. According to this notion, an evolving knowledge base at some state s, consists of a tuple $\langle \mathcal{P}_s, SU_s \rangle$ where $\mathcal{P}_s = P_1 \oplus ... \oplus P_s$ is a dynamic logic program (DLP), and SU_s is the self update, i.e. a specification that partially encodes its future evolution. At each state transition, the knowledge base receives a set of external updates (EU_{s+1}) and perceives a set of external observations (EO_{s+1}). The self and external updates are combined, evaluated against the dynamic logic program and external observations, to determine the next state of the evolving knowledge base $\langle \mathcal{P}_{s+1}, SU_{s+1} \rangle$:

$$\langle \mathcal{P}_s, SU_s \rangle \overset{\langle EU_{s+1}, EO_{s+1} \rangle}{\longrightarrow} \langle \mathcal{P}_{s+1}, SU_{s+1} \rangle$$

To specify such knowledge bases, we need an update language capable of not only specifying the assertions and retractions of the object level rules in the DLP, but also capable of updating the behaviour specified by the self update. One way to extend the existing languages of updates in order to express such statements, is to allow the update commands not only to specify the set of logic program rules that belong to the KB produced by the "current" state transition, but to also specify a set of commands that belong to the self update that will govern the next state transition, i.e. we need commands to assert and retract the **assert** and **retract** commands, and we need to assert and retract these, in turn, i.e., we need nested (or embedded) commands.

Given that $\mathcal{P}_s$ encodes the object level knowledge and SU_s encodes the behaviour, we need to define a language capable of updating them both. To this purpose, we introduce the *Knowledge And Behaviour Update Language* (*KABUL*) as a language to fully specify such *Evolving Knowledge Bases.*

Even though the main motivation behind the introduction of *DLP* was to represent the evolution of knowledge in time, the relationship between the different states can encode other aspects of a system. In fact, since its introduction, *DLP* (and *LUPS*) has been employed to represent a stock of features of a system, some of which explored in this work, namely as a means to represent and reason about the evolution of knowledge in time; combine rules learnt by a diversity of agents; reason about updates of agents' beliefs; model agent interaction; model and reason about actions; resolve inconsistencies in metaphorical reasoning. The common property among these applications of *DLP* is that the states associated with the given set of theories encode a single one of several possible representational dimensions (e.g. time, hierarchies, domains,...). This is so inasmuch *DLP* is defined for linear sequences of states alone.

For example, *DLP* can be used to model the relationship of a hierarchical related group of agents, and *DLP* can be used to model the evolution of a single agency over time. But *DLP*, as it stands, cannot deal with both settings at once, and model the evolution of one such group of agents over time. An instance of such a multi-dimensional scenario can be found in legal reasoning, where the legislative agency is divided conforming to a hierarchy of power, governed by the principle *Lex Superior (Lex Superior Derogat Legi Inferiori)* according to which the rule issued by a higher hierarchical authority overrides the one issued by a lower one, and the evolution of law in time is governed by the principle *Lex Posterior (Lex Posterior Derogat Legi Priori)* according to which the rule enacted at a later point in time overrides the earlier one. *DLP* can be used to model each of these principles separately, by using the sequence of states to represent either the hierarchy or time, but is unable to cope with both at once when they interact.

In order to overcome this limitation, we introduce *Multi-dimensional Dynamic Logic Programming* ($\mathcal{MDLP}$). According to $\mathcal{MDLP}$, a generalization of *DLP*, knowledge is given by a set of logic programs, indexed by collections of states organized into arbitrary acyclic directed graphs (*DAG*s) representing precedence relations. $\mathcal{MDLP}$ assigns semantics to sets and subsets of logic programs, depending on how they stand in relation to one another, as defined by the acyclic digraph (*DAG*) that represents the states and their configuration. The extra flexibility afforded by the *DAG* allows $\mathcal{MDLP}$ to provide a semantic framework for the representation, in a unified manner and with precise declarative and procedural semantics, to not only knowledge represented by logic programs related according to some hierarchy (possibly involving multiple inheritance), but also to represent its inner dynamics, i.e. its evolution in time, as well as any other aspect of a knowledge system that is representable in *DLP*. By dint of such natural generalization, $\mathcal{MDLP}$ affords extra expressiveness, thereby enlarging the latitude of logic programming applications unifiable under a single framework. The generality and flexibility provided by a *DAG* ensures a wide scope and variety of new possibilities. By virtue of the newly added characteristics of multiplicity and composition, $\mathcal{MDLP}$ provides a "societal" viewpoint in Logic Programming, important in these web and agent days, for combining knowledge in general.

Whereas $\mathcal{MDLP}$ provides a declarative and procedural semantics of a sequence of program updates, based on a hierarchy determined by a *DAG,* as it was the case with *DLP,* it does not provide any language for the specification of such multi-dimensional updates, which depend on the knowledge acquired in the intervening states and on the topology of the *DAG.* It also does not provide any language for the specification (and possible updating) of the precedence topology itself. To address this issue, we extend *KABUL* with the powerful capability of specifying and updating evolving knowledge bases which enjoy the extra capabilities provided by $\mathcal{MDLP}$.

This last piece of the puzzle, which embeds all previously introduced ones, allows the specification, with a precise semantical characterization, of rather elaborate *Evolving Knowledge Bases* with features such as the abilities to:

- combine knowledge from different sources;
- specify external updates to the knowledge of each individual source;
- relate the sources of knowledge according to elaborate precedence relations;
- update such precedence relations;
- specify and update the evolution of such precedence relations;
- specify and update the internal behaviour of the knowledge base;
- access and reason about external observations;
- specify multiple entities (sub-agents), within an evolving knowledge base, each independently carrying out part of the internal behaviour;
- specify and update precedence relations among such sub-agents;

1.3 The Route

The remainder of this work is structured as follows:

Chapter 2 - Logic Programming For Non-Monotonic Reasoning: Along this Chapter we provide a bird's-eye view of the field of *Logic Programming for Non-Monotonic Reasoning.* We start with a brief historical perspective before presenting the syntax and semantics of logic programs used throughout this work. In particular, we present a class of logic programs with default negation both in the premises and conclusions of clauses, and present its stable semantics. These programs, dubbed *generalized logic programs*, play an important role within the context of updates of knowledge bases and will constitute our main knowledge representation vehicle.

Chapter 3 - Dynamic Logic Programming: In this Chapter we investigate updates of knowledge bases represented by logic programs. In order to represent negative information we use generalized logic programs. We start by introducing the notion of an update $P \oplus U$ of one logic program P by another logic program U. Subsequently, we provide a precise semantic characterization of $P \oplus U$, and study some basic properties of program updates. In particular, we show that our update programs generalize the notion of interpretation update. We then extend this notion to compositional sequences of logic programs updates $P_1 \oplus P_2 \oplus \ldots$, introducing the paradigm of *Dynamic Logic Programming.* We also study some properties of *DLP*, present some illustrative examples and compare *DLP* with other approaches to updates.

Chapter 4 - Knowledge Update Language: Whereas DLP provides a framework and semantics to determine the meaning of sequences of logic programs, it does not provide a mechanism to construct such programs. Languages of updates accomplish this goal, and are the subject of this Chapter. We start with an overview of the language of updates LUPS [15] and its extension EPI [75]. Then we identify an intuitively incorrect behaviour of LUPS semantics and one possible, important, extension to its syntax. To address these issues, the *Knowledge Update Language* (*KUL*) is introduced and compared to its predecessors. Finally, we present some illustrative examples and show how *KUL* can be used to specify the effects of actions.

Chapter 5 - Knowledge and Behaviour Update Language: In this Chapter we extend the language of updates *KUL* with several features, the most important being the possibility to allow the knowledge base to evolve not only due to external updates but also due to self updates, thereby introducing the *Knowledge And Behaviour Update Language* (*KABUL*) that allows the specification of updates to both the object level knowledge base and to the self-updates that encode the behaviour of the knowledge base. Examples and comparisons are presented.

Chapter 6 - Multi-Dimensional Dynamic Logic Programming: In this Chapter we introduce $\mathcal{MDLP}$, a generalization of *DLP* that allows knowledge to be given by a set of logic programs, indexed by collections of states organized into arbitrary acyclic directed graphs (*DAG*s) representing precedence relations among those states. Several illustrative examples are also presented.

Chapter 7 - Multi-Dimensional Update Language: In this Chapter, we extend *KABUL* with the powerful capability of specifying and updating evolving knowledge bases which enjoy the extra capabilities provided by $\mathcal{MDLP}$.

Chapter 8 - Illustrative Examples: In this Chapter we present two applications of the framework set forth, rather more elaborate than the examples proffered throughout. The first concerns the modelling of a financial advisory knowledge base which combines the advice with provenance in different advisors, together with stock market data, to produce stock acquisition recommendations. The second concerns the use of $\mathcal{MDLP}$ and *KABUL* as the basis for representing agents' epistemic states.

Chapter 9 - Concluding Remarks: In this Chapter we wrap up and conclude, pointing towards future research directions.

The best way to digest this document is to go through it in sequence. Most of the Chapters build on the previous one, and each is necessary to understand the subsequent one. The only exception concerns Chapter 6 which builds on the theories set forth in Chapter 3, and can be read before moving to Chapters 4 and 5. We have therefore the following two reading paths:

$$1 \longrightarrow 2 \longrightarrow 3 \longrightarrow 4 \longrightarrow 5 \longrightarrow 6 \longrightarrow 7 \longrightarrow 8 \longrightarrow 9$$
$$1 \longrightarrow 2 \longrightarrow 3 \longrightarrow 6 \longrightarrow 4 \longrightarrow 5 \longrightarrow 7 \longrightarrow 8 \longrightarrow 9$$

For the reader interested in the semantics of logic program modules, arranged either as a sequence or as a DAG, and who is not concerned with the way such programs are obtained, we can also suggest the following short reading path:

$$1 \longrightarrow 2 \longrightarrow 3 \longrightarrow 6$$

Appendix A contains a List of Symbols.

1.3.1 Milestones

The main contributions of this thesis, supported on extensive joint work, are:

- definition of a precise semantics for rule based updates, based on the application of the *principle of inertia* to rules rather than model literals, leading to the notion of updates based on causal rejection of rules, characterizing the result of updating a (generalized) logic program P by another (generalized) logic program U;

- introduction of the paradigm of *Dynamic Logic Programming* (*DLP*), characterizing knowledge provided by sequences of (generalized) logic programs;

- extension of *DLP* to deal with programs indexed by acyclic digraphs, introducing *Multi-dimensional Dynamic Logic Programming* ($\mathcal{MDLP}$);

- introduction of the *Knowledge and Behaviour Update Language* (*KABUL*), by specifying its syntax and *DLP* based semantics, as a framework to specify evolving knowledge bases;

- extension of *KABUL* to deal with the evolution of $\mathcal{MDLP}$ based evolving knowledge bases;

- presentation of several examples, along the entire work, to illustrate the applicability and power of all contributions;

- coherent, consolidated and progressive presentation of the above.

Several important issues could not be covered here, such as for example establishing three valued well founded semantics for updates, or integrate them with other existing non-monotonic reasoning frameworks such as preferences, revision, to name a few. Throughout this thesis we will comment on such issues, that were left unexplored, opening doors for future research paths.

1.4 About the Route

Over recent years, the notion of agency has claimed a major role in defining the trends of modern research. Influencing a broad spectrum of disciplines such as Sociology, Psychology, among others, the agent paradigm virtually invaded every sub-field of Computer Science (c.f. [114] for a survey). Although commonly implemented by means of imperative languages, mainly for reasons of efficiency, the agent concept has recently increased its influence in the research and development of computational logic based systems. Since efficiency is not always the crucial issue, but clear specification and correctness is, *Logic Programming* and *Non-monotonic Reasoning* have been revived back into the spotlight [4, 114, 123, 160, 208, 211].

The *Logic Programming* paradigm provides a well-defined, general, integrative, encompassing, and rigorous framework for systematically studying computation, be it syntax, semantics, procedures, or attending implementations, environments, tools, and standards. *LP* approaches problems, and provides solutions, at a sufficient level of abstraction so that they generalize from problem domain to problem domain. This is afforded by the nature of its very foundation in logic, both in substance and method, and constitutes one of its major assets. To this accrues the recent significant improvements in the efficiency of *Logic Programming* implementations for *Non-monotonic Reasoning* [69, 176, 216, 231]. Besides allowing for a unified declarative and procedural semantics, eliminating the traditional wide gap between theory and practice, the use of several and quite powerful results in the field of non-monotonic extensions to *Logic Programming (LP)*, such as belief revision, inductive learning, argumentation, preferences, abduction, etc.[211] can represent an important composite added value to the design of rational agents. These results, together with the improvement in efficiency, allow the referred mustering of *Logic Programming* and *Non-monotonic Reasoning* to accomplish a felicitous degree of combination between reactive and rational behaviours of agents, the *Holy Grail* of modern *Artificial Intelligence*, whilst preserving clear and precise specification enjoyed by declarative languages.

Until recently, *Logic Programming* could be seen as a good representation language for static knowledge. If we are to move to a more open and dynamic environment, typical of the agency paradigm, we need to consider ways of representing and integrating knowledge from different sources which may evolve in time. Moreover, an agent not only comprises knowledge about each state, but also some form of knowledge about the transitions between states. This knowledge about state transitions can represent the agent's knowledge about the environment's (or other agents') evolution, as well as its own behaviour and evolution.

The introduction of Evolving Knowledge Bases allows for a unified declarative specification of such states, state transitions and their evolution, whilst preserving the underlying Logic Programming based representation, thus making it amenable to be the melting pot for combining existing non-monotonic extensions to Logic Programming. We therefore hope that this work contributes to the opening of *Logic Programming for Non-monotonic Reasoning* to these otherwise unreachable dynamic worlds, typical of the agency paradigm.

Chapter 2

Logic Programming for Non-Monotonic Reasoning

In this chapter we provide a birds-eye view of the field of Logic Programming for Non-Monotonic Reasoning. We start with a brief historical perspective before presenting the syntax and semantics of logic programs, used throughout this work. In particular, we define a class of logic programs with default negation both in the premises and conclusions of clauses, and present its stable semantics. These programs, dubbed generalized logic programs, *play an important role within the context of updates of knowledge bases and will constitute our main knowledge representation vehicle. Parts of this Chapter appeared in [5–8].*

2.1 Introduction

The basic paradigm used throughout this work is Logic Programming, in particular its use for Knowledge Representation and Non-Monotonic Reasoning. In this Chapter we provide the reader with a brief overview of this area of research, with particular emphasis on the definitions and results that will be used subsequently.

Following this Introduction, we set Logic Programming for Non-Monotonic Reasoning in context, with a brief historical perspective with pointers to relevant literature. Subsequently, we present the syntax of logic programs. In Sections 2.4 and 2.5 we present the stable model semantics for several classes of logic programs. In Section 2.6 we set forth a general class of logic programs, not introduced in the previous sections, whose main characteristic is in allowing its rules to employ default negation both in the premises as well as in the conclusions. We extend the stable model semantics for this class of programs, dubbed generalized logic programs, that constitute the basic knowledge representation paradigm used throughout this work. In Section 2.7 we briefly mention some other relevant issues in the context of logic programming. The overview in this Chapter is partially based on those appearing in [27, 65, 145, 189].

2.2 Brief Historical Perspective

The field of logic programming for knowledge representation and non-monotonic reasoning, by now a very well established research area, confirmed by the recent large amount of dedicated international meetings and publications (e.g. [14, 23, 43, 62, 63, 66–68, 71, 72, 83, 90, 112, 126, 128, 147, 150, 152–154, 156, 167, 173, 177, 180, 188, 214, 215, 217, 221, 226]), can, nowadays, be seen as the merging of two initially distinct areas of research: that of non-monotonic reasoning and that of logic programming.

Since the mid-fifties there has been a strong intent to use logic-based languages for representing and reasoning about knowledge. The advantages of such were originally expressed by John McCarthy [161] and later rephrased in [164] as follows:

> Expressing information in declarative sentences is far more modular than expressing it in segments of computer programs or in tables. Sentences can be true in a much wider context than programs can be used. The supplier of a fact does not have to understand much about how the receiver functions or how or whether the receiver will use it. The same fact can be used for many purposes, because the logical consequences of collections of facts can be available.

This idea was developed by many researchers using the classical logic of the predicate calculus, at first, because of its well defined semantics together with a well understood inference mechanism and an expressive power capable of representing mathematical knowledge. Soon they realized that the monotonic characteristic of such theories, whereby the addition of new axioms proved in them never leads to the loss of previously proved theorems, was inadequate to represent common-sense reasoning which is inherently non-monotonic: we are constantly forced to withdraw conclusions in the face of new information. This led to the investigation on a new class of logics - non-monotonic logics - of which, the most well known are circumscription [144, 162, 163], default logic [205] and non-monotonic modal logics [165, 166, 170]. For more on the early work on non-monotonic reasoning permit us to suggest the collection of papers [99], the survey [206], the book [22] and the papers [40, 100, 169, 207].

Simultaneously, other researchers were investigating the idea of combining logic, as a representation language, with the theory of automated deduction. Early relevant work is due to Kowalski [119, 120] and Colmerauer et al. [48] who defined and implemented the first PROLOG interpreter, based on a model theoretic, fixpoint and operational semantics for the Horn-clause fragment. This was the beginning of the paradigm of Logic Programming. The late 1970's also witnessed the beginning of the development of the formal foundations of Logic Programming, in particular with the work of van Emden and Kowalski [82] on the least model semantics, the first PROLOG compiler [225], Clark's work on program completion [47] and Reiter's work on the closed world assumption [204], leading to the formalization of *negation-as-finite-failure* in PROLOG. The first book devoted to the foundations of logic Programming appeared in 1984 [148, 149].

Logic Programming introduced in Computer Science the important concept of declarative, as opposed to procedural programming. A procedural language can be seen as one to specify "*how*", whereas a declarative language is one to specify "*what*".

According to this declarative view, summarized by Kowalski [120] as $Algorithm = \mathcal{L}ogic + \mathcal{C}ontrol$, a programmer should only be concerned with the declarative meaning of the program, while the procedural aspects of its execution should be handled automatically.

Even though non-monotonic reasoning and logic programming shared many common intuitions and goals, for a long period of time there were no strong bridges between the two communities.

At some point, there was a separation in research directions in the Logic Programming community: on one hand, the PROLOG community was actively working towards providing PROLOG with efficient engines as well as equipping it with enough features to make it a competing full fledged programming language, often at the cost of losing its clear declarative semantics. On the other hand, investigation on logic programming languages and their declarative semantics continued, by now with a major contribution from people more interested in knowledge representation and non-monotonic reasoning. This line of research diverged from the "classical" logic programming inasmuch as the prime concerned had been shifted from modelling negation-as-finite-failure, to rather develop new semantics more suitable for knowledge representation. This can be traced back to 1986, to the Workshop on the Foundations of Deductive Databases and Logic Programming organized by Jack Minker [168] at the behest of John McCarthy, in particular to the presentation of the stratified [24] and perfect [190] semantics which, although still important for the "classical" logic programming community, were clearly inspired by non-monotonic reasoning.

Since then, most of the effort in finding the intended semantics for logic programs has been devoted to the meaning of several forms of negation.

The late 1980's and early 1990's witnessed the introduction of two main semantics for the class of normal logic programs i.e. logic programs with default negation in rule bodies, namely the two-valued stable model semantics [91] and the three-valued well founded semantics [89].

The declarative nature of logic programming together with its amenability to implementation made it an important candidate for knowledge representation, based on the so called "logical approach to knowledge representation". The use of logic programming as a knowledge representation and non-monotonic reasoning tool brought the need for a mechanism to explicitly declare falsity, first proposed in [179]. This led to the introduction of a symmetric kind of negation which may assume several names (classical, pseudo, strong, explicit) corresponding to different properties and distinct applicabilities [11, 19, 21, 70, 92–94, 109, 121, 122, 178, 179, 185–187, 196, 223, 224]. Again, several semantics were set forth for this extended class of programs [195] of which we highlight the answer set semantics [92] as an extension of the stable model semantics and WFSX [183] as an extension of the well founded semantics.

This class of so called extended logic programs has been fundamental in bridging the gap between logic programming and non-monotonic formalisms such as circumscription, default logic and non-monotonic modal logics, these bridges allowing for a high degree of cross fertilization between both fields. For an overview the reader is referred to [169].

During the 1990's a considerable amount of research has been devoted to extend the class of logic programs to allow for disjunctive information. As shown in [78–80], formalisms that allow for disjunctive information are more expressive and more natural to use for they permit direct translation of disjunctive statements often found in natural language and informal specifications. Several semantics for disjunctive logic programs have been proposed, and we refer the interested reader to the papers [35–37, 59, 78–80, 93, 191–193, 195, 196, 209].

The theoretical work on the field of logic programming for non-monotonic reasoning led to new programming paradigms which triggered a considerable amount of effort in implementations. Of the newly developed systems we highlight the system SMODELS developed by Ilkka Niemelä et al. [176, 218] and the system DLV developed by Nicola Leone et al. [69, 81] both representing the answer-set programming paradigm, and the XSB-Prolog developed by David S. Warren et al. [203, 231] using the well founded semantics.

Throughout the remainder of this Chapter we will overview the main definitions related to logic programming for non-monotonic reasoning, while introducing others, that will be used throughout this work. This overview is by no means exhaustive and we refer the interested reader to the previously cited papers and, in particular to the survey papers [25, 27, 65, 145, 169, 189, 200]

2.3 Language of Logic Programs

By an alphabet $\mathcal{A}$ of a language $\mathcal{L}$ we mean a (finite or countably infinite) disjoint set of constants, predicate symbols with associated arity, and function symbols with associated arity. The sets of constant and predicate symbols are assumed to be non-empty. In addition, any alphabet is assumed to contain a countably infinite set of distinguished variable symbols. A *term* over $\mathcal{A}$ is defined recursively as either a variable, a constant or an expression of the form $f(t_1, ..., t_n)$, where f is a function symbol, with arity n, of $\mathcal{A}$, and t_i's are terms. A term is called *ground* if it does not contain variables. The set of all ground terms of $\mathcal{A}$ is called the *Herbrand universe* of $\mathcal{A}$.

An *atom* over $\mathcal{A}$ is an expression of the form $p(t_1, ..., t_n)$, where p is a predicate symbol, with arity n, of $\mathcal{A}$, and the t_i's are terms. An atom is called *ground* if all of its terms are ground. The set of all ground atoms of $\mathcal{A}$ is called the *Herbrand base* of $\mathcal{A}$. An *objective literal* over $\mathcal{A}$ is either an atom A or an atom preceded by the symbol $-$ i.e. $-A$, representing the explicit negation of A. The former is referred to as a *positive objective literal* while the later is referred to as a *negative objective literal.* The set of all ground objective literals of $\mathcal{A}$ is called the *Extended Herbrand base* of $\mathcal{A}$. A *default objective literal* over $\mathcal{A}$ is an objective literal preceded by the symbol "*not*" that represents default negation, i.e. it is either a *default positive literal (or default literal)* $not\,A$ or a *default negative literal* $not\ -A$. A *literal* over $\mathcal{A}$ is either a positive objective literal (or atom) or a default positive literal (or default literal)[1]. An *extended literal* over $\mathcal{A}$ is either an objective literal or a default objective literal.

A literal is called *ground* if it does not contain variables.

Definition 1 (Logic Program) *A* logic program *is a countable set of rules (or clauses) of the form:*

$$L \leftarrow L_1, ..., L_m$$

where, L and each L_i are extended literals.

We assume that the alphabet $\mathcal{A}$ used to write a program P consists precisely of all the constants, and predicate and function symbols that explicitly appear in P. The Herbrand base of P, denoted by $\mathcal{H}(P)$, is the (Extended) Herbrand base of $\mathcal{A}$.

By grounded version of a logic program P we mean the (possibly infinite) set of grounded rules obtained from P by substituting in all possible ways each of the variables in P by elements of its Herbrand universe.

[1]Note that some authors use the notion of *literal* to refer to either an *objective literal* or a *default objective literal.*

If r is a rule of the form $L \leftarrow L_1, ..., L_m$, by the head of r, denoted by $H(r)$, we mean L and by the body of r, denoted by $B(r)$, we mean $L_1, \ldots, L_m$. If $m = 0$ the rule is referred to as a fact and the rule symbol $\leftarrow$ may be dropped.

2.4 Model Theory

Throughout this work, we restrict ourselves to Herbrand interpretations and models, thus dropping the qualification Herbrand. Thus, without loss of generality [189], we treat programs as propositional objects where rules with variables are to be viewed as "schemata" that represent their ground instances.

Definition 2 (Interpretation) *By a* (two-valued) interpretation I *of a logic program* P *we mean a set of extended literals*

$$I = T \cup not\, F$$

such that $T \cup F = \mathcal{H}(P)$ *and* $T \cap F = \{\}$[2]. *If* $F = \{a_1, ..., a_m\}$, *by* $not\, F$ *we mean* $\{not\, a_1, ..., not\, a_m\}$. *The set* T *contains all objective literals which are true in* I *(i.e. those that belong to* I*), and the set* F *contains all objective literals which are false in* I *(i.e. those that do not belong to* I*). The 2-valued designation comes from the fact that* $T \cup F = \mathcal{H}(P)$ *and* $T \cap F = \{\}$ *i.e. a value* true *or* false *is assigned to every ground objective literal. Given an interpretation* I *we define:*

$$I^+ = \{A \in \mathcal{H}(P) : A \in I\} = T$$
$$I^- = \{not\, A : A \in \mathcal{H}(P),\ not\, A \in I\} = \{not\, A : A \in \mathcal{H}(P),\ A \notin I\} = not\, F$$

Definition 3 (Satisfaction) *Let* I *be a (2-valued) interpretation of a logic program* P. *We say that*

- *I satisfies an extended literal L, denoted by $I \models L$, iff $L \in I$.*
- *I satisfies the conjunction $L_1, \ldots, L_n$, denoted by $I \models L_1, \ldots, L_n$, iff $I \models L_1$, ..., and $I \models L_n$.*
- *I satisfies the rule $L \leftarrow L_1, \ldots, L_n$, denoted by $I \models (L \leftarrow L_1, \ldots, L_n)$, iff whenever $L_1, \ldots, L_n$ is satisfied by I then L is also satisfied by I.*

The notion of model of a logic program is:

Definition 4 (Model) *By a (2-valued)* model I *of a logic program* P *we mean a (2-valued) interpretation of* P *that satisfies all of its rules.*

Next we define an ordering among interpretations and models:

Definition 5 (Classical ordering) *If* $I_1 = T_1 \cup not\, F_1$ *and* $I_2 = T_2 \cup not\, F_2$ *are two interpretations with respect to a logic program. Then we say that* $I_1 \preceq_T I_2$ *if* $T_1 \subseteq T_2$. *If* $\mathcal{I}$ *is a collection of interpretations, then an interpretation* $I \in \mathcal{I}$ *is called* minimal *in* $\mathcal{I}$ *if there is no interpretation* $J \in \mathcal{I}$ *such that* $J \preceq_T I$ *and* $I \neq J$. *An interpretation* I *is called* least *in* $\mathcal{I}$ *if* $I \preceq_T J$ *for any other interpretation* $J \in \mathcal{I}$. *A model* M *of a logic program* P *is called minimal (resp. least) if it is minimal (resp. least) among all models of* P.

[2] For our purposes, to make the definitions in other Chapters somehow simpler, we use this slightly non-standard definition of interpretation where default literals appear explicitly.

2.5 Declarative Semantics of Logic Programs

We need to associate with any logic program a precise meaning, or semantics, in order to provide a declarative specification. A declarative semantics provides a mathematically precise characterization of the meaning of a program, in a way that is procedurally independent, context free, easy to manipulate, exchange and reason about [189].

Finding a proper declarative semantics is one of the most important tasks, yet one of the hardest ones. The difficulty of this task stems from the fact that there is no precise set of conditions that a semantics must satisfy, but rather only a general agreement that it must obey the somewhat fuzzy common sense and intuition. Nevertheless, some desirable properties have been identified in [60, 61] providing a framework to classify and study declarative semantics of logic programs.

There are several ways in which one can define declarative semantics of logic programs, the two most common being *proof-theoretic* and *model-theoretic* (a combination of both has been used in [124] and [85]. According to the model-theoretic way of defining a semantics, which will be used throughout this work, to each program we assign one, or a set of, intended models. In the remainder of this Chapter we describe the Stable Models semantics for several classes of logic programs.

2.5.1 Definite Logic Programs

The first class of logic programs that will be addressed is that of Definite Logic Programs. Such programs do not allow any form of negation in their rules, and are formally defined as follows:

Definition 6 (Definite Logic Program) *A* definite logic program *is a countable set of rules (or clauses) of the form:*

$$L \leftarrow L_1, ..., L_m$$

where, L and each L_i are atoms.

For the case of definite logic programs there is a consensus as to what the model theoretic semantics should be. It is based on the idea of minimizing positive information (true atoms) as much as possible, restricting it to the facts explicitly implied by the program, making everything else false, i.e. it is based on the notion of closed world assumption. The following theorem ensures that all definite logic programs have a unique least model.

Theorem 1 *[82] Every definite logic program P has a unique least model M.*

Based on this result, the least model semantics was defined:

Definition 7 (Least Model Semantics) *[82] By the least model semantics of a definite logic program P we mean the semantics determined by the least model M of P.*

The least model semantics has a fixed point characterization based on the following operator:

Definition 8 (The van Emden-Kowalski Operator) *[82] Let P be a definite logic program and M an interpretation. Then*

$$\begin{aligned} T_P(M) = \{L \mid L \leftarrow L_1, \ldots, L_n \in P \textit{ and } \{L_1, \ldots, L_n\} \subseteq M\} \cup \\ \cup \{not\, L \mid \nexists L \leftarrow L_1, \ldots, L_n \in P \textit{ and } \{L_1, \ldots, L_n\} \subseteq M\} \end{aligned}$$

The van Emden-Kowalski Operator is also known as the immediate consequence operator, or simply the T_P operator.

Theorem 2 *[82] The van Emden-Kowalski Operator has the least fixed point, which coincides with the least model. Moreover, the least fixed point can be obtained by iterating the operator T_P, starting from the smallest interpretation $I_0 = \{\} \cup not\,\mathcal{H}(P)$, until a fixed point is achieved, in at most ω steps, i.e.*

$$least\,(P) = T_P^{\uparrow\omega}$$

We denote the least model of a definite logic program P by $least\,(P)$. If $A \in least\,(P)$ we say that $P \vdash A$.

2.5.2 Normal Logic Programs

The next class of programs allow the use of default negation in the premises of their rules. These programs are dubbed Normal Logic Programs and are formally defined as follows:

Definition 9 (Normal Logic Program) *A* normal logic program *is a countable set of rules (or clauses) of the form:*

$$L \leftarrow L_1, ..., L_m$$

where, L is an atom and each L_i is a literal.

In [91], the authors introduce the so-called "stable model semantics". Informally, when one assumes true some set of (hypothetical) default literals, and false all the others, some consequences follow according to the semantics of definite programs [82]. If the consequences completely corroborate the hypotheses made, then they form a stable model. Formally:

Definition 10 (Gelfond-Lifschitz operator) *[91] Let P be a normal logic program and I a 2-valued interpretation. The GL-transformation of P modulo I is the program $\frac{P}{I}$ obtained from P by performing the following operations:*

- *Remove from P all rules containing a default literal not A such that $A \in I$;*
- *Remove from all remaining rules all default literals.*

Since the resulting program $\frac{P}{I}$ is a definite program, it has a unique least model. We define $\Gamma(I) = least\left(\frac{P}{I}\right)$.

It can be shown that fixed points of the Gelfond-Lifschitz operator Γ for a normal logic program P are always models of P.

Proposition 3 *Fixed points of the Gelfond-Lifschitz operator Γ for a normal logic program P are minimal models of P.*

This result led to the definition of stable model semantics:

Definition 11 (Stable model semantics) *A 2-valued interpretation I of a logic program P is a stable model of P iff $\Gamma(I) = I$.*

An atom A of P is true under the stable model semantics iff A belongs to all stable models of P.

2.5.3 Extended Logic Programs

Several authors have recently shown the importance of including, beside default negation, a symmetric kind of negation $-$ in logic programs. For the motivation for such extension, the reader is referred to [11, 19, 21, 70, 92–94, 109, 121, 122, 178, 179, 185–187, 196, 223, 224].

Definition 12 (Extended Logic Program) *An* extended logic program *is a countable set of rules (or clauses) of the form:*

$$L \leftarrow L_1, ..., L_m$$

where, L is an objective literal and each L_i is an extended literal.

Introduced in [92], the answer-set semantics is the first semantics defined for extended logic programs. It is a generalization of the stable model semantics for the language of such programs.

Definition 13 (Extended Gelfond-Lifschitz operator) *[92] Let P be an extended logic program and I a 2-valued interpretation. The GL-transformation of P modulo I is the program $\frac{P}{I}$ obtained from P by performing the following operations:*

- *Remove from P all rules containing a default objective literal $not\, L$ such that $L \in I$;*
- *Remove from all remaining rules all default objective literals.*

Since the resulting program $\frac{P}{I}$ is a definite program, it has a unique least model. If $least\left(\frac{P}{I}\right)$ contains a pair of complementary objective literals $(A, -A)$, then $\Gamma(I) = \mathcal{H}$. Otherwise, $\Gamma(I) = least\left(\frac{P}{I}\right)$.

Definition 14 (Answer-set semantics) *[92] A 2-valued interpretation I of an extended logic program P is an answer-set of P iff $\Gamma(I) = I$.*

An objective literal L of P is true under the answer-set semantics iff L belongs to all answer-sets of P; L is false if $-L$ is true; otherwise L is unknown.[3]

2.6 Generalized Logic Programs

As we have informally seen before, in an update setting we need to express that some atom is to become false after the update is performed, i.e. we need some form of negation in the heads of logic program clauses. While extended logic programs [19, 21, 92] already allow for a symmetric kind of negation, which can also appear in the conclusions of rules, using only such kind of symmetric negation, to negate an atom after an update, would cost us the loss of the expressive power afforded by using both kinds of negations jointly.

For a given atom A, we want to be able to express any of the following (consistent) epistemic states:

1. that A is true and $-A$ is false corresponding to the interpretation $\{A, not\, -A\}$;

[3] In the remainder of this work, we say that an objective literal L is false in an answer-set M if L doesn't belong to M.

2. that $-A$ is true and A is false corresponding to the interpretation $\{-A, not\, A\}$;

3. that both A and $-A$ are false corresponding to the interpretation $\{not\, A, not\; -A\}$.

Furthermore, we want to be able to express an update that specifies the transition between any two pairs of these epistemic states. In particular, we want make a distinction between a transition from the state represented by $\{A, not\; -A\}$ to each of the states $\{-A, not\, A\}$ and $\{not\, A, not\; -A\}$. The former can be read as a transition between a state where A is true to a state where A is explicitly false (i.e. $-A$ is true). The latter can be read as a transition from the same state but to a new state where neither A nor $-A$ are true, i.e. they are both false by default. For comprehensive studies on the differences between the epistemic meaning of both kinds of negations and their use for knowledge representation, the reader is referred to [19, 27, 189].

Let us informally illustrate this by means of an example. Suppose we have a logic program consisting of the following clauses:

$$\begin{aligned} cross &\leftarrow -train \\ stop &\leftarrow train \\ listen &\leftarrow not\, train \end{aligned}$$

whose intuitive meaning is: one should cross if there is evidence that a train is not approaching; one should stop if there is evidence that a train is approaching; one should listen if there is no evidence that a train is approaching. Consider a situation where a train is approaching, represented by the clause:

$$train \leftarrow$$

After this train has passed by, we want to update our knowledge to an epistemic state where we don't have evidence that a train is approaching. If this was accomplished with the (update) clause:

$$-train \leftarrow$$

we would cross the tracks at the subsequent state, risking being killed by another train that was approaching. We, therefore, need to express an update stating that all past evidence for an atom is to be removed. This can be accomplished by allowing default negation in the heads of clauses. In the previous example, the intended update would be expressed by the clause:

$$not\, train \leftarrow$$

In order to represent such *negative* information in logic programs and in their updates, we need more general logic programs that allow default negation $not\, A$ not only in premises of their clauses but also in their heads. We call such programs *generalized logic programs*.

Symmetry in logic programs, in particular what concerns the use of default negation in the heads of rules has long been a source of contention. Since the common reading for a default literal $not\, A$ is that $not\, A$ should be assumed by default i.e., $not\, A$ should be true if there is no evidence for A, it may seem somehow odd to state, by means of the head of a rule, that A is defaultly false. Note here the difference between saying that A is false, in which case strong negation should be employed, and saying that A is false by default. Without taking a stand in such contention, at least for the case of a single logic program, we argue that for the case of updates of logic programs such defaultly negated atoms in the heads of rules have a reading according to which such atoms should be false, by default, *again*. In this interpretation, the "*again*" constitutes the novelty, making no sense in the case of single logic programs, that render this class of generalized logic programs more than necessary, essential. We also claim that logic program updates constitute the *killer application* for generalized logic programs.

Logic programs have also been extended to include integrity constraints (denials). An integrity constraint is a rule with an empty head or, according to an alternative notation, with the symbol $\perp$ in the head:

$$\perp \leftarrow L_1, ..., L_m$$

Informally, such rule states that its body cannot be satisfied by a model. To determine the stable models of a program with integrity constraints, one first determines the set of stable model composed of all rules that are not integrity constraints and then discard those models that violate any of the integrity constraints. In [111], the authors show that there is an embedding of generalized logic programs by normal logic programs with integrity constraints, the later being obtained from the former by replacing any rule of the form

$$not\, A \leftarrow L_1, ..., L_m$$

with the integrity constraint

$$\perp \leftarrow L_1, ..., L_m, A$$

Even though this result holds for the case of a single generalized logic program, in updates the head *not* s cannot be moved freely into the body, to obtain simple denials: there is inescapable pragmatic information in specifying exactly which *not* literal figures in the head, namely the one being turned *defaultly false* when the body holds true, and thus it is not indifferent that any other (positive) body literal in the denial could be moved to the head. For example, in an update setting, the rule $not\, a \leftarrow b$ should be different from the rule $not\, b \leftarrow a$: the first states that a is to be deleted whenever b is true while the latter states that b is to be deleted whenever a is true. In single generalized programs, as proven in [111], these two rules are equivalent (and are also equivalent to the denial $\leftarrow a, b$).

In this section we introduce generalized logic programs and extend the stable model semantics of normal logic programs [91] to this broader class of programs. In [110, 146], the authors present a generalization of the answer set semantics to the class of disjunctive logic programs allowing for two forms of negation (*not* and $-$) both in the premises and in the conclusions of clauses. The class of generalized logic programs can be viewed as a special case of those introduced earlier in [110, 146]. While our definition is different and seems to be simpler than the one used in [110, 146], when restricted to the language that we are considering, the two definitions can be shown to be equivalent. It should be stressed that the class of generalized logic programs differs from the class of programs with the so called *"classical"* negation [92] which allow the use of *strong* rather than *default* negation in their heads. In Section 2.6.3 we extend generalized logic programs with strong negation, introducing generalized extended logic programs.

2.6.1 Language

It will be convenient to *syntactically* represent generalized logic programs as *propositional Horn theories*. In particular, we will deal with a default literal $not\, A$ as a standard propositional variable. To this purpose, consider an arbitrary set of propositional variables, $\mathcal{K}$, whose names do not begin with a "*not*". By the propositional language $\mathcal{L}_{\mathcal{K}}$ *generated* by the set $\mathcal{K}$ we mean the language $\mathcal{L}$ whose set of propositional variables consists of:

$$\{A : A \in \mathcal{K}\} \cup \{not\, A : A \in \mathcal{K}\}$$

Note that even though we will deal with both A and $not\, A$ as standard propositional variables, i.e. as atoms, we keep the previous designation according to which: A is an atom, $not\, A$ is a default literal, and both A and $not\, A$ are literals.

Over this language, as before, we define interpretations:

Definition 15 (Interpretation) *By a (2-valued)* interpretation *M of $\mathcal{L}_{\mathcal{K}}$ we mean any set of literals from $\mathcal{L}_{\mathcal{K}}$ that satisfies the following condition:*

- *for any A in $\mathcal{K}$,* precisely one *of the literals A or $not\, A$ belongs to M.*

As before, given an interpretation M we define:

$$M^+ = \{A \in \mathcal{K} : A \in M\}$$
$$M^- = \{not\, A : A \in \mathcal{K},\ not\, A \in M\} = \{not\, A : A \in \mathcal{K},\ A \notin M\}$$

Definition 16 (Generalized Logic Program) *By a* generalized logic program *(GLP) P in the language $\mathcal{L}_{\mathcal{K}}$ we mean a finite or infinite set of propositional Horn clauses (or rules) of the form:*

$$L \leftarrow L_1, \ldots, L_n$$

where L and L_i are literals from $\mathcal{L}_{\mathcal{K}}$ and $n \geq 0$. If all the literals L appearing in heads of clauses of P are atoms, then we say that the logic program P is normal. *As before, if r is a clause (or rule), by the head of r, denoted by $H(r)$, we mean L and by the body of r, denoted by $B(r)$, we mean $L_1, \ldots, L_n$. If $H(r) = A$ (resp. $H(r) = not\, A$) then $not\, H(r) = not\, A$ (resp. $not\, H(r) = A$). If $n = 0$ the rule is referred to as a fact and the rule symbol $\leftarrow$ may be dropped.*

Consequently, from a syntactic standpoint, a logic program is simply viewed as a definite logic program. However, its *semantics* significantly differs from the semantics of classical propositional theories and is determined by the class of stable models defined below.

2.6.2 Semantics

Definition 17 (Stable models of generalized logic programs) *We say that a (2-valued) interpretation M of $\mathcal{L}_{\mathcal{K}}$ is a stable model of a generalized logic program P if M is the least model of the Horn theory $P \cup M^-$:*

$$M = least\left(P \cup M^-\right)$$

or, equivalently, if $M^+ = \{A : A$ is an atom and $P \cup M^- \vdash A\}$.

We use $SM\,(P)$ to denote the set of all stable models of P.

Example 3 *Consider the program P consisting of the following rules:*

$$\begin{aligned} a &\leftarrow not\, b \\ not\, d &\leftarrow not\, c, a \\ c &\leftarrow b \\ d &\leftarrow not\, e \\ e &\leftarrow not\, d \\ g &\leftarrow a \end{aligned}$$

and let $\mathcal{K} = \{a, b, c, d, e, g\}$. *This program has precisely one stable model:*

$$M = \{a, e, g, not\, b, not\, c, not\, d\}$$

To see that M *is stable we simply observe that:*

$$M = least\,(P \cup \{not\, b, not\, c, not\, d\})\,.$$

Where $least\,(P \cup \{not\, b, not\, c, not\, d\})$ *can be obtained with the* T_P *operator, as follows:*

$$\begin{aligned} T^{\uparrow 0}_{P\cup\{not\, b, not\, c, not\, d\}} &= \{\} \\ T^{\uparrow 1}_{P\cup\{not\, b, not\, c, not\, d\}} &= \{a, e, not\, b, not\, c, not\, d\} \\ T^{\uparrow 2}_{P\cup\{not\, b, not\, c, not\, d\}} &= \{a, e, g, not\, b, not\, c, not\, d\} \\ T^{\uparrow 2}_{P\cup\{not\, b, not\, c, not\, d\}} &= T^{\uparrow 3}_{P\cup\{not\, b, not\, c, not\, d\}} = least(P \cup \{not\, b, not\, c, not\, d\}) \end{aligned}$$

On the other hand, the interpretation $N = \{not\, a, not\, e, b, c, d, g\}$ *is not a stable model because:*

$$N \neq least\,(P \cup \{not\, e, not\, a\})$$

Where $least\,(P \cup \{not\, e, not\, a\})$ *is:*

$$\begin{aligned} T^{\uparrow 0}_{P\cup\{not\, e, not\, a\}} &= \{\} \\ T^{\uparrow 1}_{P\cup\{not\, e, not\, a\}} &= \{d, not\, e, not\, a\} \\ T^{\uparrow 2}_{P\cup\{not\, e, not\, a\}} &= T^{\uparrow 1}_{P\cup\{not\, e, not\, a\}} = least(P \cup \{not\, e, not\, a\}) \end{aligned}$$

Following an established tradition, whenever convenient we will be omitting the default literals when describing interpretations and models. Thus the above model M will be simply listed as $M = \{a, e, g\}$.

Definition 18 (Consistency) *A generalized logic program is consistent iff it has at least one stable model.*

Throughout, by the *semantics* of a generalized logic program we mean the stable semantics.

Definition 19 *Let* P *be a generalized logic program. Let* $L_1, \ldots, L_n$ *be a conjunction of literals. We say that* $P \models_{sm} L_1, \ldots, L_n$ *iff*

$$L_1 \in \bigcap_{M \in SM(P)} M \wedge \ldots \wedge L_n \in \bigcap_{M \in SM(P)} M$$

We also say that two generalized logic programs in a given language $\mathcal{L}$ are *semantically equivalent* if they have the same set of stable models.

Definition 20 (Gelfond-Lifschitz Transformation $\frac{P}{M}$) *Given a generalized logic program P and an interpretation M, by the* Gelfond-Lifschitz transform *of P with respect to M we mean a generalized logic program $\frac{P}{M}$ obtained from P by:*

- *removing from P all clauses which contain default literals $not\, A$, in their bodies, such that $A \in M$;*
- *removing default literals $not\, A$ from the bodies of all the remaining clauses.*

Clearly, the above definition extends the notion of the Gelfond-Lifschitz transform (cf. Definition 10) from the class of normal programs to the class of generalized logic programs. The following proposition easily follows from the definition of stable models.

Proposition 4 *An interpretation M of $\mathcal{L}_{\mathcal{K}}$ is a stable model of a generalized logic program P if and only if*

$$M^{+} = \left\{A : A \in \mathcal{K} \text{ and } \frac{P}{M} \vdash A\right\}$$

and

$$M^{-} \supseteq \left\{not\, A : A \in \mathcal{K} \text{ and } \frac{P}{M} \vdash not A\right\}$$

Clearly, the second condition in the above proposition is always vacuously satisfied for normal programs. Since the first condition characterizes stable models of normal programs [91], we immediately obtain:

Proposition 5 *The class of stable models of generalized logic programs extends the class of stable models of normal programs. More precisely, an interpretation is a stable model of a normal program in the sense of Definition 17 if and only if it is a stable model in the sense of* Gelfond-Lifschitz *[91].*

2.6.3 Adding Strong Negation

We now show that it is easy to add *strong negation* $-A$ ([19, 21, 92]) to generalized logic programs. This demonstrates that the class of generalized logic programs is at least as expressive as the class of logic programs with strong negation. It also allows us to update logic programs with strong negation and to use strong negation in updating programs.

Let $\mathcal{K}$ be an arbitrary set of propositional variables. In order to add strong negation to the language $\mathcal{L} = \mathcal{L}_{\mathcal{K}}$ we just augment the set $\mathcal{K}$ with new propositional symbols $\{-A : A \in \mathcal{K}\}$, obtaining the new set $\mathcal{K}^*$, and consider the extended language $\mathcal{L}^* = \mathcal{L}_{\mathcal{K}^*}$. Atoms $A, -A \in \mathcal{K}^*$, are called *objective literals* while the atoms $not\, A$ and $not\, -A$ are called *default objective literals*. We dub elements of $\mathcal{L}_{\mathcal{K}^*}$ extended literals.

Definition 21 (Generalized Extended Logic Program) *By a* generalized extended logic program (GELP) *P in the language $\mathcal{L}^*$ we mean a finite or infinite set of propositional Horn clauses of the form:*

$$L \leftarrow L_1, \ldots, L_n$$

where L and L_i are extended literals from $\mathcal{L}^*$. If all the extended literals L appearing in heads of clauses of P are objective literals, then we say that the logic program P is an extended logic program (ELP).

Its *semantics* is determined by the class of stable models defined below.

Definition 22 (Extended Interpretation) *By a (2-valued)* extended interpretation *M of $\mathcal{L}^*$ we mean any set of extended literals from $\mathcal{L}^*$ that satisfies the following condition:*

- *for any A in $\mathcal{K}^*$,* precisely one *of A or not A belongs to M.*

As before, given an extended interpretation M we define:

$$M^+ = \{A \in \mathcal{K}^* : A \in M\}$$
$$M^- = \{not\, A : A \in \mathcal{K}^*,\ not\, A \in M\} = \{not\, A : A \in \mathcal{K}^*,\ A \notin M\}$$

As for the case of generalized logic programs, by a (2-valued) *extended model* M of a generalized extended logic program P we mean a (2-valued) extended interpretation of P that satisfies all of its clauses. An extended interpretation (resp. model) M is called *consistent* if for any A in $\mathcal{K}$, $\{A, -A\} \not\subseteq M$. A program is called *consistent* if it has a consistent model. A model M is considered *smaller* than a model N if the set of objective literals of M is properly contained in the set of objective literals of N. A model of P is called *minimal* if there is no smaller model of P. A model of P is called *least* if it is the smallest model of P.

Before we define the stable models of such generalized extended logic programs, we will define the expanded version of one such program:

Definition 23 (Expanded generalized extended logic programs) *Let P be a generalized extended logic program. The expanded generalized extended logic program of P, P^{exp}, is obtained from P by adding, for each rule r such that $H(r) \in \mathcal{K}^*$, the rule*

$$not\ - H(r) \leftarrow B(r)$$

i.e.

$$P^{exp} = P \cup \{not\ - H(r) \leftarrow B(r) : r \in P, H(r) \in \mathcal{K}^*\}$$

where $- - A = A$.

Definition 24 (Stable models of generalized extended logic programs) *We say that a (2-valued) extended interpretation M of $\mathcal{L}^*$ is a stable model of a generalized extended logic program P if M is the least model of the Horn theory $P^{exp} \cup M^-$:*

$$M = least\left(P^{exp} \cup M^-\right)$$

Example 4 *Consider the generalized extended logic program P consisting of the following rules:*

$$\begin{array}{ll} a \leftarrow not\, b & not\, d \leftarrow not\, c, a \\ not\, c \leftarrow not\, g & d \leftarrow not\, e \\ e \leftarrow not\, d & -g \leftarrow not\, h \\ not\, h \leftarrow -g & \end{array}$$

and let $\mathcal{K} = \{a, b, c, d, e, g, h\}$. *The expanded program* P^{exp} *consists of the following rules:*

$$\begin{array}{lll} a \leftarrow not\, b & not\, d \leftarrow not\, c, a & not\ -a \leftarrow not\, b \\ not\, c \leftarrow not\, g & d \leftarrow not\, e & not\ -d \leftarrow not\, e \\ e \leftarrow not\, d & -g \leftarrow not\, h & not\, g \leftarrow not\, h \\ not\, h \leftarrow -g & & not\ -e \leftarrow not\, d \end{array}$$

This program has precisely one stable model, namely

$$M = \left\{ \begin{array}{c} a, e, -g, not\ -a, not\ -e, not\ -b, not\ -c, \\ not\ -h, not\, g, not\, h, not\, b, not\, c, not\, d, not\ -d \end{array} \right\}$$

To see that M *is stable we simply observe that:*

$$M = least\left(P^{exp} \cup \left\{ \begin{array}{c} not\ -a, not\ -e, not\ -b, not\ -c, not\ -h, \\ not\, g, not\, h, not\, b, not\, c, not\, d, not\ -d \end{array} \right\} \right) \tag{2.1}$$

Even though the semantics of stable models for extended generalized logic programs could have been defined in a way such that the expansion of the program was not needed, the definition here set forth will greatly facilitate the inclusion of strong negation within the framework of logic program updating, as will become clear below.

Remark 6 *From now on, when we mention generalized extended logic programs we always assume their expanded versions, as per Definition 23.*

As mentioned before, the class of extended generalized logic programs can be viewed as a special case of a yet broader class of programs introduced earlier in [110, 146]. We review here the characterization of "generalized answer sets" of [146] given by [110], restricted to the non-disjunctive fragment of their language. We start with the notion of extended answer set of a definite extended logic program with denials (i.e. rules with empty heads, or integrity constraints):

Definition 25 (Answer sets) *[92, 146] Let* P *be a definite extended logic programs with denials, i.e.* P *is a set of rules of the form (where* L *and* L_i *are* objective *literals):*

$$\begin{array}{r} L \leftarrow L_1, \ldots, L_n \\ \leftarrow L_1, \ldots, L_n \end{array}$$

A consistent extended interpretation M *is an answer set of* P *iff* M *is the minimal set satisfying each rule from* P*, i.e. if the rule is of the form* $L \leftarrow L_1, \ldots, L_n$ *then if* $\{L_1, \ldots, L_n\} \subseteq M$*, then* $L \in M$*; if the rule is of the form* $\leftarrow L_1, \ldots, L_n$*, then* $\{L_1, \ldots, L_n\} \nsubseteq M$.

We can now define the generalized answer sets.

Definition 26 (Generalized Answer Sets) *[110, 146] Let* P *be a generalized extended logic program and* M *an extended interpretation. The reduct* P^M *is the definite extended logic programs with denials obtained as follows (where* L *and* L_i *are* objective *atoms):*

- *removing from* P *all clauses which contain default premises* $not\, L$ *such that* $L \in M$*;*

- *removing default premises not L from all the remaining clauses.*
- *replacing all rules with default heads, of the form not $L \leftarrow L_1, \ldots, L_n$, with the denial $\leftarrow L_1, \ldots, L_n$ if $L \in M$;*
- *removing all remaining rules with default heads.*

M is a generalized answer set of P iff M is an answer set of P^M.

While our definition is different and seems to be simpler than the one used in [146], when restricted to the language that we are considering as per Definition 26, the two definitions are equivalent.

Proposition 7 *The class of stable models of generalized extended logic programs coincides with the class of generalized answer sets. More precisely, an interpretation is a stable model of a generalized extended logic programs in the sense of Definition 24 if and only if it is an extended answer set in the sense of Definition 26 [110, 146].*

Proof. *(Sketch) The important points to remark are:*

- *the rules added to the original generalized extended logic program P, to obtain its expanded version P^{exp}, ensure that any interpretation M that satisfies*

$$M = least\left(P^{exp} \cup M^-\right)$$

be consistent. Note that if M was not consistent, then for some atom A we would have that $\{A, -A\} \subseteq M$. Then, there would be at lease one rule r in P (and in P^{exp}) such that $H(r) = A$ and $B(r) \subseteq M$. But if such rule exists in P, then the rule r' such that $H(r') = not\ -A$ and $B(r') = B(r)$ would also exist in P^{exp}, and thus $not\ -A \in least\left(P^{exp} \cup M^-\right)$, i.e. $\{not\ -A, -A\} \subseteq M$, violating the initial assumption that M was an interpretation.

- *the minimality of models and satisfaction of the denials in Def. 25, after being transformed from those rules with default objective literals in their heads, is ensured by the least $\left(P^{exp} \cup M^-\right)$ where L and not L are both treated as independent propositional variables, and the requirement that M be an interpretation, i.e. both L and not L cannot simultaneously belong to it.*

■

2.7 Concluding Remarks

In this Chapter we have put Logic Programming for Non-Monotonic Reasoning in perspective and have overviewed the relevant definitions that will be used throughout the remainder of this work. We have presented the class of generalized logic programs that will constitute the basic underlying knowledge representation framework used throughout, and redefined its stable model semantics in a way that will facilitate the setting forth of the paradigm of logic program updates.

Note however that what has been presented constitutes only a summary of a small fragment of what has been recently explored in this area. Although answer-set programming, alone, has been experiencing a steady growth as a novel programming paradigm, a great amount of effort has been devoted to study other paradigms, among which, the most important are those of abductive logic programming, inductive logic programming and constraint logic programming, as well as combinations of them. Although such paradigms are outside the scope of this work, we shall not conclude without providing the interested reader with the references [86, 113, 115, 129, 158, 172, 210] which constitute good entry points to explore these new fields of research.

Chapter 3

Dynamic Logic Programming

In this chapter we investigate updates of knowledge bases represented by logic programs. In order to represent negative information, we use generalized logic programs which allow default negation not only in rule bodies but also in their heads. We start by introducing the notion of an update $P \oplus U$ of one logic program P by another logic program U. Subsequently, we provide a precise semantic characterization of $P \oplus U$, and study some basic properties of program updates. In particular, we show that our update programs generalize the notion of interpretation update. We then extend this notion to compositional sequences of logic programs updates $P_1 \oplus P_2 \oplus \ldots$, introducing the paradigm of dynamic logic programming. *This paradigm significantly facilitates modularization of logic programming, and thus modularization of non-monotonic reasoning as a whole. Specifically, suppose that we are given a set of logic program modules, each describing a different state of our knowledge of the world. Different states may represent different time points or different sets of priorities or perhaps even different viewpoints. Consequently, program modules may contain mutually contradictory as well as overlapping information. The role of the dynamic program update is to employ the mutual relationships existing between different modules to precisely determine, at any given module composition stage, the declarative as well as the procedural semantics of the combined program resulting from the modules. We also study some properties of* dynamic logic programming *and present some illustrative examples. Parts of this chapter appeared in [5–8, 140].*

3.1 Introduction

When dealing with modifications to a knowledge base represented by a propositional theory, two kinds of abstract frameworks have been distinguished both by Keller and Winslett in [117] and by Katsuno and Mendelzon in [116]. One, *theory revision*, deals with incorporating new knowledge about a static world. The other deals with changing worlds, and is known as *theory update*. In this work, we are concerned with theory update only, in the context of logic programming. For insight on the subject of theory revision, the reader is referred to [3, 10, 11, 33, 87, 88, 184, 202, 229, 230].

Most of the work conducted so far in the field of logic programming has focused on representing *static* knowledge, i.e., knowledge that does not evolve with time. This is a serious drawback when dealing with *dynamic knowledge bases* in which not only the *extensional* part (the set of facts) changes dynamically but so does the *intensional* part (the set of rules).

In this chapter we investigate updates of knowledge bases represented by logic programs. In order to represent negative information, we use *generalized logic programs* which allow default negation not only in rule bodies but also in their heads. The updates are far more expressive than a mere insertion and deletion of facts. They can be specified by means of arbitrary program rules and thus they themselves are logic programs. Consequently, our approach demonstrates how to update one generalized logic program P (the initial program) by another generalized logic program U (the updating program), obtaining as a result a new, updated logic program $P \oplus U$.

Several authors have addressed the issue of updates of logic programs and deductive databases (see e.g. [12, 56, 102, 103, 157, 194, 197]), most of them following the so called *"interpretation update"* approach, originally proposed in [116, 228]. This approach is based on the idea of reducing the problem of finding an update of a knowledge base DB by another knowledge base U to the problem of finding updates of its individual interpretations (models[1]). More precisely, a knowledge base DB' is considered to be the update of a knowledge base DB by U if the set of models of DB'coincides with the set of updated models of DB, i.e., "the set of models of DB'" = "the set of updated models of DB". The update of models is governed by the update rules specified in U, and also by inertia applied to those literals of the models not directly affected by the update program. Thus, according to the interpretation update approach, the problem of finding an update of a *deductive* database DB is reduced to the problem of finding individual updates of all of its *relational instantiations* (models) M. Unfortunately, such an approach suffers, in general, from several important drawbacks:

- In order to obtain the update DB' of a knowledge base DB one has to first compute all the models M of DB (typically, a daunting task) and then individually compute their (possibly multiple) updates M_U by U. An update M_U of a given interpretation M is obtained by changing the status of only those literals in M that are *"forced"* to change by the update U, while keeping all the other literals intact by *inertia* (see e.g. [157, 194, 197]).

- The updated knowledge base DB' is not defined directly but, instead, it is indirectly characterized as a knowledge base whose models coincide with the set of all updated models M_U of DB. In general, there is therefore no natural way of computing[2] DB' because the only straightforward candidate for DB' is the typically intractably large knowledge base DB'' consisting of all clauses that are entailed by all the updated models M_U of DB.

- Most importantly, while the *semantics* of the resulting knowledge base DB' indeed represents the *intended* meaning when just the *extensional* part of the knowledge base DB (the set of facts) is being updated, it leads to strongly *counter-intuitive* results when also the *intensional* part of the database (the set of rules) undergoes change, as the following example shows.

[1] The notion of a model depends on the type of considered knowledge bases and on their semantics. Here, we are considering (generalized) logic programs under the stable model semantics.

[2] In fact, in general such a database DB' may not exist at all.

Example 5 *Consider the logic program P consisting of the following rules:*

$$\begin{aligned} sleep &\leftarrow not\, tv\_on \\ tv\_on &\leftarrow \\ watch\_tv &\leftarrow tv\_on. \end{aligned}$$

Clearly $M = \{tv\_on, watch\_tv\}$ is its only stable model. Suppose now that the update U states that there is a power failure, and if there is a power failure then the TV is no longer on, as represented by the logic program U:

$$\begin{aligned} not\, tv\_on &\leftarrow power\_failure \\ power\_failure &\leftarrow \end{aligned}$$

According to the above mentioned interpretation approach to updating, we would obtain $M_U = \{power\_failure, watch\_tv\}$ as the only update of M by U. This is because $power\_failure$ needs to be added to the model and its addition forces us to make tv_on false. As a result, even though there is a power failure, we are still watching TV. However, by inspecting the initial program and the updating rules, we are likely to conclude that since "$watch\_tv$" was true only because "tv_on" was true, the removal of "tv_on" should make "$watch\_tv$" false by default. Moreover, one would expect "$sleep$" to become true as well. Consequently, the intended model of the update of P by U is the model $M'_U = \{power\_failure, sleep\}$.

Suppose now that another update U_2 follows, described by the logic program:

$$not\, power\_failure \leftarrow$$

stating that power is back up again. We should now expect the TV to be on again. Since power was restored, i.e. "$power\_failure$" is false, the rule "$not\, tv\_on \leftarrow power\_failure$" of U should have no effect and the truth value of "tv_on" should be obtained by inertia from the rule "$tv\_on \leftarrow$ " of the original program P.

In [12] the authors addressed the first two of the drawbacks mentioned above. They showed how to directly construct, given a logic program P, another logic program P' whose partial stable models are exactly the interpretation updates of the partial stable models of P. This eliminates both of these drawbacks (in the case when knowledge bases are logic programs) but it does not eliminate the third, *most important* drawback. Let us look at another example:

Example 6 *Consider the logic program:*

$$\begin{aligned} free &\leftarrow not\, jail \\ jail &\leftarrow jail\_for\_euthanasia \\ jail\_for\_euthanasia &\leftarrow euthanasia \end{aligned}$$

whose only stable model is $M = \{free\}$. Suppose now that the update U states that "$euthanasia$" becomes true, i.e. $U = \{euthanasia \leftarrow\}$. According to the interpretation approach to updating, we would obtain $\{free, euthanasia\}$ as the only update of M by U. However, by inspecting the initial program and the update, we are likely to conclude that, since "$free$" was true because "$jail$" could be assumed false, which was the case because "$euthanasia$" was false, now that "$euthanasia$" became true "$jail\_for\_euthanasia$"

and "jail" should also have become true, and "free" should be removed from the conclusions.

Suppose now that the law changes, so that euthanasia no longer implies going to jail. That could be described by the new (update) program:

$$U_2 = \{not\, jail\_for\_euthanasia \leftarrow euthanasia\}$$

We should now expect "jail" to become false and so "free" to become true (again).

Why are we obtaining these somewhat unintuitive results? To answer this question we must first consider the role of inertia in updates.

Newton's first law, also known as the law of inertia, states that: *"every body remains at rest or moves with constant velocity in a straight line, unless it is compelled to change that state by an unbalanced force acting upon it"* (adapted from [174]). Commonsense often tends to interpret this law as things keeping as they are unless some kind of force is applied to them. This is true but it doesn't exhaust the meaning of the law. It is the result of all applied forces that governs the outcome. Take a body to which several forces are applied, and which is in a state of equilibrium due to those forces cancelling out. Later one of those forces is removed and the body starts to move.

The same kind of behaviour presents itself when updating programs. Before obtaining the truth value, by inertia, of those elements not directly affected by the update program, one should verify whether the truth of such elements is not indirectly affected by the updating of other elements.

This example illustrates that, when updating knowledge bases, it is not sufficient to just consider the truth values of literals figuring in the heads of its rules because the truth value of their rule bodies may also be affected by the updates of other literals. In other words, it suggests that the *principle of inertia* should be applied not just to the individual literals in an interpretation but rather to the *entire rules of the knowledge base.* And all the more so in Logic Programming because rules encode directional information concerning the entailment: contrapositives are not warranted as in classical logic, but must be stated on their own if so desired. The import of directionality is even more patent when updating is involved: The final update rule of the example states that if you assist in euthanasia you will not be in jail for it, but it does not purport to assert the contrapositive, i.e. that if you are not in jail for euthanasia then you will not have assisted it. In the sequel, use of negated heads interpreted as deletion will be elaborated upon.

The above example also leads us to another important observation, namely, that the notion of an update DB' of one knowledge base DB by another knowledge base U should not just depend on the *semantics* of the knowledge bases DB and U, as it is the case with interpretation updates, but that it should also depend on their *syntax.* This is best illustrated by the following, even simpler, example:

Example 7 *Consider the logic program P:*

$$innocent \leftarrow not\, found\_guilty$$

whose only stable model is $M = \{innocent\}$, because $found\_guilty$ is false by default. Suppose now that the update U states that the person has been found guilty, represented by the following rule:

$$found\_guilty \leftarrow$$

Using the interpretation approach, we would obtain $M_U = \{innocent, found\_guilty\}$ *as the only update of* M *by* U *thus leading us to the counter-intuitive conclusion that the person is both innocent and guilty. This is because* $found\_guilty$ *must be added to the model* M *and yet its addition does not force us to make innocent false. However, it is intuitively clear that the interpretation* $M_U^{'} = \{found\_guilty\}$, *stating that the person is guilty but no longer presumed innocent, should be the only model of the updated program. Observe, however, that the program* P *is* semantically equivalent *to program* P' *consisting of the following rule:*

$$innocent \leftarrow$$

because the programs P *and* P' *have exactly the same set of stable models, namely the model* M. *Nevertheless, while the model* $M_U = \{innocent, found\_guilty\}$ *is not the intended model of the update of* P *by* U *it is in fact the only reasonable model of the update of* P' *by* U.

In this chapter we investigate the problem of updating knowledge bases represented by generalized logic programs and we propose a new solution to this problem that attempts to eliminate the drawbacks of the previously proposed approaches. Specifically, given one generalized logic program P (the so called initial program) and another logic program U (the updating program) we define a new generalized logic program $P \uplus U$ called the *update* of P by U. The definition of the updated program $P \uplus U$ does not require any computation of the models of either P or U and is in fact obtained by means of a simple, *linear-time* transformation of the programs P and U. As a result, the update transformation can be accomplished very efficiently and its *implementation* is quite straightforward.

Due to the application of the inertia principle not just to literals but to entire program rules, the semantics of our updated program $P \uplus U$ avoids the drawbacks of interpretation updates and it seems to properly represent the intended semantics. As mentioned above, the updated program $P \uplus U$ does not just depend on the *semantics* of the programs P and U, as it was the case with interpretation updates, but it also depends on their *syntax*. In order to make the meaning of the updated program clear and easily verifiable, we provide a *complete characterization* of the semantics of update operation of P by U denoted by $P \oplus U$.

Nevertheless, while our notion of program update significantly differs from the notion of interpretation update, it coincides with the latter (as originally introduced in [157] under the name of *revision program* and later reformulated in the language of logic programs in [194, 197]) when the initial program P is purely *extensional*, i.e., when the initial program is just a set of facts. Our definition also allows significant flexibility and can be easily modified to handle updates which incorporate *contradiction removal* or specify different inertia rules. Consequently, our approach can be viewed as introducing a general dynamic logic programming *framework for updating logic programs* which can be suitably modified to make it fit different application domains and requirements.

Finally, we extend the notion of program updates to sequences of programs, defining the so called *dynamic program updates*. The idea of dynamic updates is very simple and quite fundamental. Suppose that we are given a set of program modules P_s, indexed by different states of the world s. Each program P_s contains some knowledge that is supposed to be true at the state s. Different states may represent different time periods or different sets of priorities or perhaps even different viewpoints. Consequently, the individual program modules may contain mutually contradictory as well as overlapping information. The role of the dynamic program update $\biguplus\{P_s : s \in \mathcal{T}\}$ is to use the mutual relationships existing between different states (as specified by the order relation) to precisely determine, at any given state s, the *declarative* as well as the (transformational based) *procedural* semantics of the combined program, composed of all modules.

Consequently, the notion of a dynamic program update supports the important paradigm of *dynamic logic programming*. Given individual and largely *independent* program modules P_s describing our knowledge at different states of the world (for example, the knowledge acquired at different times), the dynamic program update $\biguplus\{P_s : s \in \mathcal{T}\}$ specifies the exact meaning of the union of these programs. Dynamic programming significantly facilitates *modularization* of logic programming and, thus, modularization of non-monotonic reasoning as a whole. Whereas traditional logic programming has concerned itself mostly with representing static knowledge, we show how to use logic programs to represent dynamically changing knowledge.

The remainder of this Chapter is structured as follows: In Section 3.2 we investigate the problem of updating a logic program P by another logic program U. In Section 3.3 we introduce the notion of dynamic logic programming. In Section 3.5 we draw some comparisons with related work. We close the Chapter with a Section devoted to some concluding remarks and open issues.

3.2 Logic Program Updates

In this Section we investigate the problem of updating a logic program P by another logic program U. It is structured as follows: In Section 3.2.1 we provide a complete characterization of the semantics of $P \oplus U$ and in Section 3.2.3 we study their basic properties. In Section 3.2.2 we provide an equivalent characterization of $P \oplus U$ based on a syntactical transformation.

3.2.1 Declarative Semantics

In this section we provide a complete semantic characterization of update programs $P \oplus U$ by describing their stable models. This characterization shows precisely how the semantics of the update program $P \oplus U$ depends on the syntax and semantics of the programs P and U.

When we generalize the notion of update, from interpretations to the new case where we want to actually update programs, the resulting update program should be made to depend only on the initial program and on the update program, and not on any specific initial interpretation. An interpretation should be a model of the (original) logic program updated by another (update) logic program if the truth of each of its literals is either supported by a rule of the update program with a body that is satisfied by the interpretation or, in case there isn't one, by a rule of the original program whose conclusion is not contravened by the update program. In case there are no rules with a body that is satisfied by the interpretation, for some atom A, in either of the logic programs, its default negation, i.e. *not* A, is assumed. We refer to the set of such default literals as the *set of defaults*.

Another way to view program updating, and in particular the role of inertia, is to say that the rules of the original program carry over to the updated program, due to inertia, instead of the truth of interpretation literals like in interpretation based updates, just in case they are not overruled by the update program. This is to be preferred because the rules encode more information than the literals. Inertia of literals is a special case of rule inertia since literals can be coded as factual rules.

To achieve rule inertia we start by defining the sub program of the initial program which contains the rules that should persist in the updated program due to inertia. We use this program together with the update program and the set of defaults to characterize $P \oplus U$.

We now formalize these notions and define:

Definition 27 (Conflicting Rules) *We say that two rules r and r' are conflicting, denoted by $r \bowtie r'$, iff $H(r) = not\, H(r')$.*

Definition 28 *Let P and U be generalized logic programs in the language $\mathcal{L} = \mathcal{L}_K$. For any interpretation M of the language $\mathcal{L}$ define:*

$$\begin{aligned} Rejected\,(M) &= \{r \mid r \in P, \exists r' \in U, r \bowtie r', M \models B(r),\ M \models B(r')\} \\ Defaults\,(M) &= \{not\, A \mid \nexists r \in P \cup U : H(r) = A \wedge M \models B(r)\} \\ Residue\,(M) &= P \cup U - Rejected\,(M) \end{aligned}$$

The set $Defaults(M)$ contains default negations $not\, A$ of all *unsupported* atoms A in M, i.e., atoms that have the property that the body of every clause from $P \cup U$ with the head A is false in M. Consequently, negation $not\, A$ of these unsupported atoms A can be assumed by default. The set $Rejected\,(M) \subseteq P$ represents the set of clauses of the original program P that are *rejected* (or contradicted) by the update program U and the interpretation M. The residue $Residue(M)$ consists of all clauses in the union $P \cup U$ of programs P and U that were *not* rejected by the update program U. Note that all the three sets depend on the interpretation M as well as on the *syntax* of the programs P and U.

Now we are able to describe the semantics of $P \oplus U$ by providing a complete characterization of its stable models.

Definition 29 (Stable Models of $P \oplus U$) *Let P and U be generalized logic programs in the language $\mathcal{L}$. An interpretation M of the language $\mathcal{L}$ is a stable model of $P \oplus U$ if and only if M satisfies the condition:*

$$M = least(P \cup U - Rejected\,(M) \cup Defaults\,(M)) \tag{3.1}$$

or, equivalently:

$$M = least(Residue\,(M) \cup Defaults\,(M))$$

Example 8 *Consider the programs P and U from Example 5:*

$$\begin{aligned} P:\ & sleep \leftarrow not\, tv\_on \\ & tv\_on \leftarrow \\ & watch\_tv \leftarrow tv\_on \\ \\ U:\ & not\ tv\_on \leftarrow power\_failure \\ & power\_failure \leftarrow \end{aligned} \tag{3.2}$$

Let $M = \{power\_failure, sleep\}$. As for conflicting rules we have that:

$$tv\_on \leftarrow \quad \bowtie \quad not\ tv\_on \leftarrow power\_failure$$

We obtain:

$$
\begin{aligned}
Rejected\,(M) &= \{tv\_on \leftarrow\} \\
Residue\,(M) &= \left\{ \begin{array}{l} sleep \leftarrow not\, tv\_on \\ watch\_tv \leftarrow tv\_on \\ not\, tv\_on \leftarrow power\_failure \\ power\_failure \leftarrow \end{array} \right\} \\
Defaults\,(M) &= \{not\, watch\_tv\}
\end{aligned}
$$

and thus it is easy to see that

$$M = least(Residue\,(M) \ \cup \ Defaults\,(M)).$$

Consequently, M is a stable model of $P \oplus U$. In fact, it is the only stable model of this program.

3.2.2 Transformational Semantics

In this Section we present a program transformation that given two generalized logic programs, the original program P and the update U, produces a generalized logic program whose stable models will be in a one to one relationship with the previously characterized stable models of $P \oplus U$. The resulting program will be written in an expanded language, which we start by defining.

Suppose that $\mathcal{K}$ is an arbitrary set of propositional variables, and P and U are two generalized logic programs in the language $\mathcal{L} = \mathcal{L}_{\mathcal{K}}$. By $\widehat{\mathcal{K}}$ we denote the following superset of $\mathcal{K}$:

$$\widehat{\mathcal{K}} = \mathcal{K} \cup \{A^-,\ A_P,\ A_{\overline{P}}^-,\ A_U,\ A_{\overline{U}}^- : A \in \mathcal{K}\}. \tag{3.3}$$

This definition assumes that the original set $\mathcal{K}$ of propositional variables does not contain any of the newly added symbols of the form $A^-, A_P, A_{\overline{P}}^-, A_U, A_{\overline{U}}^-$ so that they are all disjoint sets of symbols. If $\mathcal{K}$ contains any such symbols then they have to be *renamed* before the expansion of $\mathcal{K}$ takes place. We denote by $\widehat{\mathcal{L}} = \mathcal{L}_{\widehat{\mathcal{K}}}$ the expansion of the language $\mathcal{L} = \mathcal{L}_{\mathcal{K}}$ generated by $\widehat{\mathcal{K}}$. We are now ready to present the transformation:

Definition 30 (Program Updates Transformation) *Let P and U be generalized programs in the language $\mathcal{L}$. We call P the original program and U the updating program. By the update of P by U we mean the generalized logic program $P \uplus U$, which consists of the following clauses in the expanded language $\widehat{\mathcal{L}}$:*

(RP) Rewritten original program clauses:

$$A_P \leftarrow B_1, \ldots, B_m, C_1^-, \ldots, C_n^- \tag{3.4}$$
$$A_{\overline{P}}^- \leftarrow B_1, \ldots, B_m, C_1^-, \ldots, C_n^- \tag{3.5}$$

for any clause:

$$A \ \leftarrow B_1,\ \ldots,\ B_m,\ \ not\, C_1,\ \ldots,\ not\, C_n,$$

respectively,

$$not\, A \ \ \leftarrow B_1,\ \ldots,\ B_m,\ not\, C_1,\ \ldots,\ not\, C_n,$$

in the original program P. The rewritten clauses are obtained from the original ones by replacing atoms A (respectively, the default literals not A) occurring in their heads by the atoms A_P (respectively, A_P^-) and by replacing negative premises not C by C^-.
The role of the new meta-level atoms A_P and A_P^- is to indicate the fact that these clauses originally came from the program P. Moreover, as we will demonstrate below, the new atoms A^- serve as meta-language representation of the default literals not A.

(RU) Rewritten updating program clauses:

$$A_U \leftarrow B_1, \ldots, B_m, C_1^-, \ldots, C_n^- \tag{3.6}$$
$$A_U^- \leftarrow B_1, \ldots, B_m, C_1^-, \ldots, C_n^- \tag{3.7}$$

for any clause:

$$A \;\leftarrow B_1,\;\ldots,\;B_m,\;\; not\, C_1,\;\ldots,\; not\, C_n,$$

respectively,

$$not\, A \;\;\leftarrow B_1,\;\ldots,\;B_m,\; not\, C_1,\;\ldots,\; not\, C_n,$$

in the updating program U. The rewritten clauses are obtained from the original ones by replacing atoms A (respectively, the default literals not A) occurring in their heads by the atoms A_U (respectively, A_U^-) and by replacing negative premises not C by C^-.
The role of the new meta-level atoms A_U and A_U^- is to indicate the fact that these clauses originally came from the updating program U. Moreover, as we will demonstrate below, the new atoms A^- serve as meta-language representation of the default literals not A.

(UR) Update rules:

$$A \leftarrow A_U \tag{3.8}$$
$$A^- \leftarrow A_U^- \tag{3.9}$$

for all atoms $A \in \mathcal{K}$. The update rules state that an atom A must be true (respectively, false) in $P \uplus U$ if it is true (respectively, false) in the updating program U.

(IR) Inheritance rules:

$$A \leftarrow A_P, not\, A_U^- \tag{3.10}$$
$$A^- \leftarrow A_P^-, not\, A_U \tag{3.11}$$

for all atoms $A \in \mathcal{K}$. The inheritance rules say that an atom A (respectively, A^-) in the updated program $P \uplus U$ is inherited (by inertia) from the original program P provided it is not rejected (i.e., forced to be false) by the updating program U. More precisely, an atom A is true (respectively, false) in $P \uplus U$ if it is true (respectively, false) in the original program P, provided it is not made false (respectively, true) by the updating program U.

(DR) Default rules:

$$A^- \leftarrow not\, A_P, not\, A_U \tag{3.12}$$
$$not\, A \leftarrow A^- \tag{3.13}$$

for all atoms $A \in \mathcal{K}$. The first default rule states that an atom A in $P \uplus U$ is false if it is neither true in the original program P nor in the updating program U. The second says that if an atom is false then it can be assumed to be false by default. It also ensures that A and A^- cannot both be true.

Proposition 8 *Any model N of $P \uplus U$ is* coherent, *by which we mean that A is true (respectively, false) in N iff A^- is false (respectively, true) in N, for any $A \in \mathcal{K}$. In other words, every model of $P \uplus U$ satisfies the constraint $not\, A \equiv A^-$.*

Proof. Clearly, due to the second default rule, A and A^- cannot both be true in N. On the other hand, if both A and A^- are false in N then, due to the update rules, both $not\, A_U$ and $not\, A_U^-$ must be true. From the first inheritance axiom we infer that $not\, A_P$ must hold, which, in view of the first default rule, leads to a contradiction. ■

According to the above proposition, the atoms A^- can be simply regarded as *meta-level representation* of the default literals $not\, A$. Similarly, the remaining, newly added atoms, A_P, A_P^-, A_U and A_U^- serve as meta-level representation of the atoms (or their corresponding default literals) derivable from programs P and U, respectively.
When we discuss interpretations or models of the expanded language $\widehat{\mathcal{L}} = \mathcal{L}_{\widehat{\mathcal{K}}}$ we often restrict our attention to the *"relevant"* literals, i.e., to the literals from the base language $\mathcal{L} = \mathcal{L}_{\mathcal{K}}$ and thus we ignore, whenever justified, the auxiliary, meta-level atoms A^-, A_P, A_P^-, A_U and A_U^- and their corresponding default literals.

We will now show the relationship between the stable models of $P \oplus U$ and the stable models of $P \uplus U$.

Let P and U be *fixed* generalized logic programs in the language $\mathcal{L}$. Since the update program $P \uplus U$ is defined in the expanded language $\widehat{\mathcal{L}}$, we begin by first showing how interpretations of the language $\mathcal{L}$ can be naturally expanded to interpretations of the expanded language $\widehat{\mathcal{L}}$.

Since any model N of the update program $P \uplus U$ is coherent (see Proposition 8) and since the atoms A_P, A_P^-, A_U and A_U^- appear only in the heads of the rewritten program rules, if N is a minimal (in particular, stable) model of the update program $P \uplus U$ then N must satisfy, for any $A \in \mathcal{K}$:

$$\begin{array}{lll} A^- \in N & \text{iff} & not\, A \in N \\ A_P \in N & \text{iff} & \exists r \in P, H(r) = A\ , N \models B(r) \\ A_P^- \in M & \text{iff} & \exists r \in P, H(r) = not\, A\ , N \models B(r) \\ A_U \in M & \text{iff} & \exists r \in U, H(r) = A\ , N \models B(r) \\ A_U^- \in \widehat{N} & \text{iff} & \exists r \in U, H(r) = not\, A\ , N \models B(r) \end{array} \tag{3.14}$$

Accordingly, the truth or falsity in N of the atoms A^-, A_P, A_P^-, A_U and A_U^- depends only on the truth or falsity in N of the atoms A from $\mathcal{K}$. This leads us to the following definition:

Definition 31 (Expanded Interpretation) *For any interpretation M of $\mathcal{L}$ we denote by $\widehat{M}$ its expansion to an interpretation of the expanded language $\widehat{\mathcal{L}}$ defined, for* *any atom $A \in \mathcal{K}$, by the following rules:*

$$\begin{array}{lll} A^- \in \widehat{M} & \textit{iff} & not\, A \in M \\ A_P \in \widehat{M} & \textit{iff} & \exists r \in P, H(r) = A \,, M \models B(r) \\ A_P^- \in \widehat{M} & \textit{iff} & \exists r \in P, H(r) = not\, A \,, M \models B(r) \\ A_U \in \widehat{M} & \textit{iff} & \exists r \in U, H(r) = A \,, M \models B(r) \\ A_U^- \in \widehat{M} & \textit{iff} & \exists r \in U, H(r) = not\, A \,, M \models B(r) \end{array}$$

This definition immediately implies:

Proposition 9 *If N is a minimal model of the update program $P \uplus U$ and $M = N|\mathcal{L}$ is its restriction to the language $\mathcal{L}$ then $N = \widehat{M}$.*

Now we are able to state the theorem that relates the stable models of $P \oplus U$ and the stable models of $P \uplus U$.

Theorem 10 (Soundness and Completeness) *Let N be an interpretation of the language $\widehat{\mathcal{L}} = \mathcal{L}_{\widehat{\mathcal{K}}}$ and M an interpretation of the language $\mathcal{L}$, such that $N = \widehat{M}$. Then, N is a stable model of the update program $P \uplus U$ if and only if M is a stable model of $P \oplus U$.*

Proof. ($\Longrightarrow$) Suppose that N is a stable model of the update program $P \uplus U$ and let $R = (P \uplus U) \cup N^-$. From Definition 17 it follows that:

$$N = least(R) = least(\ (P \uplus U) \cup N^-). \tag{3.15}$$

Let $T = Residue\,(M) \ \cup \ Defaults\,(M)$ and let $H = least(T)$ be its least model (in the language $\mathcal{L}$). We are supposed to show that the restriction $M = N|\mathcal{L}$ of N to the language $\mathcal{L}$ coincides with H. From Proposition 9, we infer that the following equivalences hold true for every atom $A \in \mathcal{K}$:

$$A^- \in N \ \text{ iff } \ not\, A \in M \ \text{ iff } \ not\, A \in N \tag{3.16a}$$

$$\begin{aligned} A_P \in N \ \text{ iff } \ & \exists r \in P, H(r) = A \,, M \models B(r) \ \text{ iff} \\ \text{iff } \ & \exists r \in P, H(r) = A \,, N \models B(r) \end{aligned} \tag{3.16b}$$

$$\begin{aligned} A_P^- \in N \ \text{ iff } \ & \exists r \in P, H(r) = not\, A \,, M \models B(r) \ \text{ iff} \\ \text{iff } \ & \exists r \in P, H(r) = not\, A \,, N \models B(r) \end{aligned} \tag{3.16c}$$

$$\begin{aligned} A_U \in N \ \text{ iff } \ & \exists r \in U, H(r) = A \,, M \models B(r) \ \text{ iff} \\ \text{iff } \ & \exists r \in U, H(r) = A \,, N \models B(r) \end{aligned} \tag{3.16d}$$

$$\begin{aligned} A_U^- \in N \ \text{ iff } \ & \exists r \in U, H(r) = not\, A \,, M \models B(r) \ \text{ iff} \\ \text{iff } \ & \exists r \in U, H(r) = not\, A \,, N \models B(r) \end{aligned} \tag{3.16e}$$

Denote by $\mathcal{S}$ the sub-language of $\widehat{\mathcal{L}}$ that includes only propositional symbols $\{A : A \in \mathcal{K}\} \cup \{A^- : A \in \mathcal{K}\}$. By means of several simple reductions we will transform the program $R = (P \uplus U) \cup N^-$ in the language $\widehat{\mathcal{L}}$ into a simpler program Y in the language $\mathcal{S}$ so that:

The least model $J = least(Y)$ of Y is equal to the least model $N = least(R)$ of R when restricted to the language $\mathcal{S}$, i.e., $J = N|\mathcal{S}$;

The program Y in the language $\mathcal{S}$ is syntactically identical to the program $T = Residue\,(M) \ \cup \ Defaults\,(M)$ in the language $\mathcal{L}$, except that $notA$ is everywhere replaced by A^-.

First of all, we observe that from (3.16a)-(3.16e) it follows that for any $A \in \mathcal{K}$ neither A_P nor A_U belongs to N if and only if $not A \in Defaults(M)$. Accordingly, the first default rule in $R = (P \uplus U) \cup N^-$, namely, $A^- \leftarrow not\, A_P, not\, A_U$, can be replaced by the rule:

$$A^-, \text{ for all } A \in \mathcal{K} \text{ such that } not A \in Defaults(M)$$

without affecting the least model of R. As a result we obtained a transformed program R'.

From (3.16a)-(3.16e) it also follows that the inheritance rules (IR):

$$A \leftarrow A_P, not\, A_U^- \tag{3.17}$$

$$A^- \leftarrow A_P^-, not\, A_U \tag{3.18}$$

in R' can be replaced by the simpler rules:

$$A \leftarrow A_P \tag{3.19}$$

$$A^- \leftarrow A_P^- \tag{3.20}$$

without affecting the least model of R' restricted to the language $\mathcal{S}$ as long as we remove from R' all the rules:

$$A_P \leftarrow B_1, \ldots, B_m, C_1^-, \ldots, C_n^- \tag{3.21}$$

$$A_P^- \leftarrow B_1, \ldots, B_m, C_1^-, \ldots, C_n^- \tag{3.22}$$

respectively, that correspond to program rules:

$$A \leftarrow B_1, \ldots, B_m, \ not\, C_1, \ldots, \ not\, C_n,$$

$$not\, A \leftarrow B_1, \ldots, B_m, \ not\, C_1, \ldots, \ not\, C_n,$$

from P that were rejected by U, i.e., to the rules that belong to *Rejected* (M). This is due to the fact that both A_P and A_U^- (respectively, both A_P^- and A_U) are true in N if and only if there is a program clause:

$$A \leftarrow B_1, \ldots, B_m, \ not\, C_1, \ldots, \ not\, C_n,$$

respectively:

$$not\, A \leftarrow B_1, \ldots, B_m, \ not\, C_1, \ldots, \ not\, C_n,$$

in P that belongs to *Rejected* (M). Since the propositional symbols A_P and A_P^- do not appear in bodies of any other clauses from R', removing these rules from R' does not in anyway affect the truth of the propositional symbols A and A^- and thus it does not affect the least model of R' restricted to the language $\mathcal{S}$. As a result we obtain the program R''.

We can now remove all the negative facts in N^- and the default rules $not\, A \leftarrow A^-$ from R'' because they only involve propositional symbols $not\, A$ which no longer appear in bodies of any other clauses from R'' and thus do not affect the least model of R'' restricted to the language $\mathcal{S}$. As a result we obtain the program R'''.

Finally, since we are only interested in the sub-language $\mathcal{S}$, we can now safely remove from R''' all the auxiliary propositional symbols A_P and A_P^-, obtaining as a result the final program Y in the language $\mathcal{S}$ that consists of all the clauses:

$$A \leftarrow B_1, \ldots, B_m, C_1^-, \ldots, C_n^-$$

$$A^- \leftarrow B_1, \ldots, B_m, C_1^-, \ldots, C_n^-$$

corresponding to the clauses from $Residue(M) = P \cup U - Rejected(M)$ together with all the atomic facts:

$$A^-, \text{ where } notA \in Defaults(M).$$

Clearly, this program is entirely identical to the program $T = Residue(M) \cup Defaults(M)$, except that $notA$ is everywhere replaced by A^-. Consequently, the least model J of Y is identical to the least model H of T, except that $notA$ is everywhere replaced by A^-. Moreover, due to the way in which it was obtained, the least model $J = \text{Least}(Y)$ of the program Y is equal to the least model $N = \text{Least}(R)$ of R restricted to the language $\mathcal{S}$, i.e., $J = N|\mathcal{S}$. This implies that for any $A \in \mathcal{K}$:

$$\begin{array}{lllll} A \in N & \text{iff} & A \in J & \text{iff} & A \in H \\ A^- \in N & \text{iff} & A^- \in J & \text{iff} & notA \in H \end{array}$$

We conclude that $M = N|\mathcal{L} = H$, because from (3.16a) it follows that $notA \in N$ iff $A^- \in N$. This completes the proof of the implication from left to right.

The converse implication is established in a completely analogous way. ■

Example 9 *Consider again the programs P and U from Example 5:*

$$\begin{array}{ll} P: & sleep \leftarrow not\, tv\_on \\ & tv\_on \leftarrow \\ & watch\_tv \leftarrow tv\_on \\ \\ U: & not\ tv\_on \leftarrow power\_failure \\ & power\_failure \leftarrow \end{array} \tag{3.23}$$

According to Definition 30, $P \uplus U$ is:

$$P \uplus U = (RP) \cup (RU) \cup (UR) \cup (IR) \cup (DR)$$

where:

$$\begin{array}{ll} RP: & sleep_P \leftarrow tv\_on^- \\ & tv\_on_P \leftarrow \\ & watch\_tv_P \leftarrow tv\_on \\ \\ RU: & tv\_on_U^- \leftarrow power\_failure \\ & power\_failure_U \leftarrow \end{array} \tag{3.24}$$

It is easy to verify that $M = \{power\_failure, sleep\}$ is the only stable model (restricted to relevant atoms) of $P \uplus U$. Indeed, $power\_failure$ follows from the second clause of (RU) and from the Update Rules (UR). Now from power_failure, the first rule of (RU) and the Update Rules (UR) we deduce tv_on^- and thus also not tv_on. From the first rule of (RP) we infer $sleep_P$ and from the Inheritance Rules (IR) we deduce sleep. Finally, $watch\_tv^-$ and not watch_tv follow from the default rules.

3.2.3 Properties

In this section we study the basic properties of program updates.

Proposition 11 *If M is a stable model of $P \oplus U$ then M is a stable model of $Residue(M) = P \cup U - Rejected(M)$.*

Proof. *Since $Defaults(M) \subseteq M^-$, we conclude that the condition*

$$M = least(Residue(M) \cup Defaults(M)) \tag{3.25}$$

clearly implies the condition:

$$M = least(Residue(M) \cup M^-) \tag{3.26}$$

this condition, according to Proposition 4, is equivalent to the model M being a stable model of $Residue(M) = P \cup U - Rejected(M)$. ■

In general, the converse of the above implication does not hold. This is because (3.25) states that the model M is *determined* not just by the set M^- of all default literals $not\, A$ but rather by the generally smaller set $Defaults(M)$ of negations of unsupported atoms.

Example 10 *Let P contain only the fact $A \leftarrow$, let U contain only the clause $not\, A \leftarrow not\, A$ and let $M = \{not\, A\}$. Since $Residue(M) = U$ clearly M is a stable model of $Residue(M)$ and thus satisfies the condition (3.26). However, since $Defaults(M) = \emptyset$ the interpretation M does not satisfy (3.25) and thus M is not a stable model of $P \oplus U$. In fact, $M = \{A\}$ is the only stable model of $P \oplus U$.*

The semantics of $P \oplus U$ is always weaker than or equal to the semantics of the union $P \cup U$ of programs P and U:

Proposition 12 *If M is a stable model of the union $P \cup U$ of programs P and U then M is a stable model of $P \oplus U$.*

Proof. *If $Rejected(M) = \emptyset$ then the two conditions (3.25) and (3.26) above coincide because then M is a model of $Residue(M) = P \cup U$ and thus $Defaults(M) = M^-$. In particular, $Rejected(M) = \emptyset$ if M is a stable model of $P \cup U$* ■

Of course, the converse of the above result does not hold, otherwise updates would simply amount to the union of programs. In particular, the union $P \cup U$ may be a contradictory program with no stable models.

Example 11 *Consider again the programs P and U from Example 5. It is easy to see that $P \cup U$ is contradictory.*

Proposition 13 *Let $\emptyset$ denote the empty program. M is a stable model of $P \oplus \emptyset$ iff M is a stable model of $\emptyset \oplus P$ iff M is a stable model of P.*

Proof. *If either P or U is empty then, for any interpretation M, $Rejected(M) = \emptyset$.* ■

Proposition 14 *M is a stable model of $P \oplus P$ iff M is a stable model of P.*

Proof. *If P is equal to U, then $Residue(M) = P = U$.* ■

In general, we have $Rejected(M) = \emptyset$ if there are no conflicting rules. We obtain:

Proposition 15 *If P and U do not contain conflicting rules, i.e. $\nexists r \in P, r' \in U : r \bowtie r'$, then M is a stable model of $P \cup U$ iff M is a stable model of $P \oplus U$.*

Proof. *Immediate by Definitions 28 and 29.* ■

Corollary 16 *If both P and U are normal programs (or if both have only clauses with default literals not A in their heads) then M is a stable model of $P \cup U$ iff M is a stable model of $P \oplus U$. Thus, in this case the semantics of $P \oplus U$ also coincides with the semantics of the union $P \cup U$ of programs P and U.*

In particular, this last proposition states that the update of two programs written in disjoint languages is semantically equivalent to the union of both programs.

The definition of *Rejected* (M) can be simplified by dropping the condition that the body of the rejected rules be satisfied by the interpretation being considered. Note that such rules do not affect the least model since

$$least\,(P) = least\,(P - \{r\}) \quad \text{if} \quad least\,(P) \nvDash B(r)$$

We then have the following simplified characterization of the stable models of $P \oplus U$.

Proposition 17 (Stable Models of $P \oplus U$ (Alternative Characterization)) *Let P and U be generalized logic programs in the language $\mathcal{L}$. An interpretation M of the language $\mathcal{L}$ is a stable model of $P \oplus U$ if and only if M satisfies the condition:*

$$M = least(Residue\,(M) \cup Defaults\,(M)) \tag{3.27}$$

where:

$$\begin{aligned} Rejected\,(M) &= \{r \mid r \in P, \exists r' \in U, r \bowtie r',\ M \models B(r')\} \\ Defaults\,(M) &= \{not\,A \mid \nexists r \in P \ \cup \ U : H(r) = A \wedge M \models B(r)\} \\ Residue\,(M) &= P \ \cup \ U - Rejected\,(M) \end{aligned}$$

Proof. *The extra rules in the set Rejected (M) are precisely those rules r of P for which there is a conflicting rule in U, with a body satisfied by M, but whose body (of r) is not satisfied by M, i.e. they are inactive rules and their presence or absence is irrelevant.* ■

Program Updates Generalize Interpretation Updates

In this section we show that *interpretation updates*, originally introduced under the name *"revision programs"* by Marek and Truszczynski [157], and subsequently given a somewhat simpler characterization by Przymusinski and Turner [194, 197], constitute a special case of program updates. First, we briefly recap their original definition.

Definition 32 (Revision Programs) *[157]Let $\mathcal{K}$ be a set of propositions. An in-rule, is any expression of the form:*

$$in(A_0) \leftarrow in(A_1), ..., in(A_m), out(A_{m+1}), ..., out(A_n) \tag{3.28}$$

where $A_i \in \mathcal{K}$, $0 \leq i \leq n$.
An out-rule, is any expression of the form:

$$out(A_0) \leftarrow in(A_1), ..., in(A_m), out(A_{m+1}), ..., out(A_n) \tag{3.29}$$

where $A_i \in \mathcal{K}$, $0 \leq i \leq n$.
A collection of in-rules and out-rules is called a revision program.

Revision programs can syntactically be viewed as logic programs. However they are assigned with a special update semantics. In order to present the semantics we first need the definition of the necessary change determined by a revision program.

Definition 33 (Necessary Change) *[157]Let U be a revision program with least model M. The* necessary change *determined by U is the pair (I_U, O_U), where*

$$I_U = \{a : in(a) \in M\}$$
$$O_U = \{a : out(a) \in M\}$$

Intuitively, atoms in I_U are those that must be added and atoms in O_U are those that must be deleted. If $I_U \cap O_U = \{\}$ then U is said coherent.

And the semantics of U-justified update is defined in the following way:

Definition 34 (U-justified revision) *[157]Let U be a revision program and $I_i = I_i^+ \cup I_i^-$ and $I_u = I_u^+ \cup I_u^-$ two interpretations. The reduct $U_{I_u|I_i}$ with respect to I_i and I_u is obtained by the following operations:*

1. *Removing from U all rules whose body contains some $in(a)$ and $a \notin I_u$;*
2. *Removing from U all rules whose body contains some $out(a)$ and $a \in I_u$;*
3. *Removing from the body of any remaining rules of U all $in(a)$ such that $a \in I_i$;*
4. *Removing from the body of any remaining rules of U all $out(a)$ such that $a \notin I_i$.*

Let (I, O) be the necessary change determined by $U_{I_u|I_i}$. Whenever U is coherent, I_u is a U-justified revision *of I_i with respect to U if the following stability condition holds:*

$$I_u^+ = (I_i^+ - O) \cup I$$

Example 12 *Consider the revision program U and the initial interpretation I_i:*

$$U: \begin{array}{l} in(a) \leftarrow out(b) \\ out(b) \leftarrow \\ in(c) \leftarrow out(a) \end{array} \qquad I_i = \{b, not\, a, not\, c\}$$

Intuitively, the second rule will delete **b** *from I_i and as a consequence,* **a** *is inserted via the first rule. Since* **a** *was inserted, the third rule should have no effect. Thus, the U-justified revision should be:*

$$I_u = \{a, not\, b, not\, c\}$$

Indeed, if we determine the reduct $U_{I_u|I_i}$, we obtain:

$$U_{I_u|I_i}: \begin{array}{l} in(a) \leftarrow out(b) \\ out(b) \leftarrow \end{array}$$

and the necessary change is:

$$I = \{a\} \qquad O = \{b\}$$

since

$$(I_i^+ - O) \cup I = (\{b\} - \{b\}) \cup \{a\} = I_u^+$$

I_u is a U-justified revision. Any other interpretation would violate the stability condition, and so I_u is the single U-justified revision of I_i.

Here, we identify the *"revision rules"*:

$$in(A_0) \leftarrow in(A_1), ..., in(A_m), out(A_{m+1}), ..., out(A_n) \tag{3.30}$$
$$out(A_0) \leftarrow in(A_1), ..., in(A_m), out(A_{m+1}), ..., out(A_n) \tag{3.31}$$

used in [157], with the following generalized logic program clauses:

$$A_0 \leftarrow A_1, ..., A_m, not\ A_{m+1}, ..., not\ A_n \tag{3.32}$$
$$not\ A_0 \leftarrow A_1, ..., A_m, not\ A_{m+1}, ..., not\ A_n \tag{3.33}$$

Theorem 18 (Program updates generalize interpretation updates) *Let I be any interpretation and U any updating program in the language $\mathcal{L}$. Denote by P_I the generalized logic program in $\mathcal{L}$ defined by*

$$P_I = \{A\ \leftarrow : A \in I\ \} \cup \{not\ A\ \leftarrow : not\ A \in I\}$$

Then M is a stable model of $P_I \oplus U$ iff M is a U-justified revision of I with respect to U (in the sense of [157]).

Proof. In [194, 197], the authors showed that an interpretation M of $\mathcal{L}$ is an interpretation update (in the sense of [157]) of I by a program U iff M is a stable model of the following program $P(I, U)$:

Encoded interpretation I:

$$A_I \leftarrow$$

for every A such that A is in I, and ,

$$A_I^- \leftarrow$$

for every A such that *not* A is in I.

Rewritten clauses from U:

$$A \leftarrow B_1, \ldots, B_m, C_1^-, \ldots, C_n^- \tag{3.34}$$
$$A^- \leftarrow B_1, \ldots, B_m, C_1^-, \ldots, C_n^- \tag{3.35}$$

for any clause:

$$A\ \leftarrow B_1,\ \ldots,\ B_m,\ not\ C_1,\ \ldots,\ not\ C_n,$$

respectively,

$$not\ A\ \ \leftarrow B_1,\ \ldots,\ B_m, not\ C_1,\ \ldots,\ not\ C_n,$$

in the updating program U.

Inheritance rules:

$$A \leftarrow A_I, not\ A^- \tag{3.36}$$
$$A^- \leftarrow A_I^-, not\ A \tag{3.37}$$

for all atoms $A \in \mathcal{K}$.

Default rule:

$$not\ A \leftarrow A^-,$$

for all atoms $A \in \mathcal{K}$.

It is easy to see that the above program $P(I,U)$ is semantically equivalent to the program update $P_I \uplus U$ of the program P_I by the updating program U. ■

This theorem shows that when the initial program P is purely *extensional*, i.e., contains only positive or negative *facts*, then the interpretation update of P by U is semantically equivalent to $P \oplus U$.

Example 13 *In Example 12, we have the corresponding generalized logic programs:*

$$\begin{array}{llll} U: & a \leftarrow not\, b & P_{I_i}: & not\, a \leftarrow \\ & not\, b \leftarrow & & b \leftarrow \\ & c \leftarrow not\, a & & not\, c \leftarrow \end{array}$$

It is easy to check that $M = \{a, not\, b, not\, c\}$ is the only stable model of $P_{I_i} \oplus U$, corresponding to the only U-justified revision determined above.

As shown by the Examples 5 and 7, when the initial program P contains deductive rules then the two notions become significantly different.

It is easy to see that, equivalently, we could include only positive facts in the definition of the program P_I:

$$P_I = \{A \leftarrow : A \in I\}$$

thus resulting in a normal program P_I.

Adding Strong Negation

We now show that it is easy to add *strong negation* $-A$ ([19, 21, 92]) to the framework of program updates.

Definition 35 (Extended Stable Models of $P \oplus U$) *Let P and U be extended generalized logic programs in the language $\mathcal{L}^*$. A consistent extended interpretation M of the language $\mathcal{L}^*$ is a stable model of $P \oplus U$ iff M is a stable model of $P^{exp} \oplus U^{exp}$.*

I.e., in order to use strong negation in updates, one only needs to consider the expanded versions of each program and deal with complementary objective literals A and $-A$ as independent atoms.

Example 14 *Consider the following two extended generalized logic programs P and U:*

$$\begin{array}{llll} P: & a \leftarrow not\, b & U: & -a \leftarrow \\ & b \leftarrow not\, a & & not\, b \leftarrow \\ & -c \leftarrow & & not\ -c \leftarrow not\, a \\ & -d \leftarrow -c & & not\, d \leftarrow not\ -b \end{array}$$

and their expanded versions:

$$\begin{array}{lllll} P^{exp}: & a \leftarrow not\, b & not\ -a \leftarrow not\, b & U^{exp}: & -a \leftarrow \\ & b \leftarrow not\, a & not\ -b \leftarrow not\, a & & not\, b \leftarrow \\ & -c \leftarrow & not\, c \leftarrow & & not\ -c \leftarrow not\, a \\ & -d \leftarrow -c & not\, d \leftarrow -c & & not\, d \leftarrow not\ -b \\ & & & & not\, a \leftarrow \end{array}$$

The only stable model of P is:

$$M_P = \{a, not\ b, not\ c, not\ d, not\ -a, not\ -b, -c, -d\}$$

Let the extended interpretation

$$M = \{not\ a, not\ b, not\ c, not\ d, -a, not\ -b, not\ -c, not\ -d\}$$

be the candidate to be an extended stable model of the update of P by U. According to M, we have the following conflicting rules:

$$\begin{array}{lcl} a \leftarrow not\, b & \bowtie & not\, a \leftarrow \\ b \leftarrow not\, a & \bowtie & not\, b \leftarrow \\ -c \leftarrow & \bowtie & not\ -c \leftarrow not\, a \\ not\ -a \leftarrow not\, b & \bowtie & -a \leftarrow \end{array}$$

and we obtain the following set of rejected rules:

$$Rejected\,(M) = \left\{ \begin{array}{l} a \leftarrow not\, b \\ b \leftarrow not\, a \\ -c \leftarrow \\ not\ -a \leftarrow not\, b \end{array} \right\}$$

The $Residue\,(M)$ is the following set of rules:

$$\begin{array}{lll} P^{exp}: & a \leftarrow not\, b & not\ -a \leftarrow not\, b \\ & b \leftarrow not\, a & not\ -b \leftarrow not\, a \\ & -c \leftarrow & not\, c \leftarrow \\ & -d \leftarrow -c & not\, d \leftarrow -c \end{array} \qquad \begin{array}{ll} U^{exp}: & -a \leftarrow \\ & not\, b \leftarrow \\ & not\ -c \leftarrow not\, a \\ & not\, d \leftarrow not\ -b \\ & not\, a \leftarrow \end{array}$$

$$Residue\,(M) = \left\{ \begin{array}{ll} -a \leftarrow & -d \leftarrow -c \\ not\, b \leftarrow & not\ -b \leftarrow not\, a \\ not\ -c \leftarrow not\, a & not\, c \leftarrow \\ not\, d \leftarrow not\ -b & not\, d \leftarrow -c \\ not\, a \leftarrow & \end{array} \right\}$$

which, together with the set of defaults:

$$Defaults\,(M) = \{not\, c, not\, d, not\ -b, not\ -d\}$$

allows us to verify that:

$$M = least(Residue\,(M) \,\cup\, Defaults\,(M)).$$

Consequently, M is an extended stable model of $P \oplus U$. In fact, it is the only extended stable model of this program.

3.3 Dynamic Logic Programming

In this section we introduce the notion of *dynamic logic programming* $\bigoplus\{ P_s : s \in \mathcal{T}\}$ over an ordered set $\mathcal{P} = \{ P_s : s \in \mathcal{T}\}$ of logic programs which provides an important generalization of the notion of single program updates $P \oplus U$ introduced in Section 3.2.2.

The idea of dynamic updates, is simple and quite fundamental. Suppose that we are given a set of program modules P_s, indexed by different states of the world s.

Each program P_s contains some knowledge that is supposed to be true at the state s. Different states may represent different time periods or different sets of priorities or perhaps even different viewpoints. Consequently, the individual program modules may contain mutually contradictory as well as overlapping information. The role of dynamic logic programming is to use the mutual relationships existing between different states (and specified in the form of the ordering relation) to precisely determine, at any given state s, the *declarative* as well as the *procedural* semantics of the combined program, composed of all modules.

Given individual and largely *independent* program modules P_s describing our knowledge at different states of the world (for example, the knowledge acquired at different times), the dynamic logic programming specifies the exact meaning of the union of these programs. Dynamic programming significantly facilitates modularization of logic programming and, thus, modularization of non-monotonic reasoning as a whole.

Definition 36 (Dynamic Logic Program) *Let $\mathcal{L} = \mathcal{L}_{\mathcal{K}}$ be the language generated by the set of propositions $\mathcal{K}$. A* Dynamic Logic Program $\mathcal{P}$ *is a finite or infinite sequence of generalized logic programs in the language $\mathcal{L}$, $\{ P_s : s \in \mathcal{T}\}$, indexed by the finite or infinite set $\mathcal{T} = \{1, 2, \ldots, n, \ldots\}$ of natural numbers. We will call elements s of the set $\mathcal{T} \cup \{0\}$* states *and we will refer to* 0 *as the* initial state. *If the set $\mathcal{T}$ has a largest element s, we refer to it as* max. *Instead on natural numbers we can use any totally ordered set of states that is well founded.*

3.3.1 Declarative Semantics

We want to characterize the models of $\mathcal{P}$ at any given state. To this purpose, we will keep to the basic intuition of the single update, whereby an interpretation is a stable model of the update of a program P by a program U iff it is a stable model of a program consisting of the rules of U together with the subset of rules of P comprised by those that are not rejected, i.e.do not carry over by inertia due to their being overridden by update program U. For the case of a sequence of logic programs, we generalize the notion of rejection to comprise all rules of any logic program in the sequence such that there is a rule belonging to a "newer" logic program that overrides it. All rules, from all logic programs in the sequence, that are not rejected will contribute to determining the stable models. Accordingly, the set of defaults must be generalized to include default negations *not* A of all *unsupported* atoms A in the interpretation being considered, i.e., atoms that have the property that the body of every clause from all logic programs in the sequence with the head A is false in such interpretation.

Definition 37 (Stable models of a DLP at state s.) *Let $\mathcal{P} = \{ P_t : t \in \mathcal{T}\}$ be a* Dynamic Logic Program, *let $s \in \mathcal{T}$. An interpretation M_s is a* stable model of $\mathcal{P}$ at state s, *iff:*

$$M_s = least\left(\left[\rho\left(\mathcal{P}\right)_s - Reject\left(\mathcal{P}, s, M_s\right)\right] \cup Default\left(\rho\left(\mathcal{P}\right)_s, M_s\right)\right) \tag{3.38}$$

where

$$\rho\left(\mathcal{P}\right)_s = \bigcup_{i \le s} P_i \tag{3.39}$$

$$Reject\left(\mathcal{P}, s, M_s\right) = \{r \in P_i \mid \exists r' \in P_j, i < j \le s, r \bowtie r' \wedge M_s \vDash B(r')\} \tag{3.40}$$

$$Default\left(\rho\left(\mathcal{P}\right)_s, M_s\right) = \{not\, A \mid \nexists r \in \rho\left(\mathcal{P}\right)_s : (H(r) = A) \wedge M_s \vDash B(r)\} \tag{3.41}$$

By $SM\left(\bigoplus_s \mathcal{P}\right)$ we mean the set of all stable models of $\mathcal{P}$ at state s. If some literal or conjunction of literals ϕ holds in all stable models of $\mathcal{P}$ at state s, we write $\bigoplus_s \mathcal{P} \models_{sm} \phi$. If $s = max$ we simply omit the reference and write $\bigoplus \mathcal{P} \models_{sm} \phi$. Similarly, if $s = max$, instead of $SM\left(\bigoplus_s \mathcal{P}\right)$ we write $SM\left(\bigoplus \mathcal{P}\right)$, or simply $SM\left(\mathcal{P}\right)$ and instead of $\rho\left(\mathcal{P}\right)_s$ we simply write $\rho\left(\mathcal{P}\right)$.

Intuitively, the set $Reject\left(\mathcal{P}, s, M_s\right)$ contains those rules belonging to a program indexed by a state i that are overridden by the head of another rule belonging to a program indexed by a "newer" state j with true body. $\rho\left(\mathcal{P}\right)_s$ contains all rules of all programs that are indexed by a state up to and including state s, i.e. all rules until the current state s. The set $Default\left(\rho\left(\mathcal{P}\right)_s, M_s\right)$ contains default negations $not\, A$ of all unsupported atoms A, i.e., those atoms A for which there is no rule in $\rho\left(\mathcal{P}\right)_s$ whose body is true in M_s. Note that, in this definition, we follow the simplification set forth in Proposition 17 thus not requiring that the bodies of rejected rules be satisfied by the interpretation. It could be easily shown that adding the condition $M_s \models B(r)$ to the set of conditions in $Reject\left(\mathcal{P}, s, M_s\right)$ would not cause any change to the results.

Example 15 *Let $\mathcal{P} = \{P_1, P_2, P_3\}$, where P_1, P_2 and P_3 are as follows:*

$$\begin{array}{rl} P_1: & sleep \leftarrow not\, tv\_on \\ & watch\_tv \leftarrow tv\_on \\ & tv\_on \leftarrow \\ P_2: & not\, tv\_on \leftarrow power\_failure \\ & power\_failure \leftarrow \\ P_3: & not\, power\_failure \leftarrow \end{array}$$

Let $s = 3$ and $M_3 = \{tv\_on, watch\_tv, not\, sleep, not\, power\_failure\}$. We obtain:

$$Reject\left(\mathcal{P}, 3, M_3\right) = \{power\_failure \leftarrow\}$$

$$\rho\left(\mathcal{P}\right)_3 - Reject\left(\mathcal{P}, 3, M_3\right) = \left\{ \begin{array}{l} sleep \leftarrow not\, tv\_on \\ watch\_tv \leftarrow tv\_on \\ tv\_on \leftarrow \\ not\, tv\_on \leftarrow power\_failure \\ not\, power\_failure \leftarrow \end{array} \right\}$$

$$Default\left(\rho\left(\mathcal{P}\right)_3, M_3\right) = \{not\, sleep\}$$

and, thus, it is easy to see that

$$M_3 = least(\rho\left(\mathcal{P}\right)_3 - Reject\left(\mathcal{P}, 3, M_3\right) \cup Default\left(\rho\left(\mathcal{P}\right)_3, M_3\right)).$$

Consequently, M_3 is a stable model of $\mathcal{P}$ at state 3. In fact, it is the only stable model of $\mathcal{P}$ at state 3. The reader can check that, as intended, $\mathcal{P}$ has the single stable model at state 1:

$$M_1 = \{tv\_on, watch\_tv, not\, sleep, not\, power\_failure\}$$

and $\mathcal{P}$ has the single stable model at state 2:

$$M_2 = \{not\, tv\_on, not\, watch\_tv, sleep, power\_failure\}$$

Moreover, $\mathcal{P}$ at state 1 is semantically equivalent to P_1 and $\mathcal{P}$ at state 2 is semantically equivalent to $P_1 \oplus P_2$.

3.3.2 Properties

In this section we study the basic properties of program updates. We start by establishing that the previously introduced notion of updating one logic program by another one is a particular case of DLP. Subsequently, after presenting two other basic results, we turn our attention to the issue of equivalence between DLPs. We define two distinct notions of equivalence between DLPs:

Equivalence: this strong notion of equivalence states that two DLPs are *equivalent* iff their semantics coincide at every of their past, present or future states, i.e. not only their semantics must coincide at each of their states but it must also coincide when both programs are updated with the same arbitrary sequences of programs.

Update Equivalence: this weaker notion of equivalence states that two DLPs are *update equivalent* iff their semantics only coincide at every future state.

The importance of studying such notions of equivalence resides mostly in the importance of somehow establishing ways to simplify a DLP. Since, in most practical situations, we are not concerned with past states, we are particularly interested in establishing (preferably syntactical) ways to reduce the size of a DLP, whilst preserving *update equivalence.* There are two main ways to reduce the size of a DLP: *state condensing* and *state simplification.* By state condensing we mean combining two (or more) past states into a single one. By state simplification we mean reducing the size of each of the programs in the DLP. Most of this Section will be devoted to these issues. In particular, we establish that it is not possible to define a general state condensing operator that combines any two (or more) consecutive programs into a single one written in the same language. Nevertheless, even without such general state condensing operator, there are several situations where state condensing is possible, some of which we will explore. We also set forth several state simplification operations that preserve update equivalence. In a subsequent section, we will present a syntactical transformation that, given a DLP, produces a single generalized logic program, written in an extended language, whose semantics coincides with the semantics of the DLP.

As we've mentioned, we start by relating DLP with the single update case. Since the sets $Rejected\,(M)$ and $Defaults\,(M)$ (in Proposition 17) are particular cases of the sets $Reject\,(\mathcal{P}, s, M_s)$ and $Default\,(\rho\,(\mathcal{P})_s\,, M_s)$for $s = 2$, we immediately obtain:

Proposition 19 *Let P_1 and P_2 be arbitrary generalized logic programs and let $\mathcal{T}= \{1,2\}$. The dynamic logic program $\mathcal{P} =\{P_1, P_2\}$ is semantically equivalent to $P_1 \oplus P_2$.*

Proof. *For $s = 2$ we have:*

$$\begin{aligned} Reject\,(\mathcal{P}, 2, M_2) &= \{r \in P_i \mid \exists r' \in P_j, i < j \leq 2, r \bowtie r' \wedge M_2 \models B(r')\} = \\ &= \{r \in P_1 \mid \exists r' \in P_2, r \bowtie r' \wedge M_2 \models B(r')\} = \\ &= Rejected\,(M_2) \ \ \textit{(as in Proposition 17)} \end{aligned}$$

$$\rho\,(\mathcal{P})_2 = \bigcup_{i \leq 2} P_i = P_1 \cup P_2$$

$$\begin{aligned} Default\,(\rho\,(\mathcal{P})_2\,, M_2) &= \{not\,A \mid \nexists r \in \rho\,(\mathcal{P})_2 : (H(r) = A) \wedge M_2 \models B(r)\} = \\ &= \{not\,A \mid \nexists r \in P_1 \cup P_2 : (H(r) = A) \wedge M_2 \models B(r)\} = \\ &= Defaults\,(M_2) \end{aligned}$$

$$\rho(\mathcal{P})_2 - Reject(\mathcal{P}, 2, M_2) = P \cup U - Rejected(M_2) = Residue(M_2)$$

Therefore, we have that:

$$\begin{aligned} & M_2 = least([\rho(\mathcal{P})_2 - Reject(\mathcal{P}, 2, M_2)] \cup Default(\rho(\mathcal{P})_2, M_2)) \quad iff \\ iff \ & M_2 = least(Residue(M_2) \cup Defaults(M_2)) \end{aligned}$$

which completes the proof. ■

Before we continue, we introduce some notation. Suppose that $\mathcal{T} = \{s_1, ..., s_n\}$ and $\mathcal{P} = \{P_s : s \in \mathcal{T}\}$ is a sequence of generalized logic programs, indexed by the elements of $\mathcal{T}$. Instead of $\mathcal{P}$ we often use $\bigoplus \mathcal{P}$ or $P_{s_1} \oplus ... \oplus P_{s_n}$. If $s_i \in \mathcal{T}$, by $\bigoplus_{s_i} \mathcal{P}$ we mean $P_{s_1} \oplus ... \oplus P_{s_i}$. If P is a logic program, by $\mathcal{P} \oplus P$ we mean the Dynamic Logic Program $P_{s_1} \oplus ... \oplus P_{s_n} \oplus P$. Conversely, by $P \oplus \mathcal{P}$ we mean the Dynamic Logic Program $P \oplus P_{s_1} \oplus ... \oplus P_{s_n}$. If $\mathcal{P}' = P_{s'_1} \oplus ... \oplus P_{s'_n}$, by $\mathcal{P} \oplus \mathcal{P}'$ we mean $P_{s_1} \oplus ... \oplus P_{s_n} \oplus P_{s'_1} \oplus ... \oplus P_{s'_n}$.

We start with a rather trivial, but nevertheless important, proposition according to which an update by an empty program does not change the stable models of a dynamic logic program:

Proposition 20 *Let $\mathcal{P}$ be a Dynamic Logic Program. Then*

$$SM(\mathcal{P}) = SM(\mathcal{P} \oplus \emptyset) = SM(\emptyset \oplus \mathcal{P})$$

where $\emptyset$ denotes an empty program.

Proof. *Since the empty program does not affect the set $Reject(\mathcal{P}, s, M_s)$ nor the set $Default(\rho(\mathcal{P})_s, M)$, and does not contribute with any rules to the set $\rho(\mathcal{P})_s$. For example, to prove that $SM(\mathcal{P}) = SM(\mathcal{P} \oplus \emptyset)$ let $\mathcal{P} = P_1 \oplus ... \oplus P_n$ and $\mathcal{P}' = P_1 \oplus ... \oplus P_n \oplus P_{n+1}$ such that $P_{n+1} = \{\}$. An interpretation M_{n+1} is a stable model of $\mathcal{P}'$ at state $n+1$ iff*

$$M_{n+1} = least\left(\left[\rho(\mathcal{P}')_{n+1} - Reject(\mathcal{P}', n+1, M_{n+1})\right] \cup Default\left(\rho(\mathcal{P}')_{n+1}, M_{n+1}\right)\right)$$

By Definition 37 we have that $\rho(\mathcal{P}')_{n+1} = \rho(\mathcal{P})_n$, $Reject(\mathcal{P}', n+1, M_{n+1}) = Reject(\mathcal{P}, n, M_{n+1})$ and $Default\left(\rho(\mathcal{P}')_{n+1}, M_{n+1}\right) = Default(\rho(\mathcal{P})_n, M_{n+1})$. Therefore, M_{n+1} is a stable model of $\mathcal{P}'$ at state $n+1$ iff

$$M_{n+1} = least([\rho(\mathcal{P})_n - Reject(\mathcal{P}, n, M_{n+1})] \cup Default(\rho(\mathcal{P})_n, M_{n+1}))$$

which is the condition for M_{n+1} to be a stable model of $\mathcal{P}$ at state n, i.e. M_{n+1} is a stable model of $\mathcal{P}'$ at state $n+1$ iff M_{n+1} is a stable model of $\mathcal{P}$ at state n. The proof of the other equality is similar. ■

The next proposition states that in order to determine the semantics of some DLP at some state s, one needs not consider those programs indexed by states higher than s, i.e. the future does not affect the present.

Proposition 21 *Let $\mathcal{P} = P_1 \oplus ... \oplus P_n$ be a dynamic logic program. Then, for any state i, $1 \leq i \leq n$,*

$$SM\left(\bigoplus_i \mathcal{P}\right) = SM(P_1 \oplus ... \oplus P_i)$$

Proof. *In the condition for being a stable model at state s, all its variable elements involved, namely the sets $\rho(\mathcal{P})_s$, $Reject(\mathcal{P}, s, M)$ and $Default(\rho(\mathcal{P})_s, M)$, and the condition that all considered programs P_i are such that $i \leq s$.* ■

We now define two notions of equivalence between dynamic logic programs. The first and most obvious notion of equivalence states, intuitively, that two dynamic logic programs indexed by the same set of states are equivalent if and only if their stable models coincide for all their states and, if both are updated by the same arbitrary sequence of logic programs, their stable models will still coincide. This notion of equivalence between two dynamic logic programs requires *past* and *future* semantical equivalence between them. Formally:

Definition 38 (Equivalence between Dynamic Logic Programs) *Consider two Dynamic Logic Programs, $\mathcal{P} = \{P_s : s \in \mathcal{T}\}$ and $\mathcal{P}' = \{P'_s : s \in \mathcal{T}\}$. We say that $\mathcal{P}$ and $\mathcal{P}'$ are* equivalent, *denoted by $\mathcal{P} \equiv \mathcal{P}'$ iff the following two conditions hold:*

1. *For every $s \in \mathcal{T}$ it holds that*

$$SM\left(\bigoplus_s \mathcal{P}\right) = SM\left(\bigoplus_s \mathcal{P}'\right)$$

2. *For every Dynamic Logic Program $\mathcal{Q} = Q_1 \oplus ... \oplus Q_n$, and every state $i, 1 \leq i \leq n$, it holds that*

$$SM\left(\mathcal{P} \oplus Q_1 \oplus ... \oplus Q_i\right) = SM\left(\mathcal{P}' \oplus Q_1 \oplus ... \oplus Q_i\right)$$

Note that the requirement that both dynamic logic programs be indexed by the same set of states $\mathcal{T}$ could be dropped. Instead, we could allow $\mathcal{P}$ and $\mathcal{P}'$ to be indexed by different state sets $\mathcal{T}$ and $\mathcal{T}'$, as long as there is a suitable mapping function between them. For simplicity, we assume them to be indexed by the same set of states. We start with a proposition establishing the requirements for $\equiv$ to be, in fact, an equivalence relation i.e., $\equiv$ is symmetric, reflexive and transitive:

Proposition 22 *Let $\mathcal{P}$, $\mathcal{P}'$, $\mathcal{P}''$ be three Dynamic Logic Programs. Then:*

Symmetry: *if $\mathcal{P} \equiv \mathcal{P}'$ then $\mathcal{P}' \equiv \mathcal{P}$;*

Reflexivity: $\mathcal{P} \equiv \mathcal{P}$;

Transitivity: *if $\mathcal{P} \equiv \mathcal{P}'$ and $\mathcal{P}' \equiv \mathcal{P}''$ then $\mathcal{P} \equiv \mathcal{P}''$.*

Proof. *Since $\equiv$ is only based on $=$, namely on equality between sets of stable models, and $=$ obeys symmetry, reflexivity and transitivity, then so does $\equiv$.* ■

Proposition 23 *Let $\mathcal{P}$, $\mathcal{P}'$, $\mathcal{P}''$ be three Dynamic Logic Programs. If $\mathcal{P} \equiv \mathcal{P}'$ then $(\mathcal{P}' \oplus \mathcal{P}'') \equiv (\mathcal{P} \oplus \mathcal{P}'')$.*

Proof. *Immediately follows from the definition of equivalence.* ■

This rather strong notion of equivalence may be conceptually interesting to establish classes of programs that can be replaced by one another, while keeping the past, present and future semantics. Nevertheless it seems more important, from our point of view, to study classes of programs that share the same future (and present) semantics, not necessarily sharing the same past semantics. This is particularly important when we want to somehow simplify a long dynamic logic program, possibly with a different semantics if queried at some past states, but guaranteeing that such simplified DLP will yield exactly the same results as the original one, if updated by any arbitrary sequence of programs, i.e. we may not be interested in the past, as long as the future is the same. For this, we define a weaker notion of equivalence, namely, *update equivalence.*

Definition 39 (Update Equivalence between Dynamic Logic Programs) *Let $\mathcal{P}$ and $\mathcal{P}'$ be two Dynamic Logic Programs. We say that, $\mathcal{P}$ and $\mathcal{P}'$ are* update equivalent, *denoted by $\mathcal{P}\overset{\oplus}{\equiv}\mathcal{P}'$ iff for every Dynamic Logic Program $\mathcal{Q} = Q_1 \oplus ... \oplus Q_n$ and every state $i, 1 \leq i \leq n$, it holds that*

$$SM\left(\mathcal{P} \oplus Q_1 \oplus ... \oplus Q_i\right) = SM\left(\mathcal{P}' \oplus Q_1 \oplus ... \oplus Q_i\right)$$

This definition states that two sequences of GLP's are *update equivalent* iff their stable models coincide after an arbitrary number of updates with arbitrary GLP's.

Again, we start with a proposition establishing the requirements for $\overset{\oplus}{\equiv}$ to be, in fact, an equivalence relation i.e., $\overset{\oplus}{\equiv}$ is symmetric, reflexive and transitive:

There follow two basic properties of equivalence:

Proposition 24 *Let $\mathcal{P}$, $\mathcal{P}'$, $\mathcal{P}''$ be three Dynamic Logic Programs. Then:*

Symmetry: *if $\mathcal{P}\overset{\oplus}{\equiv}\mathcal{P}'$ then $\mathcal{P}'\overset{\oplus}{\equiv}\mathcal{P}$;*

Reflexivity: *$\mathcal{P}\overset{\oplus}{\equiv}\mathcal{P}$;*

Transitivity: *if $\mathcal{P}\overset{\oplus}{\equiv}\mathcal{P}'$ and $\mathcal{P}'\overset{\oplus}{\equiv}\mathcal{P}''$ then $\mathcal{P}\overset{\oplus}{\equiv}\mathcal{P}''$.*

Proof. *As for the case of equivalence between DLPs, since $\overset{\oplus}{\equiv}$ is only based on $=$, namely on equality between sets of stable models, it obeys symmetry, reflexivity and transitivity.* ∎

Clearly we have that if $\mathcal{P} \equiv \mathcal{P}'$ then $\mathcal{P}\overset{\oplus}{\equiv}\mathcal{P}'$.

We will now study some basic properties related to this equivalence definition.

The following proposition says that if two sequences of GLPs are update equivalent then their stable models must coincide at their *max* states.

Proposition 25 *Let $\mathcal{P}$ and $\mathcal{P}'$ be two Dynamic Logic Programs. If $\mathcal{P}\overset{\oplus}{\equiv}\mathcal{P}'$ then $SM(\mathcal{P}) = SM(\mathcal{P}')$.*

Proof. *Just make $\mathcal{Q} = \{Q_1\} = \{\emptyset\}$ in Definition 39 and use Proposition 20.* ∎

Proposition 26 *Let $\mathcal{P}$, $\mathcal{P}'$ be two Dynamic Logic Programs. Then, the following hold:*

$$(\mathcal{P} \oplus \emptyset) \overset{\oplus}{\equiv} \mathcal{P}$$
$$(\emptyset \oplus \mathcal{P}) \overset{\oplus}{\equiv} \mathcal{P}$$
$$(\mathcal{P} \oplus \emptyset \oplus \mathcal{P}') \overset{\oplus}{\equiv} (\mathcal{P} \oplus \mathcal{P}')$$

Proof. *Trivial since the empty program does not contribute with any rules nor to the sets $Reject(\_,\_,\_)$ and $Default(\_,\_)$.* ∎

Proposition 27 *Let $\mathcal{P}$, $\mathcal{P}'$ be two Dynamic Logic Programs. If for every dynamic logic program $\mathcal{P}''$, it holds that $(\mathcal{P} \oplus \mathcal{P}'') \overset{\oplus}{\equiv} (\mathcal{P}' \oplus \mathcal{P}'')$, then $\mathcal{P}\overset{\oplus}{\equiv}\mathcal{P}'$.*

Proof. *In particular, $(\mathcal{P} \oplus \mathcal{P}'') \overset{\oplus}{\equiv} (\mathcal{P}' \oplus \mathcal{P}'')$ holds for $\mathcal{P}'' = \emptyset$. Then, from Proposition 26 it follows that $\mathcal{P}\overset{\oplus}{\equiv}\mathcal{P}'$.* ∎

Proposition 28 *Let $\mathcal{P}$ be a dynamic logic program. Let $P^{\mathcal{K}}$ and $P^{\,not\,\mathcal{K}}$ be two generalized logic programs defined as follows:*

$$P^{\mathcal{K}} = \{A \leftarrow : A \in \mathcal{K}\}$$
$$P^{\,not\,\mathcal{K}} = \{not\, A \leftarrow : A \in \mathcal{K}\}$$

Let $\mathcal{P}'$ be the dynamic logic program such that $\mathcal{P}' = P^{\mathcal{K}} \oplus P^{\,not\,\mathcal{K}} \oplus \mathcal{P}$. Then $\mathcal{P} \stackrel{\oplus}{\equiv} \mathcal{P}'$.

Proof. *To prove that $\mathcal{P} \stackrel{\oplus}{\equiv} \mathcal{P}'$ we need to prove that for an arbitrary DLP $\mathcal{Q}$ and all its states, we have that $SM(\mathcal{P} \oplus \mathcal{Q}) = SM\left(P^{\mathcal{K}} \oplus P^{\,not\,\mathcal{K}} \oplus \mathcal{P} \oplus \mathcal{Q}\right)$. Since $\mathcal{P} \oplus \mathcal{Q}$ are both arbitrary, we can just prove that for an arbitrary $\mathcal{P}$ and its maximal state s, the semantics coincide, i.e. $SM(\mathcal{P}) = SM\left(P^{\mathcal{K}} \oplus P^{\,not\,\mathcal{K}} \oplus \mathcal{P}\right)$. An interpretation M is a stable model of $\mathcal{P}$ iff:*

$$M = least\left(\left[\rho(\mathcal{P}) - Reject(\mathcal{P}, s, M)\right] \cup Default\left(\rho(\mathcal{P})_s, M\right)\right) \tag{3.42}$$

An interpretation M is a stable model of $\mathcal{P}'$ iff:

$$M = least\left(\left[\rho(\mathcal{P}') - Reject(\mathcal{P}', s, M)\right] \cup Default\left(\rho(\mathcal{P}')_s, M\right)\right) \tag{3.43}$$

We want to prove that M satisfies 3.42 iff it satisfies 3.43. First of all note that $Default\left(\rho(\mathcal{P}')_s, M\right) = \{\}$ because for every $A \in \mathcal{K}$ there is at least a rule r in $\rho(\mathcal{P}')$ such that $H(r) = A$ and $M \vDash B(r)$, namely rule $A \leftarrow \in P^{\mathcal{K}}$. If we separate the set $\rho(\mathcal{P}') - Reject(\mathcal{P}', s, M)$ into three disjoint sets according to the origin of its rules, we have:

$$\begin{aligned}\rho(\mathcal{P}') - Reject(\mathcal{P}', s, M) = {} & \left[\rho(\mathcal{P}) - Reject(\mathcal{P}, s, M)\right] \cup \\ & \cup \left[P^{\mathcal{K}} - Reject^*(P^{\mathcal{K}})\right] \cup \\ & \cup \left[P^{\,not\,\mathcal{K}} - Reject^*(P^{\,not\,\mathcal{K}})\right]\end{aligned}$$

Since $Reject^*(P^{\mathcal{K}}) = P^{\mathcal{K}}$ because for every rule in $P^{\mathcal{K}}$ there is one rule from $P^{\,not\,\mathcal{K}}$ that rejects it, we have that $P^{\mathcal{K}} - Reject^*(P^{\mathcal{K}}) = \{\}$ and since

$$Reject^*(P^{\,not\,\mathcal{K}}) = \{not\, A \leftarrow : \exists r \in \rho(\mathcal{P}), H(r) = A \wedge M \vDash B(r)\}$$

we have that $P^{\,not\,\mathcal{K}} - Reject^*(P^{\,not\,\mathcal{K}}) = Default\left(\rho(\mathcal{P})_s, M\right)$, it follows that M is a stable model of $\mathcal{P}'$ iff

$$M = least\left(\left[\rho(\mathcal{P}) - Reject(\mathcal{P}, s, M)\right] \cup Default\left(\rho(\mathcal{P})_s, M\right)\right)$$

i.e., iff it is a stable model of $\mathcal{P}$, and therefore, $\mathcal{P} \stackrel{\oplus}{\equiv} \mathcal{P}'$. ■

Corollary 29 *Let $\mathcal{P}$ be a dynamic logic program and s one of its states. Let $\mathcal{P}'$ be the dynamic logic program such that $\mathcal{P}' = P^{\mathcal{K}} \oplus P^{\,not\,\mathcal{K}} \oplus \mathcal{P}$. An interpretation M is a stable model of $\mathcal{P}'$ at state s iff*

$$M = least\left(\rho(\mathcal{P}') - Reject(\mathcal{P}', s, M)\right)$$

Proof. *As we have seen in the proof of Proposition 28, $Default\left(\rho(\mathcal{P}')_s, M\right) = \{\}$.*

■

The next theorem establishes that, in order to have update equivalence between two DLP's $\mathcal{P}$ and $\mathcal{P}'$, i.e. that any future updates will produce the same result, one only needs to show that their semantics coincide for any arbitrary update with a single generalized logic. i.e.

$$\nexists P : SM(\mathcal{P} \oplus P) \neq SM\left(\mathcal{P}' \oplus P\right) \Rightarrow \mathcal{P} \overset{\oplus}{\equiv} \mathcal{P}'$$

which, together with the definition of update equivalence, allows us to conclude

$$\nexists P : SM(\mathcal{P} \oplus P) \neq SM\left(\mathcal{P}' \oplus P\right) \Leftrightarrow \mathcal{P} \overset{\oplus}{\equiv} \mathcal{P}'$$

Theorem 30 *Let $\mathcal{P}$ and $\mathcal{P}'$ be two Dynamic Logic Programs. If $SM(\mathcal{P} \oplus P) = SM(\mathcal{P}' \oplus P)$ for every generalized logic program P, then $\mathcal{P} \overset{\oplus}{\equiv} \mathcal{P}'$.*

Before we prove the theorem, we start by proving the following lemma:

Lemma 31 *Let $\mathcal{P} = P_1 \oplus ... \oplus P_i$ be a Dynamic Logic Program. If M is a stable model of $\mathcal{P}' = \mathcal{P} \oplus P_j \oplus P_k$ then M is a stable model of $\mathcal{P}'' = \mathcal{P} \oplus P_{jk}$ where:*

$$P_{jk} = P_k \cup [P_j - Reject^*(P_j, P_k, M)]$$

and

$$Reject^*(P_j, P_k, M) = \{r \in P_j \mid \exists r' \in P_k, H(r) = not\, H(r') \wedge M \models B(r')\}$$

Proof. *We start the proof by defining a set of rejected rules belonging to a set of GLPs of a DLP, by another set of GLPs of the same DLP. Let $\mathcal{P} = \{P_s : s \in \mathcal{T}\} = P_1 \oplus ... \oplus P_i$ be a DLP with $\mathcal{T} = \{1, ..., i\}$. Then:*

$$Reject^*(\mathcal{P}_m, \mathcal{P}_n, M) = \left\{ \begin{array}{c} r \in P_h \in \mathcal{P}_m \mid \exists r' \in P_j \in \mathcal{P}_n, j > h, \\ H(r) = not\, H(r') \wedge M \models B(r') \end{array} \right\} \tag{3.44}$$

where $\mathcal{P}_m, \mathcal{P}_n \subseteq \mathcal{P}$. If $\mathcal{P}_m$ or $\mathcal{P}_n$ are singletons, then we simply write its element instead of the set as argument of the set $Reject^*(\_,\_,\_)$. Also for simplicity, we often write the multiset of $\mathcal{P}_m$ or $\mathcal{P}_n$ instead of $\mathcal{P}_m$ or $\mathcal{P}_n$, assuming the origin of rules implicit.

Let $\mathcal{P} = P_1 \oplus ... \oplus P_i$. Let $\mathcal{P}' = \mathcal{P}_i \oplus P_j \oplus P_k$. Let M be a stable model of $\mathcal{P}'$ at state k. Then

$$M = least\left([\rho(\mathcal{P}') - Reject(\mathcal{P}', k, M)] \cup Defaults(\rho(\mathcal{P}'), M)\right) \tag{3.45}$$

where

$$Reject(\mathcal{P}', k, M) = \{r \in P_i \mid \exists r' \in P_j, i < j \leq k, H(r) = not\, H(r') \wedge M \models B(r')\}$$

$$Default(\rho(\mathcal{P}'), M) = \{not\, A \mid \nexists r \in \rho(\mathcal{P}') : (H(r) = A) \wedge M_s \models B(r)\}$$

are as per Def.37. Note that $Reject(\mathcal{P}', k, M) = Reject^*\left(\mathcal{P}', \mathcal{P}', M\right)$. We can rewrite this as:

$$\begin{aligned} Reject^*\left(\mathcal{P}', \mathcal{P}', M\right) &= Reject^*(\mathcal{P}, \mathcal{P}, M) \cup Reject^*(\mathcal{P}, P_k, M) \cup \\ &\cup Reject^*(\mathcal{P}, P_j - Reject^*(P_j, P_k, M), M) \cup \\ &\cup Reject^*(\mathcal{P}, Reject^*(P_j, P_k, M), M) \cup \\ &\cup Reject^*(P_j, P_k, M) \end{aligned}$$

The set $Defaults(\rho(\mathcal{P}'), M)$ *can also be rewritten as:*

$$Defaults(\rho(\mathcal{P}'), M) = Defaults(\rho(\mathcal{P}), M) \cap Defaults(P_k, M) \cap \\ \cap Defaults((P_j - Reject^*(P_j, P_k, M)), M) \cap \\ \cap Defaults(Reject^*(P_j, P_k, M), M)$$

Since

$$\rho(\mathcal{P}') = \rho(\mathcal{P}) \cup P_k \cup (P_j - Reject^*(P_j, P_k, M)) \cup Reject^*(P_j, P_k, M)$$

We can now rewrite 3.45 and obtain:

$$M = least\left(\begin{array}{c}\left[\begin{array}{c}\left(\begin{array}{c}\rho(\mathcal{P}) - Reject^*(\mathcal{P}, \mathcal{P}, M) - Reject^*(\mathcal{P}, P_k, M) - \\ -Reject^*(\mathcal{P}, P_j - Reject^*(P_j, P_k, M), M) - \\ -Reject^*(\mathcal{P}, Reject^*(P_j, P_k, M), M)\end{array}\right) \cup \\ \cup (P_j - Reject^*(P_j, P_k, M)) \cup P_k\end{array}\right] \cup \\ \cup \left(\begin{array}{c}Defaults(\rho(\mathcal{P}), M) \cap Defaults(P_k, M) \cap \\ \cap Defaults((P_j - Reject^*(P_j, P_k, M)), M) \cap \\ \cap Defaults(Reject^*(P_j, P_k, M), M)\end{array}\right)\end{array}\right) \tag{3.46}$$

Let us now turn to $\mathcal{P}'' = \mathcal{P} \oplus P_{jk}$. *An interpretation* M *is a stable model of* $\mathcal{P} \oplus P_{jk}$ *iff*

$$M = least([\rho(\mathcal{P}'') - Reject(\mathcal{P}'', jk, M)] \cup Defaults(\rho(\mathcal{P}''), M)) \tag{3.47}$$

where

$$P_{jk} = P_k \cup [P_j - Reject^*(P_j, P_k, M)]$$

Note that $Reject(\mathcal{P}'', jk, M) = Reject^*(\mathcal{P}'', \mathcal{P}'', M)$. *We can rewrite this as:*

$$Reject^*(\mathcal{P}'', \mathcal{P}'', M) = Reject^*(\mathcal{P}, \mathcal{P}, M) \cup Reject^*(\mathcal{P}, P_k, M) \cup \\ \cup Reject^*(\mathcal{P}, P_j - Reject^*(P_j, P_k, M), M)$$

The set $Defaults(\rho(\mathcal{P}''), M)$ *can also be rewritten as:*

$$Defaults(\rho(\mathcal{P}''), M) = Defaults(\rho(\mathcal{P}), M) \cap Defaults(P_k, M) \cap \\ \cap Defaults((P_j - Reject^*(P_j, P_k, M)), M)$$

Since

$$\rho(\mathcal{P}'')_{jk} = \rho(\mathcal{P}) \cup P_k \cup (P_j - Reject^*(P_j, P_k, M))$$

We can now rewrite 3.47 and obtain:

$$M = least\left(\begin{array}{c}\left[\begin{array}{c}\left(\begin{array}{c}\rho(\mathcal{P}) - Reject^*(\mathcal{P}, \mathcal{P}, M) - Reject^*(\mathcal{P}, P_k, M) - \\ -Reject^*(\mathcal{P}, P_j - Reject^*(P_j, P_k, M), M)\end{array}\right) \cup \\ \cup (P_j - Reject^*(P_j, P_k, M)) \cup P_k\end{array}\right] \cup \\ \cup \left(\begin{array}{c}Defaults(\rho(\mathcal{P}), M) \cap Defaults(P_k, M) \cap \\ \cap Defaults((P_j - Reject^*(P_j, P_k, M)), M)\end{array}\right)\end{array}\right) \tag{3.48}$$

We need to show that if M *satisfies* (3.46) *then* M *also satisfies* (3.48). *Let* Π *be:*

$$\Pi = \left[\begin{array}{c}\left(\begin{array}{c}\rho(\mathcal{P}) - Reject^*(\mathcal{P}, \mathcal{P}, M) - Reject^*(\mathcal{P}, P_k, M) - \\ -Reject^*(\mathcal{P}, P_j - Reject^*(P_j, P_k, M), M)\end{array}\right) \cup \\ \cup (P_j - Reject^*(P_j, P_k, M)) \cup P_k\end{array}\right]$$

and Δ *be:*

$$\Delta = \left(\begin{array}{c} Defaults(\rho(\mathcal{P}), M) \cap Defaults(Reject^*(P_j, P_k, M), M) \cap \\ \cap Defaults(P_k, M) \cap Defaults((P_j - Reject^*(P_j, P_k, M)), M) \end{array} \right)$$

then (3.46) *reduces to:*

$$M = least\left([\Pi - Reject^*(\mathcal{P}, Reject^*(P_j, P_k, M), M)] \cup \Delta\right) \tag{3.49}$$

and (3.48) *reduces to:*

$$M = least\left(\Pi \cup \Delta \cup \Delta'\right) \tag{3.50}$$

where

$$\Delta' = \left\{ \begin{array}{c} not\, A \mid \exists r \in Reject^*(P_j, P_k, M): \\ : (H(r) = A) \wedge (M \vDash B(r)) \wedge (not\, A \notin \Delta) \end{array} \right\} \tag{3.51}$$

Let us start from (3.49)*. The set* $Reject^*(\mathcal{P}, Reject^*(P_j, P_k, M), M)$ *is given by:*

$$\begin{array}{l} Reject^*(\mathcal{P}, Reject^*(P_j, P_k, M), M) = \\ = \left\{ \begin{array}{c} r \in P_n \mid \exists r' \in Reject^*(P_j, P_k, M), 1 \le n \le i, \\ H(r) = not\, H(r') \wedge M \vDash B(r') \end{array} \right\} = \\ = \left\{ \begin{array}{c} r \in P_n \mid \exists r' \in P_j, \exists r'' \in P_k, 1 \le n \le i, \\ H(r') = not\, H(r'') \wedge M \vDash B(r'') \wedge \\ \wedge H(r) = not\, H(r') \wedge M \vDash B(r') \end{array} \right\} \end{array}$$

From this we can infer that:

$$\forall r \in Reject^*(\mathcal{P}, Reject^*(P_j, P_k, M), M), \exists r'' \in P_k : H(r) = H(r'') \wedge M \vDash B(r'')$$

Since $P_k \subseteq \Pi$ *and* $Reject^*(\mathcal{P}, Reject^*(P_j, P_k, M), M) \cap P_k = \emptyset$*, we have that for every rule* r *in* $Reject^*(\mathcal{P}, Reject^*(P_j, P_k, M), M)$ *there is a rule* r'' *in* $\Pi - Reject^*(\mathcal{P}, Reject^*(P_j, P_k, M), M)$ *such that* $M \vDash B(r'')$, $H(r) = H(r'')$ *and therefore,* $H(r) \in M$*.*

We can therefore add the set of rules $Reject^*(\mathcal{P}, Reject^*(P_j, P_k, M), M)$ *in* (3.49) *without affecting the least model. The equation* (3.49) *can be reduced to*

$$M = least\left(\Pi \cup \Delta\right)$$

We have proven that

$$M = least\left([\Pi - Reject^*(\mathcal{P}, Reject^*(P_j, P_k, M), M)] \cup \Delta\right) \text{ iff } M = least\left(\Pi \cup \Delta\right)$$

It remains to be proved that

$$M = least\left(\Pi \cup \Delta \cup \Delta'\right) \text{ if } M = least\left(\Pi \cup \Delta\right)$$

For every $not\, A \in \Delta'$*, from* (3.51)*, there is a rule* r' *in* Π *(originated in* P_k*) such that* $H(r') = not\, A$ *and* $M \vDash B(r)$*. Therefore, for every* $not\, A \in \Delta'$ *we have that* $not\, A \in M$ *and* $not\, A \in least\left(\Pi \cup \Delta\right)$*, i.e.* $\Delta' \subseteq least\left(\Pi \cup \Delta\right)$*. From* $M = least\left(\Pi \cup \Delta\right)$ *and* $\Delta' \subseteq least\left(\Pi \cup \Delta\right)$ *it follows that* $M = least\left(\Pi \cup \Delta \cup \Delta'\right)$*.* ■

Proof of Theorem 30. Let $\mathcal{Q} = Q_1 \oplus ... \oplus Q_n \oplus ...$ be an arbitrary DLP. Let P be an arbitrary GLP. We want to prove that:

$$\forall P : SM\left(\mathcal{P} \oplus P\right) = SM\left(\mathcal{P}' \oplus P\right) \Rightarrow \forall \mathcal{Q} : SM\left(\mathcal{P} \oplus \mathcal{Q}\right) = SM\left(\mathcal{P}' \oplus \mathcal{Q}\right)$$

Let $\mathcal{Q}^n = Q_1 \oplus ... \oplus Q_n, 1 \le n$.

We will prove by induction on n (the number of states of $\mathcal{Q}$). Note that for $\mathcal{Q} = \{\}$ it is proved by Proposition 25.

- $n = 1$:

$\mathcal{Q}^1 = Q_1$

$$\forall P : SM(\mathcal{P} \oplus P) = SM\left(\mathcal{P}' \oplus P\right) \Rightarrow \forall Q_1 : SM(\mathcal{P} \oplus Q_1) = SM\left(\mathcal{P}' \oplus Q_1\right)$$

just make $P = Q_1$.

- step:

By induction hypothesis ($n > 1$),

$$\forall P : SM(\mathcal{P} \oplus P) = SM\left(\mathcal{P}' \oplus P\right) \Rightarrow$$
$$\Rightarrow \forall \mathcal{Q}^{n-1} : SM\left(\mathcal{P} \oplus \mathcal{Q}^{n-1}\right) = SM\left(\mathcal{P}' \oplus \mathcal{Q}^{n-1}\right) \tag{3.52}$$

and we want to prove that

$$\forall P : SM(\mathcal{P} \oplus P) = SM\left(\mathcal{P}' \oplus P\right) \Rightarrow \forall \mathcal{Q}^n : SM(\mathcal{P} \oplus \mathcal{Q}^n) = SM\left(\mathcal{P}' \oplus \mathcal{Q}^n\right)$$

Without loss of generality (Proposition 28) we will replace $\mathcal{P}$ with $P^{\mathcal{K}} \oplus P^{\,not\,\mathcal{K}} \oplus \mathcal{P}$ and $\mathcal{P}'$ with $P^{\mathcal{K}} \oplus P^{\,not\,\mathcal{K}} \oplus \mathcal{P}'$, but keeping the designations $\mathcal{P}$ and $\mathcal{P}'$ for simplicity. Suppose that M is an interpretation such that M is a stable model of $\mathcal{P} \oplus \mathcal{Q}^n$, i.e. a stable model of $\mathcal{P} \oplus Q_1 \oplus ... \oplus Q_n$ Then, by Lemma 31, M is also a stable model of $\mathcal{P} \oplus Q_1 \oplus ... \oplus Q_{n-2} \oplus Q$ where Q is defined as follows:

$$Q = Q_n \cup [Q_{n-1} - Reject^*(Q_{n-1}, Q_n, M)]$$

and (as by 3.44):

$$Reject^*(Q_{n-1}, Q_n, M) = \{r \in Q_{n-1} \mid \exists r' \in Q_n, H(r) = not\, H(r') \wedge M \vDash B(r')\}$$

But since $Q_1 \oplus ... \oplus Q_{n-2} \oplus Q$ is a DLP of size $n-1$, then, by the induction hypothesis (3.52), M is also a stable model of $\mathcal{P}' \oplus Q_1 \oplus ... \oplus Q_{n-2} \oplus Q$. Then $M = least(\Phi)$ where

$$\begin{aligned}\Phi = &\left(\begin{array}{c} \rho(\mathcal{P}') - Reject^*(\mathcal{P}', \mathcal{P}', M) - \\ -Reject^*(\mathcal{P}', \mathcal{Q}^{n-2}, M) - Reject^*(\mathcal{P}', Q_n, M) - \\ -Reject^*(\mathcal{P}', (Q_{n-1} - Reject^*(Q_{n-1}, Q_n, M), M)) \end{array}\right) \cup \\ \cup &\left(\begin{array}{c} \rho(\mathcal{Q}^{n-2}) - Reject^*(\mathcal{Q}^{n-2}, \mathcal{Q}^{n-2}, M) - \\ -Reject^*(\mathcal{Q}^{n-2}, Q_n, M) - \\ -Reject^*(\mathcal{Q}^{n-2}, (Q_{n-1} - Reject^*(Q_{n-1}, Q_n, M), M)) \end{array}\right) \cup \\ \cup &(Q_{n-1} - Reject^*(Q_{n-1}, Q_n, M), M) \cup \\ \cup &Q_n\end{aligned}$$

where:

$$\mathcal{Q}^{n-2} = Q_1 \oplus ... \oplus Q_{n-2}$$

Let

$$\begin{aligned}\Pi' &= \rho(\mathcal{P}') - Reject^*\left(\mathcal{P}', \mathcal{P}', M\right) - Reject^*\left(\mathcal{P}', \mathcal{Q}^{n-2}, M\right) - \\ &- Reject^*\left(\mathcal{P}', Q_n, M\right) - Reject^*\left(\mathcal{P}', (Q_{n-1} - Reject^*(Q_{n-1}, Q_n, M), M)\right) \\ \Psi &= \rho\left(\mathcal{Q}^{n-2}\right) - Reject^*\left(\mathcal{Q}^{n-2}, \mathcal{Q}^{n-2}, M\right) - Reject^*\left(\mathcal{Q}^{n-2}, Q_n, M\right) - \\ &- Reject^*\left(\mathcal{Q}^{n-2}, (Q_{n-1} - Reject^*(Q_{n-1}, Q_n, M), M)\right) \\ \Omega &= (Q_{n-1} - Reject^*(Q_{n-1}, Q_n, M), M) \cup Q_n\end{aligned}$$

Then:

$$M = least\,(\Pi' \cup \Psi \cup \Omega)$$

We want to prove that M is also a stable model of $\mathcal{P}' \oplus \mathcal{Q}^n$. This is so iff:

$$M = least\,((\Pi' \cup \Psi \cup \Omega) - \Pi'') \tag{3.53}$$

where:

$$\Pi'' = Reject^*\left(\mathcal{P}', Reject^*\left(Q_{n-1}, Q_n, M\right), M\right) \cup \tag{3.54}$$

$$\cup Reject^*\left(\mathcal{Q}^{n-2}, Reject^*\left(Q_{n-1}, Q_n, M\right), M\right) = \tag{3.55}$$

$$= \left\{ \begin{array}{c} r \in (\Pi' \cup \Psi) \mid \exists r' \in Reject^*\left(Q_{n-1}, Q_n, M\right), \\ , H(r) = not\, H(r') \wedge M \vDash B(r') \end{array} \right\} = \tag{3.56}$$

$$= \left\{ \begin{array}{c} r \in (\Pi' \cup \Psi) \mid \exists r'' \in Q_n, \exists r' \in Q_{n-1}, H(r) = H(r'')\wedge \\ \wedge H(r') = not\, H(r'') \wedge M \vDash B(r') \wedge M \vDash B(r'') \end{array} \right\} \tag{3.57}$$

From this we can conclude that for every rule in Π'' there is at least one rule in Q_n, and therefore in $(\Pi' \cup \Psi \cup \Omega) - \Pi''$ with the same head and true body:

$$\forall r \in \Pi'', \exists r'' \in Q_n : H(r) = H(r'') \wedge M \vDash B(r'')$$

and that for every rule in Π'' such that $H(r) = A$ (resp. $H(r) = not\, A$), M contains A (resp. $not\, A$):

$$\forall r \in \Pi'', H(r) \in M$$

Since M is a stable model of $\mathcal{P} \oplus \mathcal{Q}^n$, is satisfies the condition:

$$M = least\,((\Pi''' \cup \Psi \cup \Omega) - \Pi'''')$$

where Π''' (resp. Π'''') is obtained as Π' (resp. Π'') but replacing $\mathcal{P}'$ with $\mathcal{P}$.

We need to prove that if $M = least\,(\Pi' \cup \Psi \cup \Omega)$ (and also $M = least\,((\Pi''' \cup \Psi \cup \Omega) - \Pi''''))$ then $M = least\,((\Pi' \cup \Psi \cup \Omega) - \Pi'')$. Suppose that $M \neq least\,((\Pi' \cup \Psi \cup \Omega) - \Pi'')$. Let $M' = least\,((\Pi' \cup \Psi \cup \Omega) - \Pi'')$. Then $M' \subseteq M$. Let $Y = M - M'$. Let L be such that $L \in T_{(\Pi''' \cup \Psi \cup \Omega) - \Pi''''}(M')$ and $L \notin M'$. Then $L \in Y$. If such element does not exist then, of course, $M = M'$. Then there would be one (or more) rules r in Π'' such that $H(r) = L$ and $B(r) \subseteq M'$; and there would not be any rules in $(\Psi - \Pi'') \cup \Omega$ such that $H(r) = L$ and $B(r) \subseteq M'$:

$$\nexists r \in (\Psi - \Pi'') \cup \Omega : H(r) = L \wedge B(r) \subseteq M' \tag{3.58}$$

Since $L \in T_{(\Pi''' \cup \Psi \cup \Omega) - \Pi''''}(M')$, there is at least one rule in $(\Pi''' \cup \Psi \cup \Omega) - \Pi''''$ such that $H(r) = L$ and $B(r) \subseteq M'$. But since we have that $\Pi''' - \Pi''''$ does not contain any rules r' with $H(r') = L$, the rule r must be in $(\Psi - \Pi'''') \cup \Omega$. But since $\Psi - \Pi'''' = \Psi - \Pi''$, such rule would also exist in $(\Psi - \Pi'') \cup \Omega$, thus violating 3.58. Therefore, L cannot exist and $M = M'$.

We have proved that if M is a stable model of $\mathcal{P} \oplus \mathcal{Q}^n$ then M is a stable model of $\mathcal{P}' \oplus \mathcal{Q}^n$. But the converse also holds because everything is symmetrical, i.e. M is a stable model of $\mathcal{P}' \oplus \mathcal{Q}^n$ then M is a stable model of $\mathcal{P} \oplus \mathcal{Q}^n$, thus completing the proof of the Theorem. ■

Corollary 32 *Let $\mathcal{P}$ and $\mathcal{P}'$ be two Dynamic Logic Programs. Then:*

$$\nexists P : SM\,(\mathcal{P} \oplus P) \neq SM\left(\mathcal{P}' \oplus P\right) \Leftrightarrow \mathcal{P} \overset{\oplus}{\equiv} \mathcal{P}'$$

where P is a generalized logic program.

State condensing

One of the primary objectives when defining the notion of update equivalence was, as mentioned, the desire to be able to simplify some dynamic logic programs, even at the cost of losing the semantics at past states, as long as there was the guarantee that the present and all future states would have the same semantics. If one is willing to lose the semantics at such past states, then, there would be no point in keeping the programs associated with such past states, if it were possible to condense them into one state. It would be therefore natural the quest for a syntactical operator such that, given an arbitrary sequence of logic programs, would produce another sequence so that two of its consecutive programs were condensed into a single one, written in the same language as the original ones, the resulting logic program having the property of being update equivalent to the initial sequence. The iteration of such an operator would allow the condensation of an arbitrary sequence of logic programs into a single one. We call such operators state condensing operators, generically defined as follows:

Definition 40 (State Condensing) *Let $\mathcal{L}_{\mathcal{K}}$ be an arbitrary propositional language. Let Π denote the set of all generalized logic programs that can be written with $\mathcal{L}_{\mathcal{K}}$. Let Θ be an operator with signature $\Theta : \Pi \times \Pi \rightarrow \Pi$. We say that Θ is a* state condensing operator *for $\mathcal{L}_{\mathcal{K}}$ iff for any DLP $\mathcal{P} = P_1 \oplus ... \oplus P_n$ it holds that:*

$$\mathcal{P} \overset{\oplus}{\equiv} P_1 \oplus ... \oplus P_{i-1} \oplus \Theta\left(P_i, P_{i+1}\right) \oplus P_{i+2} \oplus ... \oplus P_n$$

Unfortunately such state condensing operators, in general, do not exist, as stated by the following negative, but nevertheless important, result:

Theorem 33 *Let $\mathcal{K}$ be a set of propositions of size greater than 1. State condensing operators for $\mathcal{L}_{\mathcal{K}}$ do not exist.*

Proof. *The proof is quite simple and based on the fact that the semantics of a DLP consisting of a single generalized logic program coincides with the generalized stable model semantics of such generalized logic program. We will show an example consisting of a DLP with two states and prove that there is no single generalized logic program, written in the same language, whose stable models coincide with those of the DLP. Let $\mathcal{L} = \{a, b, not\, a, not\, b\}$ be a propositional language. Let $\mathcal{P} = P_1 \oplus P_2$ be such that:*

$$P_1 = \left\{ \begin{array}{c} a \leftarrow b \\ b \leftarrow \end{array} \right\} \qquad P_2 = \{not\, b \leftarrow not\, a\}$$

The stable models of $\mathcal{P}$ at state 2 are:

$$M_1 = \{a, b\} \qquad M_2 = \{\}$$

Any state condensing operator would have to provide a single logic program, $P_{1,2} = \Theta\left(P_1, P_2\right)$ such that $\mathcal{P} \overset{\oplus}{\equiv} P_{1,2}$. If $\mathcal{P} \overset{\oplus}{\equiv} P_{1,2}$, then $SM\left(\mathcal{P}\right) = SM\left(P_{1,2}\right)$. But there is no generalized logic program whose stable models are M_1 and M_2. This is so because of minimality of the stable model semantics: no two models $M_1^+ \supset M_2^+$ can be stable models of the same logic program. ■

For the uninteresting case excluded by the theorem, namely with a set of propositions $\mathcal{K}$ of size 1, there is trivial state condensing operator defined as follows

Definition 41 *Let $\mathcal{K}$ be a set of propositions of size 1. Let P_i and P_{i+1} be two generalized logic programs written in $\mathcal{L}_{\mathcal{K}}$. The result of performing a state condensing of P_i and P_{i+1} is the logic program $\Theta(P_i, P_{i+1})$ defined as follows:*

- *if P_{i+1} contains a rule r such that $B(r) = \{\}$ then $\Theta(P_i, P_{i+1}) = P_{i+1}$;*
- *otherwise $\Theta(P_i, P_{i+1}) = P_i \cup P_{i+1}$.*

We have imposed that the resulting program from performing state condensing be written in the same language of the original one. In Section 3.3.3 we will explore a purely syntactical transformation that, given a DLP, produces a single generalized logic program, written in an extended language, whose stable models are in a one-to-one correspondence with the stable models of the DLP. It remains an open problem to address the issue of finding what is the smaller extended language required to allow the definition of such state condensing operators.

Even though in general we cannot perform state condensing whilst preserving the size of the language, there are situations where it is possible to reduce the number of states of a DLP whilst, of course, preserving update equivalence. We have already seen that empty programs can be removed. We will now establish some other possibilities to reduce the number of states of a DLP.

The following proposition allows the merging of consecutive programs written in disjoint languages:

Proposition 34 *Let $\mathcal{P}$ be a dynamic logic program, P_a and P_b two logic programs written in disjoint languages. Then,*

$$(\mathcal{P} \oplus P_a \oplus P_b) \stackrel{\oplus}{\equiv} (\mathcal{P} \oplus P_b \oplus P_a) \stackrel{\oplus}{\equiv} (\mathcal{P} \oplus (P_b \cup P_a))$$

Proof. *The rules of P_b do not reject those of P_a because they are never conflicting. Conversely, those of P_a do not reject those of P_b. Since the relation between the state a (and b) and any other state is preserved by either exchanging its order or simply join them, the set of all rules, and the sets $Reject(\_,\_,\_)$ and $Default(\_,\_)$ are equal in all three situations, from which the update equivalence follows.* ■

This result can be strengthened. In fact, we only need to guarantee that there are no conflicting rules in order to merge both programs:

Proposition 35 *Let $\mathcal{P}$ be a dynamic logic program, P_a and P_b two logic programs such that*

$$\forall r_a \in P_a, r_b \in P_b : r_a \not\bowtie r_b$$

Then,

$$(\mathcal{P} \oplus P_a \oplus P_b) \stackrel{\oplus}{\equiv} (\mathcal{P} \oplus P_b \oplus P_a) \stackrel{\oplus}{\equiv} (\mathcal{P} \oplus (P_b \cup P_a))$$

Proof. *Same as for the previous proposition, i.e. the rules of P_b do not reject those of P_a because they not conflicting, and vice versa.* ■

Proposition 36 *Let $\mathcal{P}$ be a dynamic logic program, P_a and P_b two logic programs such that $P_a \subseteq P_b$. Then,*

$$(\mathcal{P} \oplus P_a \oplus P_b) \stackrel{\oplus}{\equiv} (\mathcal{P} \oplus P_b)$$

Proof. *This result can be obtained by repeatedly applying Proposition 38 until all rules in P_a have been eliminated, and then by using Proposition 26 to eliminate the resulting empty P_a.* ■

State Simplification

In this section we will address the issue of (syntactical) state simplification, i.e. reducing the size of each individual program in a DLP.

We start with a result that allows the removal of rules such that equal rules exist at subsequent states.

Proposition 37 *Let $\mathcal{P}$ be a dynamic logic program, j and m two of its states such that $j < m$. Let r be a rule such that $r \in P_m \in \mathcal{P}$ and $r \in P_j \in \mathcal{P}$. Let $\mathcal{P}'$ be the dynamic logic program obtained from $\mathcal{P}$ such that*

$$\forall P_k \in \mathcal{P}, k \neq j : P'_k = P_k \in \mathcal{P}'$$
$$P'_j = P_j - \{r\} \in \mathcal{P}'$$

Then, $\mathcal{P} \overset{\oplus}{\equiv} \mathcal{P}'$.

Proof. *Since to establish update equivalence between two dynamic logic programs we only need to consider the stable models at states (after combined with $\mathcal{Q}$) greater than their maximal states and, at those states, if r of P_m is rejected so is r of P_j and if r of P_m is not rejected, r is present when determining the least model and the presence or absence of r of P_j is irrelevant. Furthermore, the set of rejected rules is not affected by removing r of P_j because those rules that are rejected by this rule are also rejected by r of P_m. The set of defaults is trivially equal in both cases.* ■

The next proposition allows the removal of subsumed rules, i.e. rules for which there is a more recent rule for the same atom (or its default negation) whose body is a subset of the body of the rule to be eliminated.

Proposition 38 *Let $\mathcal{P}$ be a dynamic logic program, j and m two of its states such that $j < m$. Let r and r' be rules such that $r \in P_m \in \mathcal{P}$, $r' \in P_j \in \mathcal{P}$, $H(r') = H(r)$ and $B(r) \subseteq B(r')$. Let $\mathcal{P}'$ be the dynamic logic program obtained from $\mathcal{P}$ such that*

$$\forall P_k \in \mathcal{P}, k \neq j : P'_k = P_k \in \mathcal{P}'$$
$$P'_j = P_j - \{r'\} \in \mathcal{P}'$$

Then, $\mathcal{P} \overset{\oplus}{\equiv} \mathcal{P}'$.

Proof. *Let $\mathcal{P} = P_1 \oplus ... \oplus P_{j-1} \oplus P_j \oplus P_{j+1} \oplus ... \oplus P_m$. Let $r \in P_m$, $r' \in P_j$ such that $H(r') = H(r)$ and $B(r) \subseteq B(r')$ and let $\mathcal{P}' = P_1 \oplus ... \oplus P_{j-1} \oplus P'_j \oplus P_{j+1} \oplus ... \oplus P_m$ be constructed as described. Let $\mathcal{Q} = Q_{m+1} \oplus ... \oplus Q_n$ be an arbitrary DLP. We want to prove that $\forall i : m+1 \leq i \leq n$:*

$$SM\left(\mathcal{P} \oplus Q_{m+1} \oplus ... \oplus Q_i\right) = SM\left(\mathcal{P}' \oplus Q_{m+1} \oplus ... \oplus Q_i\right)$$

Again, to prove the proposition we need only prove it for the case where r belongs to the max state of $\mathcal{P}$, i.e. m. All other cases follow due to 23. Given an interpretation M_i, define:

$$Rejectedby(r', j) = \{r'' : r'' \in P_l, l < j, r'' \bowtie r', M_i \vDash B(r')\}$$

This set contains the rules that would be rejected by rule r', given an interpretation. Note that since $j < m$, $H(r') = H(r)$ and $B(r) \subseteq B(r')$, we have that $Rejectedby(r', j) \subseteq Rejectedby(r, m)$. Let $\mathcal{P}^i = \mathcal{P} \oplus Q_{m+1} \oplus ... \oplus Q_i$ and $\mathcal{P}'^i = \mathcal{P}' \oplus Q_{m+1} \oplus ... \oplus Q_i$. An interpretation M_i is a stable model of $\mathcal{P}^i$ iff:

$$M_i = least\left(\left[\rho\left(\mathcal{P}^i\right) - Reject(\mathcal{P}^i, i, M_i)\right] \cup Default\left(\rho\left(\mathcal{P}^i\right), M_i\right)\right) \tag{3.59}$$

An interpretation M_i is a stable model of $\mathcal{P}'^i$ iff:

$$M_i = least\left(\left[\rho\left(\mathcal{P}'^i\right) - Reject(\mathcal{P}'^i, i, M_i)\right] \cup Default\left(\rho\left(\mathcal{P}'^i\right), M_i\right)\right) \tag{3.60}$$

We want to prove that M_i satisfies 3.59 iff it satisfies 3.60. First let us note that $\rho\left(\mathcal{P}^i\right) = \rho\left(\mathcal{P}'^i\right) \cup \{r'\}$. Since if $H(r') = A$ and $M_i \vDash B(r')$ we also have that $H(r) = A$ and $M_i \vDash B(r)$, it follows that $Default\left(\rho\left(\mathcal{P}^i\right), M_i\right) = Default\left(\rho\left(\mathcal{P}'^i\right), M_i\right)$. The set $Reject(\mathcal{P}^i, i, M_i)$ can be decomposed in the following two disjoint sets:

$$Reject(\mathcal{P}'^i) = Reject(\mathcal{P}^i, i, M_i) \cap \rho\left(\mathcal{P}'^i\right)$$
$$Reject(r') = Reject(\mathcal{P}^i, i, M_i) \cap \{r'\}$$

We now have that M_i satisfies 3.59 iff it satisfies:

$$M_i = least\left(\left[\rho\left(\mathcal{P}'^i\right) - Reject(\mathcal{P}'^i)\right] \cup \left[\{r'\} - Reject(r')\right] \cup Default\left(\rho\left(\mathcal{P}'^i\right), M_i\right)\right) \tag{3.61}$$

We will now show that we can safely eliminate $\{r'\} - Reject(r')$ from the equation. Since $r \in \rho\left(\mathcal{P}'^i\right)$, $H(r') = H(r)$ and $B(r) \subseteq B(r')$, we have that if $r \in Reject(\mathcal{P}'^i)$, then $r' \in Reject(r')$, i.e. there is a rule in any of the programs Q_e that rejects both r and r'. If $r \notin Reject(\mathcal{P}'^i)$, then $r \in \rho\left(\mathcal{P}'^i\right) - Reject(\mathcal{P}'^i)$ and since $H(r') = H(r)$ and $B(r) \subseteq B(r')$, removing r' does not affect the least operation. We obtain that M_i satisfies 3.61 iff it satisfies:

$$M_i = least\left(\left[\rho\left(\mathcal{P}'^i\right) - Reject(\mathcal{P}'^i)\right] \cup Default\left(\rho\left(\mathcal{P}'^i\right), M_i\right)\right) \tag{3.62}$$

If we compare the sets $Reject(\mathcal{P}'^i)$ and $Reject(\mathcal{P}'^i, i, M_i)$ we see that

$$Reject(\mathcal{P}'^i) \cup Rejectedby(r', j) = Reject(\mathcal{P}'^i, i, M_i)$$

But since $Rejectedby(r', j) \subseteq Rejectedby(r, m)$ we also have that $Rejectedby(r', j) \subseteq Reject(\mathcal{P}'^i)$ (the rules rejected by r' are also rejected by r), we obtain that M_i satisfies 3.62 iff it satisfies:

$$M_i = least\left(\left[\rho\left(\mathcal{P}'^i\right) - Reject(\mathcal{P}'^i, i, M_i)\right] \cup Default\left(\rho\left(\mathcal{P}'^i\right), M_i\right)\right) \tag{3.63}$$

Since 3.63 is equal to 3.60, we have that M_i is a stable model of $\mathcal{P}^i$ iff M_i is a stable model of $\mathcal{P}'^i$ and, therefore, $\mathcal{P} \overset{\oplus}{\equiv} \mathcal{P}'$. ■

The next proposition allows the removal of all past rules for an atom A (resp. its default negation *not* A), if there is a fact for *not* A (resp. A). In conjunction with the previous Proposition, when we update with a fact for either A or *not* A we can simply eliminate all past rules for A or *not* A.

Proposition 39 *Let $\mathcal{P}$ be a dynamic logic program, j and m two of its states such that $j < m$. Let r and r' be rules such that $r \in P_m \in \mathcal{P}$, $r' \in P_j \in \mathcal{P}$, $r \bowtie r'$ and $B(r) = \emptyset$. Let $\mathcal{P}'$ be the dynamic logic program obtained from $\mathcal{P}$ such that*

$$\forall P_k \in \mathcal{P}, k \neq j : P'_k = P_k \in \mathcal{P}'$$
$$P'_j = P_j - \{r'\} \in \mathcal{P}'$$

Then, $\mathcal{P} \overset{\oplus}{\equiv} \mathcal{P}'$.

Proof. *Let* $\mathcal{P} = P_1 \oplus ... \oplus P_{j-1} \oplus P_j \oplus P_{j+1} \oplus ... \oplus P_m$. *Let* $r \in P_m$, $r' \in P_j$ *such that* $r \bowtie r'$ *and* $B(r) = \emptyset$ *and let* $\mathcal{P}' = P_1 \oplus ... \oplus P_{j-1} \oplus P_j' \oplus P_{j+1} \oplus ... \oplus P_m$ *be constructed as described. Let* $\mathcal{Q} = Q_{m+1} \oplus ... \oplus Q_n$ *be an arbitrary DLP. We want to prove that* $\forall i : m+1 \leq i \leq n$:

$$SM\left(\mathcal{P} \oplus Q_{m+1} \oplus ... \oplus Q_i\right) = SM\left(\mathcal{P}' \oplus Q_{m+1} \oplus ... \oplus Q_i\right)$$

Again, to prove the proposition we need only prove it for the case where r *belongs to the max state of* $\mathcal{P}$, *i.e.* m. *All other cases follow due to 23. Given an interpretation* M_i, *define:*

$$Rejectedby(r', j) = \{r'' : r'' \in P_l, l < j, r'' \bowtie r', M_i \vDash B(r')\}$$

Let $\mathcal{P}^i = \mathcal{P} \oplus Q_{m+1} \oplus ... \oplus Q_i$ *and* $\mathcal{P}'^i = \mathcal{P}' \oplus Q_{m+1} \oplus ... \oplus Q_i$. *An interpretation* M_i *is a stable model of* $\mathcal{P}^i$ *iff:*

$$M_i = least\left(\left[\rho\left(\mathcal{P}^i\right) - Reject(\mathcal{P}^i, i, M_i)\right] \cup Default\left(\rho\left(\mathcal{P}^i\right), M_i\right)\right) \tag{3.64}$$

An interpretation M_i *is a stable model of* $\mathcal{P}'^i$ *iff:*

$$M_i = least\left(\left[\rho\left(\mathcal{P}'^i\right) - Reject(\mathcal{P}'^i, i, M_i)\right] \cup Default\left(\rho\left(\mathcal{P}'^i\right), M_i\right)\right) \tag{3.65}$$

We want to prove that M_i *satisfies 3.64 iff it satisfies 3.65. First let us note that* $\rho\left(\mathcal{P}^i\right) = \rho\left(\mathcal{P}'^i\right) \cup \{r'\}$. *If* r' *is the only rule in* $\rho\left(\mathcal{P}^i\right)$ *such that* $H(r') = A$ *and* $M_i \vDash B(r')$, *it would cause the set* $Default\left(\rho\left(\mathcal{P}'^i\right), M_i\right)$ *to contain the default not A, that was not present in* $Default\left(\rho\left(\mathcal{P}^i\right), M_i\right)$. *But, in this situation, we have that* r *is* $not\ A \leftarrow$ *and it belongs to* $\left[\rho\left(\mathcal{P}^i\right) - Reject(\mathcal{P}^i, i, M_i)\right]$. *So we can safely replace, in 3.64, the set* $Default\left(\rho\left(\mathcal{P}^i\right), M_i\right)$ *with the set* $Default\left(\rho\left(\mathcal{P}'^i\right), M_i\right)$. *We now have that* M_i *satisfies 3.64 iff it satisfies:*

$$M_i = least\left(\left[\left(\rho\left(\mathcal{P}'^i\right) \cup \{r'\}\right) - Reject(\mathcal{P}^i, i, M_i)\right] \cup Default\left(\rho\left(\mathcal{P}'^i\right), M_i\right)\right) \tag{3.66}$$

Note that r' *always belongs to* $Reject(\mathcal{P}^i, i, M_i)$ *and does not belong to* $Reject(\mathcal{P}'^i, i, M_i)$. *Furthermore, we have that the only difference between* $\left[\left(\rho\left(\mathcal{P}'^i\right) \cup \{r'\}\right) - Reject(\mathcal{P}^i, i, M_i)\right]$ *and* $\left[\rho\left(\mathcal{P}'^i\right) - Reject(\mathcal{P}'^i, i, M_i)\right]$ *is that the later may contain rules* r''' *such that* $H(r''') = H(r)$. *But since we know that* $B(r) = \emptyset$, *the presence or absence of such rules is irrelevant when determining the least model. Therefore,* M_i *satisfies 3.65 iff it satisfies 3.66 iff it satisfies 3.64, i.e.* M_i *is a stable model of* $\mathcal{P}^i$ *iff* M_i *is a stable model of* $\mathcal{P}'^i$ *and, therefore,* $\mathcal{P} \stackrel{\oplus}{\equiv} \mathcal{P}'$. ■

3.3.3 Transformational Semantics

Definition 37 above, establishes the semantics of *Dynamic Logic Programming* by characterizing its stable models at each state. Next we present an alternative definition, based on a purely syntactical transformation that, given a *Dynamic Logic Program,* $\mathcal{P}$, produces a generalized logic program whose stable models are in a one-to-one equivalence relation with the stable models of the multi-dimensional dynamic logic program previously characterized. This linear transformation also provides a mechanism for implementing *Dynamic Logic Programming*: with a pre-processor performing the transformation, query answering is reduced to that over generalized logic programs.

By $\overline{\mathcal{K}}$ we denote the following superset of the set $\mathcal{K}$ of propositional variables:

$$\overline{\mathcal{K}} = \mathcal{K} \cup \{A^-, A_s,\ A_s^-, A_{P_s},\ A_{P_s}^- : A \in \mathcal{K},\ s \in \mathcal{T} \cup \{0\}\}.$$

As before, this definition assumes that the original set $\mathcal{K}$ of propositional variables does not contain any of the newly added symbols of the form $A^-, A_s, A_s^-, A_{P_s}, A_{P_s}^-$ so that they are all disjoint sets of symbols. If the original language $\mathcal{K}$ contains any such symbols then they have to be *renamed* before the expansion of $\mathcal{K}$ takes place. We denote by $\overline{\mathcal{L}} = \mathcal{L}_{\overline{\mathcal{K}}}$ the expansion of the language $\mathcal{L} = \mathcal{L}_{\mathcal{K}}$ generated by $\overline{\mathcal{K}}$.

Definition 42 (Dynamic Program Update) *By the dynamic program update over the sequence of updating programs $\mathcal{P} = \{P_s : s \in \mathcal{T}\}$ we mean the logic program $\biguplus\mathcal{P}$, which consists of the following clauses in the expanded language $\overline{\mathcal{L}}$:*

(RP) Rewritten program clauses:

$$A_{P_s} \leftarrow B_1, \ldots, B_m, C_1^-, \ldots, C_n^- \tag{3.67}$$
$$A_{P_s}^- \leftarrow B_1, \ldots, B_m, C_1^-, \ldots, C_n^- \tag{3.68}$$

for any clause:

$$A \leftarrow B_1, \; \ldots, \; B_m, \; not\, C_1, \; \ldots, \; not\, C_n$$

respectively, for any clause:

$$not\, A \leftarrow B_1, \; \ldots, \; B_m, \; not\, C_1, \; \ldots, \; not\, C_n$$

in the program P_s, where $s \in \mathcal{T}$. The rewritten clauses are simply obtained from the original ones by replacing atoms A (respectively, the default literals not A) occurring in their heads by the atoms A_{P_s} (respectively, $A_{P_s}^-$) and by replacing negative premises not C by C^-.

(UR) Update rules:

$$A_s \leftarrow A_{P_s} \tag{3.69}$$
$$A_s^- \leftarrow A_{P_s}^- \tag{3.70}$$

for all atoms $A \in \mathcal{K}$ and for all $s \in \mathcal{T}$. The update rules state that an atom A must be true (respectively, false) in the state $s \in \mathcal{T}$ if it is true (respectively, false) in the updating program P_s.

(IR) Inheritance rules:

$$A_s \leftarrow A_{s-1}, not\, A_{P_s}^- \tag{3.71}$$
$$A_s^- \leftarrow A_{s-1}^-, not A_{P_s} \tag{3.72}$$

for all atoms $A \in \mathcal{K}$ and for all $s \in \mathcal{T}$. The inheritance rules say that an atom A is true (respectively, false) in the state $s \in \mathcal{T}$ if it is true (respectively, false) in the previous state $s-1$ and it is not rejected, *i.e., forced to be false (respectively, true), by the updating program P_s.*

(DR) Default rules:

$$A_0^-, \tag{3.73}$$

for all atoms $A \in \mathcal{K}$. Default rules describe the initial state 0 by making all objective atoms initially false.

Observe that the dynamic program update $\biguplus\mathcal{P}$ is a normal logic program, i.e., it does not contain default literals in heads of its clauses. Moreover, only the inheritance rules contain default literals in their bodies. Also note that the program $\biguplus\mathcal{P}$ does not contain the atoms A or A^-, where $A \in \mathcal{K}$, in heads of its clauses. These atoms appear only in the bodies of rewritten program clauses. The notion of the dynamic program update $\biguplus_s\mathcal{P}$ at a given state $s \in \mathcal{T}$ changes that.

Definition 43 ***(Dynamic Program Update at a Given State)*** *Given a fixed state $s \in \mathcal{T}$, by the dynamic program update at the state s, denoted by $\biguplus_s\mathcal{P}$, we mean the dynamic program update $\biguplus\mathcal{P}$ augmented with the following:*

(CS$_s$) Current State Rules:

$$A \leftarrow A_s \tag{3.74}$$

$$A^- \leftarrow A_s^- \tag{3.75}$$

$$not\, A \leftarrow A_s^- \tag{3.76}$$

for all atoms $A \in \mathcal{K}$. Current state rules specify the current state s in which the updated program is being evaluated and determine the values of the atoms A and A^-, and the default literals not A.

Observe that although for any particular state s the program $\biguplus\mathcal{P}$ is not required to be coherent, the program update $\biguplus_s\mathcal{P}$ at the state s must be coherent (see Proposition 8).

Theorem 40 (Soundness and Completeness) *Given a* Dynamic Logic Program *$\mathcal{P}$, the generalized stable models of $\biguplus_s\mathcal{P}$, restricted to $\mathcal{L}$, coincide with the generalized stable models of $\bigoplus_s\mathcal{P}$.*

Proof. *This result immediately follows from Proposition 91 and Theorem 92 in Chapter 6, where we prove the soundness and completeness of a generalization of the definition of stable models of a DLP wrt. a generalization of the transformation to obtain program $\biguplus_s\mathcal{P}$.* ■

Next, we present an example illustrating how this transformation can be applied.

Example 16 *Let $\mathcal{P} = \{P_1, P_2, P_3\}$, where P_1, P_2 and P_3 are as follows:*

$$\begin{array}{ll} P_1: & sleep \leftarrow not\, tv\_on \\ & watch\_tv \leftarrow tv\_on \\ & tv\_on \leftarrow \\ P_2: & not\, tv\_on \leftarrow power\_failure \\ & power\_failure \leftarrow \\ P_3: & not\, power\_failure \leftarrow \end{array}$$

The dynamic program update over $\mathcal{P}$ is the logic program $\biguplus\mathcal{P} = (RP_1) \cup (RP_2) \cup (RP_3) \cup (UR) \cup (IR) \cup (DR)$, where

$$\begin{array}{ll} RP_1: & sleep_{P_1} \leftarrow tv\_on^- \\ & watch\_tv_{P_1} \leftarrow tv\_on \\ & tv\_on_{P_1} \leftarrow \\ RP_2: & tv\_on^-_{P_2} \leftarrow power\_failure \\ & power\_failure_{P_2} \leftarrow \\ RP_3: & power\_failure^-_{P_3} \leftarrow \end{array} \tag{3.77}$$

and the dynamic program update at the state s is $\biguplus_s \mathcal{P} = \biguplus \mathcal{P} \cup (CS_s)$. *Consequently, as intended,* $\biguplus_1 \mathcal{P}$ *has a single stable model* $M_1 = \{tv\_on, watch\_tv\}$; $\biguplus_2 \mathcal{P}$ *has a single stable model* $M_2 = \{sleep, power\_failure\}$ *and* $\biguplus_3 \mathcal{P}$ *has a single stable model* $M_3 = \{tv\_on, watch\_tv\}$ *(all models modulo irrelevant literals). Moreover.* $\biguplus_2 \mathcal{P}$ *is semantically equivalent to* $P_1 \biguplus P_2$.

3.3.4 Computational Complexity

In this Subsection we make some brief comments about the computational complexity of DLP. As usual in logic programming and stable model based semantics, there are four different problems to de addressed, namely:

1. deciding whether $\mathcal{P}$ has a stable model at state s;
2. deciding whether a given interpretation is a stable model of $\mathcal{P}$ at state s;
3. deciding whether a given atom is true in at least one stable model of $\mathcal{P}$ at state s;
4. deciding whether a given atom is true in all stable model of $\mathcal{P}$ at state s.

In [77], the authors have made an extensive study of the computational complexity of logic program updates. They have used a different semantical characterization for sequences of logic programs but the complexity results also hold for DLP. In a subsequent section we will compare DLP to those other existing approaches. Nevertheless, the main result in what complexity is concerned is that DLP does not add to the intrinsic complexity of the stable model semantics. The following theorem summarizes the computational complexity for the four mentioned tasks:

Theorem 41 (Computational Complexity) *Given a dynamic logic program* $\mathcal{P}$, *and one of its states s, then:*

1. *deciding whether* $\mathcal{P}$ *has a stable model at state s is* $NP-complete$;
2. *deciding whether a given interpretation is a stable model of* $\mathcal{P}$ *at state s is* P;
3. *deciding whether a given atom is true in at least one stable model of* $\mathcal{P}$ *at state s is* $NP-complete$;
4. *deciding whether a given atom is true in all stable model of* $\mathcal{P}$ *at state s is* $coNP-complete$;

Proof. *The program* $\biguplus_s \mathcal{P}$ *can be obtained in polynomial time from* $\mathcal{P}$, *given s. All the results are therefore inherited from the results from the complexity of logic programs [155].* ■

3.3.5 Other Issues

Adding Strong Negation

The introduction of strong negation to the framework of Dynamic Logic Programming is, in all, similar to the case of the single update. The extended stable models are characterized as follows:

Definition 44 (Extended Stable Models at state s) *Let $\mathcal{P} = \{P_s : s \in \mathcal{T}\}$ be a* Dynamic Logic Program *in the language $\mathcal{L}^*$ and let $s \in \mathcal{T}$. An consistent interpretation M_s is an* extended stable model of $\mathcal{P}$ at state s, *iff M_s is a* stable model of $\mathcal{P}^{exp}$ at state s *where $\mathcal{P}^{exp}$ is obtained from $\mathcal{P}$ by replacing each program $P_s \in \mathcal{P}$ by its expanded version P_s^{exp}.*

Again, in order to use strong negation in updates, one only needs to consider the expanded versions of each program and deal with complementary objective literals A and $-A$ as independent atoms.

Example 17 *Let $\mathcal{K}^* = \{a, b, c, -a, -b, -c\}$. Let $\mathcal{P} = \{P_1, P_2, P_3\}$ be the dynamic logic program such that:*

$$
\begin{array}{llllll}
P_1: & a \leftarrow not\, b & P_2: & -a \leftarrow -c & P_3: & not\ -a \leftarrow not\, b \\
 & c \leftarrow & & -c \leftarrow & & not\, b \leftarrow
\end{array}
$$

and their expanded versions:

$$
\begin{array}{llllll}
P_1^{exp}: & a \leftarrow not\, b & P_2^{exp}: & -a \leftarrow -c & P_3^{exp}: & not\ -a \leftarrow not\, b \\
 & c \leftarrow & & -c \leftarrow & & not\, b \leftarrow \\
 & not\ -a \leftarrow not\, b & & not\, a \leftarrow -c & & \\
 & not\ -c \leftarrow & & not\, c \leftarrow & &
\end{array}
$$

Let M_3 be the following consistent interpretation:

$$M_3 = \{not\ a, not\ b, not\ c, not\ -a, not\ -b, -c\}$$

According to M_3, we have the following set of rejected rules:

$$
Reject(\mathcal{P}^{exp}, 3, M_3) = \left\{ \begin{array}{l} -a \leftarrow -c \\ c \leftarrow \\ not\ -c \leftarrow \\ a \leftarrow not\, b \\ not\ -a \leftarrow not\, b \end{array} \right\}
$$

And $\rho(\mathcal{P}^{exp}) - Reject(\mathcal{P}^{exp}, 3, M_3)$ is as follows:

$$
\rho(\mathcal{P}^{exp}) - Reject(\mathcal{P}^{exp}, 3, M_3) = \left\{ \begin{array}{l} not\ -a \leftarrow not\, b \\ not\, b \leftarrow \\ -c \leftarrow \\ not\, c \leftarrow \\ not\, a \leftarrow -c \end{array} \right\}
$$

which, together with the set of defaults:

$$Default(\rho(\mathcal{P}^{exp}), M_3) = \{not\, b, not\ -b\}$$

allows us to verify that:

$$M = least((\rho(\mathcal{P}^{exp}) - Reject(\mathcal{P}^{exp}, 3, M_3)) \cup Default(\rho(\mathcal{P}^{exp}), M_3)).$$

Consequently, M_3 *is an extended stable model of* $\mathcal{P}$ *at state* 3*. In fact, it is the only extended stable model of this program.*

As the reader may notice, programs with strong negation can also be employed in the transformation of Definition 42. As in Definition 44, all that needs doing is use the expanded language $\mathcal{L}^*$ and the expanded programs $\mathcal{P}^{exp}$ instead. Since complementary objective literals A and $-A$ are treated as independent atoms, the stable models obtained from $\biguplus_s \mathcal{P}^{exp}$, modulo the newly introduced literals, coincide with those characterized by Definition 44.

Background Knowledge

Sometimes it is useful to have some kind of a *background knowledge*, i.e., knowledge that is true in every program module or state. This is true as well in the case of the taxonomy rules, which we discuss below, as well as in the general case of laws in the domain of actions and effects of action. These laws must be valid in every state and at any time (for example, the law saying that if there is no power then the TV must be off).

Rules describing background knowledge, i.e., background rules, are easily representable in dynamic logic programming: if a rule is valid in every program state, simply add that rule to every program state. However, this is not a very practical, and, especially, not a very efficient way of representing background rules. Fortunately, according to Proposition 37 in dynamic program updates at a given state s, adding a rule to every state is equivalent to adding that rule only in the state s.

Consequently, such background rules need not necessarily be added to every program state. Instead, they can simply be added at the final state s.

Dealing with Contradiction

One of the important and also very difficult issues involving dynamic updates is that of *consistency* of the updated program $P \oplus U$. As stated in Section 2, we consider a program to be *consistent* if it has at least one stable model and thus a well-defined *stable semantics*. There are two basic reasons why the updated program may not be consistent:

1. The updated generalized logic program $P \oplus U$ may contain *explicitly contradictory* information, such as A and $not\ A$, and thus not have any stable models. There are basically three cases to consider:

   (a) The contradictory information may be inherited from the original program P, which was already inconsistent, as in the example consisting of the following two programs:

   $$\begin{array}{llll} P: & a \leftarrow not\, b & \quad U: & d \leftarrow e \\ & not\, a \leftarrow not\, c & & e \leftarrow \end{array}$$

   In this case one of the possible approaches is to prevent the contradictory information from being inherited by inertia by *limiting the inheritance by inertia.* This approach is discussed in more detail in the next section.

(b) The contradictory information may be the result of the fact that the updating program U is itself contradictory, as in the example consisting of the following two programs:

$$\begin{array}{llll} P: & d \leftarrow e & U: & a \leftarrow not\, b \\ & e \leftarrow & & not\, a \leftarrow not\, c \end{array}$$

This is more difficult to eliminate because the rules of the updating program U must be, by definition, true in the updated program $P \oplus U$. One approach is to always require the updating program U to be consistent. If such a requirement is impossible to satisfy, we could accept contradiction in the current update but prevent it from proliferating further to the subsequent updates by using the approach discussed in (a).

(c) Both the original program P and the updating program U may be perfectly consistent and yet the resulting updated program may contain contradictory information, as in the example consisting of the following two programs:

$$\begin{array}{llll} P: & a \leftarrow d & U: & d \leftarrow e \\ & not\, a \leftarrow e & & e \leftarrow \end{array}$$

In this case, as in the case (a), one of the possible approaches is to prevent the contradictory information from being part of the updated program by *limiting the inheritance by inertia.* This approach is also discussed in more detail in the next subsection. Another possibility is to establish some *priorities* between different rules in order to prevent contradiction from arising in the first place.

2. Explicit contradiction, like the one discussed in (1), can only arise when the updated program contains some rules with default negation in there heads. Thus, it cannot arise when the updated program is normal. However, as is well-known, even normal logic programs may be *implicitly inconsistent* simply because they don't have any stable models. One possible way of dealing with this problem is to replace the stable semantics by the *3-valued stable*, or, equivalently, *well-founded semantics.* Every normal logic program is known to be consistent w.r.t. the well-founded semantics, i.e., it has a well-defined well-founded semantics. Defining and dealing with such three valued semantics for DLP is outside the scope of this work. Nevertheless, in [141, 143], we have shown how to perform updates under the well founded semantics, but for an update semantics other than the one presented here.

There are many other possible approaches to contradiction removal in program updates and they are part of our ongoing research in this area. However, a detailed discussion of this subject goes beyond the scope of the current work.

Limiting the Inheritance by Inertia

Inheritance rules (IR) describe *the rules of inertia*, i.e., the rules guiding the inheritance of knowledge from one state s to the next state s'. Specifically, they prevent the inheritance of knowledge that is explicitly contradicted in the new state s'. However, inheritance can be limited even further, by means of a simple modification of the inheritance rules:

Modified Inheritance Rules (IR'):

$$A_s \leftarrow A_{s-1}, not\, reject(A_{s-1}); \tag{3.78}$$
$$A_s^- \leftarrow A_{s-1}^-, not\, reject(A_{s-1}^-) \tag{3.79}$$
$$reject(A_{s-1}) \leftarrow A_{P_s}^-; \tag{3.80}$$
$$reject(A_{s-1}^-) \leftarrow A_{P_s} \tag{3.81}$$

obtained by adding new predicates $reject(A_s)$ and $reject(A_s^-)$ allowing us to specify additional restrictions on inheritance.

One important example of such additional constraints imposed on the inertia rules involves removing from the current state s' of any inconsistency that occurred in the previous state s. Such inconsistency could have already existed in the previous state s or could have been caused by the new information added at the current state s'. In order to eliminate such contradictory information, it suffices to add to the definition of *reject* the following two rules:

$$reject(A_{s-1}) \leftarrow A_{s-1}^- \tag{3.82}$$
$$reject(A_{s-1}^-) \leftarrow A_{s-1} \tag{3.83}$$

Similarly, the removal of contradictions brought about by the use of strong negation can be achieved by adding the rules:

$$reject(A_{s-1}) \leftarrow -A_{s-1} \tag{3.84}$$
$$reject(-A_{s-1}) \leftarrow A_{s-1} \tag{3.85}$$

Other conditions and applications can be coded in this way. In particular, suitable rules can be used to enact preferences, to ensure compliance with integrity constraints or to ensure non-inertiality of fluents. Also, more complex contradiction removal criteria can be similarly coded. In all such cases, the semantic characterization of program updates would have to be adjusted accordingly to account for the change in their definition. However, pursuance of this topic is outside of the scope of the present work.

3.4 Illustrative Examples

In this Section we present some examples illustrating the use of *DLP*.

3.4.1 Priority Reasoning

As mentioned in the introduction, in dynamic logic programming, logic program modules describe states of our knowledge of the world, where different states may represent different time points or different sets of priorities or even different viewpoints. Below we illustrate how to use dynamic logic programming to represent the well known problem in the domain of taxonomies by using priorities among rules.

Example 18 *Consider the well-known problem of flying birds. In this example we have several rules with different priorities. First, the animals-do-not-fly rule, which has the lowest priority; then the birds-fly rule with a higher priority; the penguins-do-not-fly rule with an even higher priority; and, finally, with the highest priority, all the rules* *describing the actual taxonomy (penguins are birds, birds are animals, etc.). This can be coded quite naturally in dynamic logic programming:*

$$\begin{array}{ll} P_1: & not\, fly(X) \leftarrow animal(X) \\ P_2: & fly(X) \leftarrow bird(X) \\ P_3: & not\, fly(X) \leftarrow penguin(X) \\ P_4: & animal(X) \leftarrow bird(X) \\ & bird(X) \leftarrow penguin(X) \\ & animal(pluto) \\ & bird(duffy) \\ & penguin(tweety) \end{array}$$

The reader can easily check that, as intended, the dynamic logic program at state 4, $\biguplus_4\{P_1, P_2, P_3, P_4\}$, has a single stable model where $fly(duffy)$ is true, and both $fly(pluto)$ and $fly(tweety)$ are false.

3.4.2 Rules and Regulations

Consider a university where it has been decided to start a periodic evaluation of faculty members based on their teaching and research activities.

At this university, it is accepted that anyone who has published many papers is considered a good researcher, and anyone whose classes are liked by the students is considered a good teacher.

At the beginning of the first evaluation period it was agreed that faculty members known to be good researchers and good teachers would receive a positive evaluation. Those not known to be strong researchers would not be positively evaluated, and those recognized as poor teachers would receive a negative evaluation. This leads us to the following program at state 1, P_1, with the obvious abbreviations, where non-ground rules stand for the set of their ground instances:

$$\begin{array}{ll} P_1: & g\_teach(X) \leftarrow students\_like(X) \\ & g\_res(X) \leftarrow many\_papers(X) \\ & g\_eval(X) \leftarrow g\_res(X), g\_teach(X) \\ & not\, g\_eval(X) \leftarrow not\, g\_res(X) \\ & -g\_eval(X) \leftarrow -g\_teach(X) \end{array}$$

Over this first evaluation period, Scott, Peter and Lisa published many papers, but not Jack. Also, a survey showed that the students liked Scott, Peter and Jack but didn't like Lisa. This knowledge leads to the following program at state 2:

$$\begin{array}{lll} P_2: & many\_papers(scott) \leftarrow & students\_like(scott) \leftarrow \\ & many\_papers(peter) \leftarrow & students\_like(peter) \leftarrow \\ & many\_papers(lisa) \leftarrow & not\, students\_like(lisa) \leftarrow \\ & not\, many\_papers(jack) \leftarrow & students\_like(jack) \leftarrow \end{array}$$

The only stable model is:

$$M_2 = \left\{ \begin{array}{c} many\_papers(scott), many\_papers(lisa), many\_papers(peter), \\ not\, many\_papers(jack), students\_like(scott), not\, students\_like(lisa), \\ students\_like(peter), students\_like(jack), g\_teach(scott), \\ not\, g\_teach(lisa), g\_teach(peter), g\_teach(jack), not\, -g\_teach(scott), \\ not\, -g\_teach(lisa), not\, -g\_teach(peter), not\, -g\_teach(jack), \\ g\_res(scott), g\_res(lisa), g\_res(peter), not\, g\_res(jack), g\_eval(scott), \\ not\, g\_eval(lisa), g\_eval(peter), not\, g\_eval(jack), not\, -g\_eval(scott), \\ not\, -g\_eval(lisa), not\, -g\_eval(peter), not\, -g\_eval(jack) \end{array} \right\}$$

Stating that both Scott and Peter receive a good evaluation; Lisa is not positively evaluated for she is not a good teacher; Jack is also not positively evaluated for he didn't publish any papers and so he is not considered a good researcher.

After this period, the evaluation board found out that one of the reasons why the students liked some of the teachers was because they missed a lot of classes. This way, they decided that anyone missing a lot of classes shouldn't be considered a good teacher. This rule was to be applied in the next evaluation period and can be represented by the following program P_3:

$$P_3: \quad not\, g\_teach(X) \leftarrow miss\_classes(X)$$

During this evaluation period, Peter missed a lot of his classes, Jack published many papers, and everything else kept as before. This leads to the following program P_4:

$$\begin{array}{ll} P_4: & miss\_classes(peter) \leftarrow \\ & many\_papers(jack) \leftarrow \end{array}$$

The only stable model is:

$$M_4 = \left\{ \begin{array}{c} many\_papers(scott), many\_papers(lisa), many\_papers(peter), \\ many\_papers(jack), not\, miss\_classes(scott), not\, miss\_classes(lisa), \\ miss\_classes(peter), not\, miss\_classes(jack), students\_like(scott), \\ not\, students\_like(lisa), students\_like(peter), students\_like(jack), \\ g\_teach(scott), not\, g\_teach(lisa), not\, g\_teach(peter), g\_teach(jack), \\ not\, -g\_teach(scott), not\, -g\_teach(lisa), not\, -g\_teach(peter), \\ not\, -g\_teach(jack), g\_res(scott), g\_res(lisa), g\_res(peter), \\ g\_res(jack), g\_eval(scott), not\, g\_eval(lisa), \\ not\, g\_eval(peter), g\_eval(jack), not\, -g\_eval(scott), \\ not\, -g\_eval(lisa), not\, -g\_eval(peter), not\, -g\_eval(jack) \end{array} \right\}$$

Note that, in what Peter's evaluation is concerned, although the students like him and he has published many papers, he is not considered a good teacher and thus doesn't have a good evaluation because he misses a lot of classes. This is so because missing a lot of classes makes the body of the rule

$$not\, g\_teach(peter) \leftarrow miss\_classes(peter)$$

true, and in turn inhibits inertia to be exerted on the rule

$$g\_teach(peter) \leftarrow students\_like(peter)$$

After this period, the evaluation board, still not happy with the criteria to evaluate the teaching skills, decided to directly evaluate some of the faculty members by means of special examinations. If a teacher has a good teaching evaluation as a result he/she is considered a good teacher. In the case of a bad teaching evaluation he/she is considered a poor teacher. This can be represented by the following update program P_5:

$$\begin{aligned} P_5 : \quad & g\_teach(X) \leftarrow g\_teach\_evaluation(X) \\ & -g\_teach(X) \leftarrow -g\_teach\_evaluation(X) \end{aligned}$$

During this evaluation period, all but Scott were directly evaluated in what their teaching skills are concerned: Peter and Lisa obtained a good teaching evaluation and Jack a negative one. Also during this period, Scott (who has always been an example to everyone) missed a lot of classes. Every other aspect was the same as in the previous evaluation period. This leads to the next update program P_6:

$$\begin{aligned} P_6 : \quad & g\_teach\_evaluation(peter) \leftarrow & -g\_teach\_evaluation(jack) \leftarrow \\ & g\_teach\_evaluation(lisa) \leftarrow & miss\_classes(scott) \leftarrow \end{aligned}$$

The only stable model is:

$$M_6 = \left\{ \begin{array}{c} many\_papers(scott), many\_papers(lisa), many\_papers(peter), \\ many\_papers(jack), miss\_classes(scott), not\, miss\_classes(lisa), \\ miss\_classes(peter), not\, miss\_classes(jack), students\_like(scott), \\ not\, students\_like(lisa), students\_like(peter), students\_like(jack), \\ not\, g\_teach\_evaluation(scott), g\_teach\_evaluation(lisa), \\ g\_teach\_evaluation(peter), not\, g\_teach\_evaluation(jack), \\ not\, -g\_teach\_evaluation(scott), not\, -g\_teach\_evaluation(lisa), \\ not\, -g\_teach\_evaluation(peter), -g\_teach\_evaluation(jack), \\ not\, g\_teach(scott), g\_teach(lisa), g\_teach(peter), not\, g\_teach(jack), \\ not\, -g\_teach(scott), not\, -g\_teach(lisa), not\, -g\_teach(peter), \\ -g\_teach(jack), g\_res(scott), g\_res(lisa), g\_res(peter), g\_res(jack), \\ not\, g\_eval(scott), g\_eval(lisa), g\_eval(peter), not\, -g\_eval(scott), \\ not\, g\_eval(jack), not\, -g\_eval(lisa), not\, -g\_eval(peter), -g\_eval(jack) \end{array} \right\}$$

Note that although Jack's students like him and he doesn't miss many classes, he is now considered a bad teacher due to a direct evaluation of his teaching skills by the board. This leads to a negative overall evaluation. In what Lisa is concerned, her teaching skills were positively evaluated and, although her students don't like her, she is considered a good teacher a receives a good overall evaluation for she is also a good researcher.

After this evaluation period the board decided that, since Scott missed a lot of classes due to an ongoing project that could lead him to win a Nobel Prize, anyone who receives such high award should be considered a good researcher and automatically receive a good evaluation. This can be represented by the following update program P_7:

$$\begin{aligned} P_7 : \quad & g\_res(X) \leftarrow nobel\_prize(X) \\ & g\_eval(X) \leftarrow nobel\_prize(X) \end{aligned}$$

It turned out that Scott indeed did receive the Nobel Prize. Also during this evaluation period, Peter didn't publish any papers. A teaching re-evaluation on Jack's teaching skills showed that, although he should not be considered a good teacher, he should not be considered a bad teacher either. Every other aspect remained the same. This leads to the update program P_8:

$$\begin{aligned} P_8 : \quad & nobel\_prize(scott) \leftarrow \\ & not\, many\_papers(peter) \leftarrow \\ & not\, -g\_teach\_evaluation(jack) \leftarrow \end{aligned}$$

The only stable model is:

$$M_8 = \left\{ \begin{array}{c} many\_papers(scott), many\_papers(lisa), not\, many\_papers(peter), \\ many\_papers(jack), miss\_classes(scott), not\, miss\_classes(lisa), \\ miss\_classes(peter), not\, miss\_classes(jack), students\_like(scott), \\ not\, students\_like(lisa), students\_like(peter), students\_like(jack), \\ nobel\_prize(scott), not\, nobel\_prize(lisa), not\, nobel\_prize(peter), \\ not\, nobel\_prize(jack), not\, g\_teach\_evaluation(scott), \\ g\_teach\_evaluation(lisa), g\_teach\_evaluation(peter), \\ not\, g\_teach\_evaluation(jack), not\ -g\_teach\_evaluation(scott), \\ not\ -g\_teach\_evaluation(lisa), not\ -g\_teach\_evaluation(peter), \\ not\ -g\_teach\_evaluation(jack), not\, g\_teach(scott), g\_teach(lisa), \\ g\_teach(peter), not\, g\_teach(jack), not\ -g\_teach(scott), \\ not\ -g\_teach(lisa), not\ -g\_teach(peter), not\ -g\_teach(jack), \\ g\_res(scott), g\_res(lisa), not\, g\_res(peter), g\_res(jack), g\_eval(scott), \\ g\_eval(lisa), not\, g\_eval(peter), not\, g\_eval(jack), not\ -g\_eval(scott), \\ not\ -g\_eval(lisa), not\ -g\_eval(peter), not\ -g\_eval(jack) \end{array} \right\}$$

Note that after a second evaluation of Jack's teaching skills, he was no longer considered a bad teacher. His overall evaluation is still not positive, but at least it is no longer negative.

In this example, if we wanted to know the effect of the new evaluation rules, added at the beginning of each period, on the evaluation record of the previous period, we could simply determine the stable models at $t = 3, 5$ and 7.

3.4.3 Metaphorical Reasoning

In modelling Computational Creativity, it is relevant to understand that a creative system must be able to work in a heterogeneous knowledge base of different domains, in such a way that it can extract and interrelate concepts apparently distant and different. Recent Metaphor Theories [30, 98, 108, 159, 222] seem to be quite promising in fulfilling this goal. These theories set forth processes to associate concepts according to an initial metaphor and yielding an interpretation. An interpretation consists in a coherent 1-to-1 mapping of elements between two domains (the *Source* and the *Target*, commonly called *Vehicle* and *Tenor*) starting from an initially chosen pair of mapped elements.

Apart from having been deeply studied along the ages, and notably being a very common process of association between domains, according to [73] and [222], Metaphor is deeply embodied in the core of our cognition, having a constant and vital role in communication [125].

In what concerns modelling Computational Creativity, metaphor may play a determinant role, since it can be used as a device for cross-domain interrelation establishment. With such a device, a system could be able to search in domains different from the one directly related to the task at hand, since there would be counterparts for some concepts (e.g. to search for new *"musical"* ideas in Visual Arts, to search for new *"computational"* concepts in Social Environments, etc.). An example of work in progress towards such a system is *Dr. Divago* [181]. In this system, knowledge is represented at two distinct levels: instancial knowledge in the form of tree-like structures (e.g. musical structures); ontological knowledge in the form of concept maps mainly describing the concepts found in instancial knowledge (e.g. generic knowledge about music). The role of Metaphor in this system is to establish correspondences between concept maps of different domains, thus allowing for transfer of information contained in instancial knowledge. The usefulness of this cross-domain mapping obviously depends much on the quality of the concept maps involved, this being the motivation leading to the development of *Clouds* [182], a module now integrated in *Dr. Divago*, aiming at helping the user in building her own concept maps by means of machine learning techniques.

In this example, within *Dr. Divago*, we extend the generation of cross-domain links such as those based on the metaphor theory of [222], to cope with the transfer of operational/procedural knowledge from one domain to another. In such cases, particularly when negative information is bought into the arena, inconsistency is a reality that has to be dealt with, as shown by the following example:

Example 19 *Consider the rule* "objects aren't big when they are in the background", *extracted from* Clouds *in the domain of Visual Arts, represented in the clausal form as:*

$$not\, big(X) \leftarrow object(X), background(X). \tag{3.86}$$

which, if we were to map it to the music domain according to the following translation:

$$\begin{aligned} big &\leadsto long \\ object &\leadsto motif \\ background &\leadsto accompaniment \end{aligned}$$

would correspond to:

$$not\, long(X) \leftarrow motif(X), accompaniment(X). \tag{3.87}$$

This can easily be proven inconsistent, at least for some instances (it is not difficult to find accompaniment motifs *that are* long, *eg. isometric motets from ars nova).*

Each metaphorical mapping will lead to the transfer of a set of rules from the *Vehicle* to the *Tenor* of which: some are redundant because equivalent rules already exist there; some, of particular interest to the creative process, yield new knowledge to the *Tenor*; some are conflicting with the knowledge already present in the *Tenor*. Although such conflicts, which may arise contradiction, are not necessarily evil, this being more evident in creative processes, we nevertheless have to detect and deal with them.

The need to detect and deal with contradiction in knowledge transfer lead us to consider the paradigm of *Dynamic Logic Programming* as a formal, while at the same time intuitive, vehicle to a solution.

In our case, the rules from the *Vehicle*, after the metaphorical mapping, should only persist if they do not lead to a contradiction by means of a rule from the *Tenor*.

Going back to the example above, let us suppose that we learn, in the music domain, the following rule:

$$long(X) \leftarrow motif(X), accompaniment(X), isometric\_motet\_element(X) \tag{3.88}$$

stating that *"the accompaniment element of an isometric motet is long"*[3]. If we were simply to consider the union of both rules, we would obtain a contradiction for all *accompaniment elements of an isometric motet.* If we were to simply consider rule 3.88, we would lose valuable information from rule 3.87 concerning *accompaniment motifs not*

[3]Also known as *Talia.*

belonging to isometric motets. Our goal is to be able to conclude that *"accompaniment elements of an isometric motet are long"*, and that *"accompaniment elements of non-isometric motets aren't long"*. That is, we would like to use rule 3.87 for those instances that do not generate a contradiction by means of rule 3.88. This is precisely the behavior of *Logic Program Updates*: to exert inertia on those rules (in this case obtained by the mapping) that are not contradicted by rules from the new domain.

As we have seen before, a metaphorical framework can be envisaged as consisting of two theories (*tenor* and *vehicle*), defined in two different languages, together with a function mapping part of the language of the *vehicle* into the language of the *tenor*. For simplicity we will consider that the mapping function is defined for all elements of the *vehicle* language. Although this is usually not the case, we could, without loss of generality, extend the language of the *tenor* with those unmapped elements from the language of the *vehicle*, and extend the mapping function accordingly.

The two theories will be represented by generalized logic programs. The mapping function between the two languages will allow the construction of a function mapping theories of one language into theories of the other language. Formally we have:

Definition 45 (Metaphorical Program Mapping) *Let $\mathcal{K}_1$ and $\mathcal{K}_2$ be two arbitrary set of propositional variables whose names do not begin with a " not". Let $\psi_{1,2}$:$\mathcal{K}_1 \rightarrow \mathcal{K}_2$ be a function, mapping elements from $\mathcal{K}_1$ into elements of $\mathcal{K}_2$. Let $\mathcal{L}_1$ (resp. $\mathcal{L}_2$) be the language obtained from $\mathcal{K}_1$ (resp. $\mathcal{K}_2$). Let $\mathcal{P}_1$ (resp. $\mathcal{P}_2$) be the set of generalized logic programs in the language $\mathcal{L}_1$ (resp. $\mathcal{L}_2$). We define the metaphorical program mapping as the function $\Psi_{1,2}$:$\mathcal{P}_1 \rightarrow \mathcal{P}_2$ such that for every $P_1 \in \mathcal{P}_1$, $\Psi_{1,2}(P_1)$ is obtained by replacing every atom A (resp. default literal not A) appearing in a rule of P_1 by $\psi_{1,2}(A)$ (resp. not $\psi_{1,2}(A)$).*

Example 20 *Let $\mathcal{K}_1$ be:*

$$\{big, object, background\}$$

and $\mathcal{K}_2$ be:

$$\{long, motif, accompaniment, isometric\_motet\_element\}$$

corresponding to the example from the introduction. Let P_1 be[4]*:*

$$not\, big(X) \leftarrow object(X), background(X).$$

and P_2 be

$$long(X) \leftarrow motif(X), accompaniment(X), isometric\_motet\_element(X).$$

Let $\psi_{1,2}$:$\mathcal{K}_1 \rightarrow \mathcal{K}_2$ be defined by:

$$\begin{aligned} \psi_{1,2}(big) &= long \\ \psi_{1,2}(object) &= motif \\ \psi_{1,2}(background) &= accompaniment \end{aligned}$$

If we apply $\Psi_{1,2}$ to P_1 we obtain $\Psi_{1,2}(P_1)$:

$$not\, long(X) \leftarrow motif(X), accompaniment(X).$$

[4]Where, as usual, rules with variables stand for the set of their ground instantiations.

Now that we have a process to transform a theory in one language (*vehicle*) into a corresponding theory in the language of the *tenor* (possibly extended with new elements), we need a way to combine this transformed theory with the theory representing the *tenor* to obtain a final theory.

This final theory will consist of the *tenor* theory together with those rules from the transformed *vehicle* theory that are not contradicted by the rules from the *tenor*. This can be seen as a process of accommodation where the rules from the transformed *vehicle* are combined with those from the *tenor*, provided they do not generate contradictions. This process is essentially equivalent to the inertia exerted on the rules of the initial program during an update. With this in mind, the definition of Metaphorical Program Update is:

Definition 46 (Metaphorical Program Update) *Let $\mathcal{K}_1$ and $\mathcal{K}_2$ be two arbitrary set of propositional variables whose names do not begin with a "not". Let $\mathcal{L}_1$ and $\mathcal{L}_2$ be the languages obtained from $\mathcal{K}_1$ and $\mathcal{K}_2$ respectively. Let P_1 and P_2 be two generalized logic programs in the languages $\mathcal{L}_1$ and $\mathcal{L}_2$ respectively. Let $\psi_{1,2}$ be a function mapping elements from $\mathcal{K}_1$ into elements of $\mathcal{K}_2$. The metaphorical program update of P_1 by P_2 given $\psi_{1,2}$, denoted by $P_1 \odot P_2$ is given by $\Psi_{1,2}(P_1) \uplus P_2$.*

The stable models of $P_1 \odot P_2$ coincide, modulo irrelevant literals, with the stable models of $\Psi_{1,2}(P_1) \oplus P_2$, and will be denoted by $SM(P_1 \odot P_2)$.

Example 21 *With P_1, P_2 and $\psi_{1,2}$ as in the previous example, the program $P_1 \odot P_2$ is:*

$$\begin{aligned}
long(X)^-_{P_1} &\leftarrow motif(X), accompaniment(X)\\
long(X)_{P_2} &\leftarrow motif(X), accompaniment(X), isometric_motet_element(X)\\
A^- &\leftarrow A^-_{P_1}, not\, A_{P_2}\\
A^- &\leftarrow not\, A_{P_1}, not\, A_{P_2}\\
A &\leftarrow A_{P_1}, not\, A^-_{P_2}\\
A^- &\leftarrow A^-_{P_2}\\
A &\leftarrow A_{P_2}\\
not\, A &\leftarrow A^-
\end{aligned}$$

where A is a proposition from $\mathcal{K}_2$ and rules for A stand for their ground instances. Note that if we were to simply join the two programs, i.e. $\Psi_{1,2}(P_1) \cup P_2$, the two rules would produce a contradiction for $X : isometric\_motet\_element(X)$. If we, on the other hand, perform a metaphorical program update of P_1 by P_2, this contradiction no longer exists. From $P_1 \odot P_2$, we are able to conclude $long(X)$ for

$$\{X : isometric\_motet\_element(X), motif(X), accompaniment(X)\}$$

and $not\, long(X)$, otherwise, as intended.

We now present a more elaborate example, based on the previous example, and discuss some important characteristics of metaphorical program updates.

Example 22 *Consider the following generalized logic program, representing some knowledge about the domain of Visual Arts*[5]*, P_1:*

$$not\, big(X) \leftarrow object(X), background(X). \quad (r_1)$$

$$tension(X) \leftarrow unbalanced(X). \quad (r_2)$$

$$contrast(X,Y) \leftarrow colour(X), colour(Y), high\_value\_difference(X,Y) \quad (r_3)$$

[5]The languages in which the programs are written are left implicit.

Now consider another generalized logic program, representing some knowledge about the domain of Music, P_2*:*

$$long(X) \leftarrow motif(X), accompaniment(X), isometric\_motet\_element(X) \quad (r_4)$$
$$tension(X) \leftarrow dissonant(X). \quad (r_5)$$

Let the metaphorical mapping be defined by the function $\psi_{1,2}:\mathcal{K}_1 \rightarrow \mathcal{K}_2$ *such that:*

$$\begin{aligned}
\psi_{1,2}(big) &= long \\
\psi_{1,2}(object) &= motif \\
\psi_{1,2}(background) &= accompaniment \\
\psi_{1,2}(tension) &= tension \\
\psi_{1,2}(unbalanced) &= dissonant \\
\psi_{1,2}(colour) &= note \\
\psi_{1,2}(high_value_difference) &= large_interval \\
\psi_{1,2}(contrast) &= contrast
\end{aligned}$$

If we apply $\Psi_{1,2}$ *to* P_1 *we obtain* $\Psi_{1,2}(P_1)$*:*

$$not\,long(X) \leftarrow motif(X), accompaniment(X). \quad (r_6)$$
$$tension(X) \leftarrow dissonant(X). \quad (r_7)$$
$$contrast(X,Y) \leftarrow note(X), note(Y), large\_interval(X,Y) \quad (r_8)$$

Looking at the rules from $\Psi_{1,2}(P_1)$ *and those from* P_2*, we can intuitively distinguish several paradigmatic cases:*

- *rule* r_6 *will be a valid rule for those instances that are not covered by rule* r_4 *as explained during the running example;*
- *rule* r_7 *will not add anything to the metaphorical update for it is the same as rule* r_5*. This represents those cases where the translated rules from the* vehicle *are already present in the* tenor*;*
- *rule* r_8 *will bring not only new relations but also new concepts to the* tenor*. This represents the most interesting case with respect to creative reasoning.*

The program $P_1 \odot P_2$ *is:*

$$long(X)^-_{P_1} \leftarrow motive(X), accompaniment(X). \quad (3.89)$$
$$tension(X)_{P_1} \leftarrow dissonant(X). \quad (3.90)$$
$$contrast(X,Y)_{P_1} \leftarrow note(X), note(Y), large\_interval(X,Y) \quad (3.91)$$
$$long(X)_{P_2} \leftarrow motif(X), accompaniment(X), isometric\_motet\_element(X) \quad (3.92)$$
$$tension(X)_{P_2} \leftarrow dissonant(X). \quad (3.93)$$

plus the corresponding ***UR***, ***IR*** *and* ***DR***. *Note that rules (3.89) through (3.93), alone, are meaningless because they only have auxiliary atoms* $(L^-_{P_1}, L_{P_2}, ...)$ *as their conclusions and there are no rules for the literals in their premisses. It is through* ***UR***, ***IR*** *and* ***DR*** *that we are able to determine the semantics of* $P_1 \odot P_2$ *with respect to the relevant literals. In the semantics of* $P_1 \odot P_2$ *we have:*

$long(X)$ *for*

$$\{X : isometric\_motet\_element(X), motif(X), accompaniment(X)\}$$

not $long(X)$ *for*

$$\{X : not\ isometric\_motet\_element(X), motif(X), accompaniment(X)\}$$

$contrast(X,Y)$ *for*

$$\{X, Y : note(X), note(Y), large\_interval(X,Y)\}$$

$tension(X)$ *for*

$$\{X : dissonant(X)\}$$

It is interesting to draw the reader's attention to some properties emerging from the definition of metaphorical program updates, and their relation to known metaphor theory characteristics. The first one is related to the very basic intuition whereby metaphors bring new knowledge into the target domain. In fact, it is easy to see that in general we have that[6]:

$$SM(P_1 \odot P_2) \neq SM(P_2) \tag{3.94}$$

$$SM(P_1) \neq SM(P_2 \odot P_1) \tag{3.95}$$

The second and very important characteristic is that of directionality which, as explained before, means that each domain has a different role and its interchange, although possibly yielding an equally valuable metaphor, will not lead to the same meaning. If we have a bijective mapping function $\psi_{1,2}$ such that $\psi_{2,1} = \psi_{1,2}^{-1}$, then, in general, we have that

$$SM(P_1 \odot P_2) \neq SM(\Psi_{1,2}(P_2 \odot P_1)) \tag{3.96}$$

If we consider, for example, P_1 to represent a set of rules from the domain of Painting, and P_2 to represent a set of rules from the domain of Music, we could have an informal interpretation of the above properties reading as:

- a painter that becomes a musician would compose music different from that of a musician (3.94);
- a painter would paint differently from a musician that became a painter (3.95);
- a painter that becomes a musician would compose music different from that of a musician that becomes a painter (if he was to map his painting rules to music composition rules) (3.96).

It would be easy to check all these properties in the previous example.

In what contradiction is concerned, it is important to mention that the metaphorical program update ($P_1 \odot P_2$), as DLP, only detects and deals with inconsistencies arising from rules from different domains. Other sources of inconsistencies can exist: P_1 can be contradictory, and so can be P_2; even in cases where P_1 and P_2 are not contradictory, $P_1 \odot P_2$ can be so, this happening when the contradiction is *'latent'* in one of the domains, and is *'brought alive'* by the metaphorical update, such as in the following example:

[6]Where by $SM(P)$ we mean the set of stable models of the program P, restricted to the relevant language ($\mathcal{L}_1$ or $\mathcal{L}_2$ depending on the case).

Example 23 *Consider the following program P_1:*

$$not\,hot(X) \leftarrow blue(X)$$
$$hot(X) \leftarrow red(X)$$

the metaphorical mapping $\psi_{1,2}$:

$$\psi_{1,2}(blue) = blues$$
$$\psi_{1,2}(red) = jazz$$
$$\psi_{1,2}(hot) = hot$$

and the program P_2:

$$jazz(Miles) \leftarrow$$
$$blues(Miles) \leftarrow$$

the metaphorical program update $P_1 \odot P_2$ is contradictory inasmuch as both $not\,hot(Miles)$ and $hot(Miles)$ are "derivable".

Nevertheless, be they important or not for our purposes, all contradictions can be detected by inspecting the truth value of the atoms A^-, A_P, A_P^-, A_U, A_U^-, etc. of the program $P_1 \odot P_2$, and dealt with either by the semantics of $P_1 \odot P_2$ itself or by other known contradiction removal techniques, e.g. [3, 10, 184].

Metaphor being a common device for communication that uses interrelationships between different domains to assess new enriched mixed concepts, it is, as we believe, a powerful source for modelling *Creativity*. The ability to search for solutions in distant domains, apparently unrelated to the actual problem, is determinant for our creative abilities [55, 104]. Metaphor theories, such as [222], can be used as cross-domain bridge establishment methods, fundamental for knowledge integration within different domains.

In this example we have explored the application of *Dynamic Logic Programming* to the problem of knowledge integration in metaphorical reasoning. The problem of resolving inconsistencies that may arise when knowledge from two different domains is combined, given a metaphorical mapping, is crucial, be it at the stage where we want to evaluate the appropriateness of the mapping function, or at a subsequent stage when we want to reason with the combined knowledge.

Quite interestingly, this combined knowledge becomes a new third domain which is not a crude sum of the original ones, but a blend of concepts and relationships among them which, in some cases, can yield potentially creative outcomes, much in the line of [220].

3.4.4 Other Examples

Dynamic Logic Programming has also been employed by others, namely as a means to combine rules learnt by a diversity of agents [127]; model agent interaction [198, 199]. Other examples can also be found in [17, 18, 20].

3.5 Comparisons

In this section we compare Dynamic Logic Programming with other somewhat related approaches to the problem of updating a logic programming based knowledge base.

These approaches can be divided into two main groups as pointed out in [77]: those based on causal rejection of rules and those not based on such form of causal rejection.

In what concerns updates based on causal rejection of rules, a group in which we can place Dynamic Logic Programming, we can find our own earlier work on the subject [130, 141–143] which, to the best of our knowledge, was the first proposal of such type of causal rejection to perform updates of logic programs. Also based on a form of causal rejection is the framework of Inheritance Programs of Buccafurri et al. [44] which, although introduced with the purpose of studying mechanisms of inheritance in logic programming, shares some similarities with logic program updates when inheritance is seen as a form of inertia. In [77], the authors have proposed a semantics for updates of logic programs with the purpose of establishing a common ground to compare and analyze such causal rejection based semantics of updates. In [77], the authors have also established a correspondence between their one proposal and the one of [44]. We could not continue without a special mention of the work of Eiter et al., reported in [77], in particular in what concerns the formal comparisons between their approach to logic program updates and the several other existing approaches, as well as establishing the few bridges with the update postulates of [116]. Some of the results presented here have been largely inspired by those established in [77].

In what refers to updates of logic programs, not based on causal rejection, we shall briefly mention and pinpoint the major characteristics of the approaches of Inoue and Sakama [212] who propose a framework to update programs through abduction, and the approach of Zhang and Foo [233] who set forth a framework to achieve updates of logic programs through priorities.

3.5.1 Updates based on Causal Rejection

We start with a brief overview of the three proposals based on some notion of causal rejection of rules.

Logic Program Updates of Leite and Pereira

The approach to update logic programs of [130, 141–143] uses sequences of update programs written in the same language as revision programs of Marek and Truszczynski. In [130], the update framework was set forth for several different classes of programs and semantics, namely for each combination of normal update programs or extended update programs and a two valued stable model semantics or a three-valued well founded semantics. As will be established, normal update programs have a one to one correspondence with generalized logic programs and extended update programs have a similar correspondence with generalized extended logic programs. Here, we only recall the most general case, where a stable semantics is used, namely for extended update programs. The case of normal update programs can be viewed as a special instance. The details of all other cases can be found in [130].

Let us assume we have a set $\mathcal{K}^*$ of propositions with strong negation as defined before.

An extended update program is simply a collection of in-rules and out-rules such as those defined in 32, which we recall here:an in-rule, is any expression of the form:

$$in(A_0) \leftarrow in(A_1), ..., in(A_m), out(A_{m+1}), ..., out(A_n)$$

where $A_i \in \mathcal{K}^*$, $0 \leq i \leq n$. An out-rule, is any expression of the form:

$$out(A_0) \leftarrow in(A_1), ..., in(A_m), out(A_{m+1}), ..., out(A_n)$$

where $A_i \in \mathcal{K}^*$, $0 \leq i \leq n$. The first step is to translate each of these programs into extended logic programs (ELP), according to the following transformation, which employs the results in [50]:

Definition 47 (Translation of extended UPs into ELPs) *[12]Let UP be an extended update program. Its* translation into the extended logic program *U, written in the language generated by $\mathcal{K}^*_{np}$, obtained by augmenting $\mathcal{K}^*$ with the set $\{L^n, L^p : L \in \mathcal{K}^*\}$ is defined as follows:*

1. *Each in-rule*

$$in(L_0) \leftarrow in(L_1), ..., in(L_m), out(L_{m+1}), ..., out(L_n) \tag{3.97}$$

where m, $n \geq 0$, and $L_i \in \mathcal{K}^*$, translates into:

$$L_0^* \leftarrow L_1, ..., L_m, not\ L_{m+1}, ..., not\ L_n \tag{3.98}$$

where $L_0^* = A^p$ if $L_0 = A$, or $L_0^* = A^n$ if $L_0 = -A$, $A \in \mathcal{K}$.

2. *Each out-rule*

$$out(L_0) \leftarrow in(L_1), ..., in(L_m), out(L_{m+1}), ..., out(L_n) \tag{3.99}$$

where m, $n \geq 0$, and $L_i \in \mathcal{K}^*$, translates into:

$$-L_0^* \leftarrow L_1, ..., L_m, not\ L_{m+1}, ..., not\ L_n \tag{3.100}$$

where $L_0^* = A^p$ if $L_0 = A$, or $L_0^* = A^n$ if $L_0 = -A$, $A \in \mathcal{K}$.

3. *For every $L \in \mathcal{K}^*$ such that $in(L)$ belongs to the head of some in-rule of UP, U contains $-L^* \leftarrow L$ where $L^* = A^n$ if $L = A$, or $L^* = A^p$ if $L = -A$, $A \in \mathcal{K}$.*

4. *For every $A \in \mathcal{K}$, U contains the rules $A \leftarrow A^p$ and $-A \leftarrow A^n$.*

Intuitively, this transformation converts an atom A into a new atom A^p and a negative objective literal $-A$ into a new atom A^n and ensures coherence. This way, there are no negative objective literals in the heads of the rules of update programs and so strong negation $-L$ can be used to code the $out(L)$ in the heads of rules, as for update programs without explicit negation. Operation 4 maps the A^n and A^p back to their original atoms.

They also define a correspondence between interpretations in both languages. Accordingly, if $M_{np} = M^+_{np} \cup M^-_{np}$ is an interpretation, of the language $\mathcal{L}^*_{np}$, the corresponding *restricted interpretation* is $M = M^+ \cup M^-$, of $\mathcal{L}^*$, where $M^+ = \{A : A \in M^+_{np},\ A \in \mathcal{K}^*\}$ and $M^- = \{A : A \in M^-_{np},\ A \in \mathcal{K}^*\}$.

Then, they present the semantics for sequences of programs, which are called justified updates. The intuition is similar to the semantics of DLP inasmuch as it is based on a notion of causal rejection of a set of rules, the semantics being the answer-sets of the union of the remaining rules. We now present the original definitions, with just a few minor modifications that do not change the semantics:

Definition 48 (Extended $\mathcal{P}$-Justified Updates at state s) *[130]Consider an ordered sequence $\mathcal{P} = \{UP_s : s \in \mathcal{T}\}$ of extended update programs UP_s, with smallest element U_{s_0}. Let $\mathcal{P}' = \{U_s : s \in \mathcal{T}\}$ be the sequence of ELPs in the language $\mathcal{L}^*_{np}$, obtained by translating each update program in $\mathcal{P}$. Let M an extended interpretation of $\mathcal{L}^*$. M is an* Extended $\mathcal{P}$-Justified Update at state t *iff there is an interpretation M_{np} of $\mathcal{L}^*_{np}$ such that M_{np} is an answer-set of*

$$\bigcup_{s_i \leq s} \mathcal{P}' - Rejected\left(M_{np}, s, \mathcal{P}'\right)$$

where:

$$Rejected\left(M_{np}, s, \mathcal{P}'\right) = \left\{r \in U_{s_1} : \exists r' \in U_{s_2}, s_1 < s_2 \leq s, r \overset{np}{\bowtie} r', M_{np} \vDash B\left(r'\right)\right\}$$

where $A \in \mathcal{K}$ and $r \overset{np}{\bowtie} r'$ iff one of the following holds:

$$H(r) = A^p \text{ and } H(r) = -A^p$$
$$H(r) = A^n \text{ and } H(r) = -A^n$$
$$H(r) = A^p \text{ and } H(r) = A^n$$
$$r' \overset{np}{\bowtie} r$$

In [130] the authors further impose that there be a non-contradictory extended $\mathcal{P}$-justified update at every state s_i, $s_0 \leq s_i \leq s$, otherwise there is no extended $\mathcal{P}$-justified update at state s. We will drop such condition since it only makes sense as an imposition on not allowing any sequence of programs to go though a contradictory state. Such update semantics was also established for the case of a three-valued semantics namely the well founded semantics, as well as for it counterpart with explicit negation, the WFSX [183]. We will not review such extensions here. The details can be found in [130].

Update Programs of Eiter et al.

Recently, in [77], the authors have proposed another framework for updates of logic programs, based on causal rejection of rules. They consider a sequence of extended logic programs, thus without default negation in the heads of clauses, and define its semantics.

According to this approach, the semantics is based on a notion of update answer-set. There follows the definition:

Definition 49 (Update Answer-Sets at state s) *[77]Let $\mathcal{P} = \{P_s : s \in \mathcal{T}\}$ be an ordered sequence of extended logic programs P_s in the language $\mathcal{L}^*$, with smallest element U_{s_0}, and M an extended interpretation of $\mathcal{L}^*$. M is an* Update Answer-Set at state s *iff M is an extended stable model of*

$$\bigcup_{s_i \leq s} \mathcal{P} - Rej\left(M, s, \mathcal{P}\right)$$

where:

$$Rej\left(M, s, \mathcal{P}\right) = \left\{ \begin{array}{c} r \in P_{s_1} \mid \exists r' \in P_{s_2} \setminus Rej\left(M, s, \mathcal{P}\right), s_1 < s_2 \leq s, \\ H\left(r\right) = -H\left(r'\right), M \vDash B\left(r'\right) \cup B\left(r\right) \end{array} \right\}$$

It is worth mentioning that, by only allowing knowledge to be represented with extended logic programs, this approach does not permit the transition between all existing epistemic states as mentioned in Chapter 2 when we motivated the introduction of generalized logic programs. Using the example presented in there, updating from a situation where we know that a train is coming, represented by the model $\{train, not\ -train\}$ to a situation where we do not know if a train is coming but we also do not know that a train is not coming, represented by the model $\{not\, train, not\ -train\}$, simply is not possible with this approach. For this we need two kinds of negations in the heads of rules. In the case of DLP, default negation in the heads is used whereas in update programs, as per the previous subsection, $out(train)$ is used for such a purpose.

There is however a natural extension of the Update Answer-Set semantics to deal with generalized (extended) logic programs, defined as follows:

Definition 50 (Generalized Update Answer-Sets at state s**)** *Let* $\mathcal{P} = \{P_s : s \in \mathcal{T}\}$ *be an ordered sequence of generalized extended logic programs* P_s *in the language* $\mathcal{L}^*$*, with smallest element* U_{s0}*, and* M *a generalized extended interpretation of* $\mathcal{L}^*$*.* M *is a* Generalized Update Answer-Set at state s *iff* M *is a generalized extended stable model of*

$$\bigcup_{s_i \leq s} \mathcal{P} - Rej^*(M, s, \mathcal{P})$$

where:

$$Rej^*(M, s, \mathcal{P}) = \left\{ \begin{array}{c} r \in P_{s_1} \mid \exists r' \in P_{s_2} \setminus Rej^*(M, s, \mathcal{P}), s_1 < s_2 \leq s, \\ r \bar{\bowtie} r', M \vDash B(r') \cup B(r) \end{array} \right\}$$

and $r \bar{\bowtie} r'$ *iff* $H(r) = not\ H(r')$ *or* $H(r) = -H(r')$*.*

Trivially both definitions coincide for the case of extended logic programs:

Proposition 42 *Let* $\mathcal{P} = \{P_s : s \in \mathcal{T}\}$ *be an ordered sequence of extended logic programs* P_s *in the language* $\mathcal{L}^*$*, with smallest element* U_{s0}*, and* M *an extended interpretation of* $\mathcal{L}^*$*.* M *is a* Generalized Update Answer-Set at state s *iff* M *is an* Update Answer-Set at state s.

Proof. *Since for extended logic programs the condition* $r \bar{\bowtie} r'$ *in the set* $Rej^*(M, s, \mathcal{P})$ *of the characterization in Theorem 43 is equivalent to* $H(r) = -H(r')$*, since there are no default objective literals in the heads of clauses, the equivalence between semantics trivially follows.* ■

Eiter et al. have also defined two other semantics based on criteria of minimality of change. As they point out, defining a purely model-based notion of minimal change does not make much sense in the context of updates, due to their intrinsic syntactical nature. Therefore, it seems more reasonable to define such criteria based on the set of rejection rules. With this in mind they have defined the following two semantics:

Definition 51 (Minimal Update Answer-Sets at state s**)** *[77] Consider an ordered sequence* $\mathcal{P} = \{P_s : s \in \mathcal{T}\}$ *of extended logic programs* P_s *in the language* $\mathcal{L}^*$*, with smallest element* U_{s0}*. An Update Answer-Set at state* s*,* M*, is minimal iff there is no Update Answer-Set at state* s M' *such that* $Rej(M', s, \mathcal{P}) \subset Rej(M, s, \mathcal{P})$*.*

Since minimal update Answer-Sets allow the violation of more recent rules in order to satisfy rules from previous updates, Eiter et al. have also defined a notion of strictly minimal update Answer-Sets:

Definition 52 (Strictly Minimal Update Answer-Sets at state s) *[77] Consider an ordered sequence $\mathcal{P} = \{P_s : s \in T\}$ of extended logic programs P_s in the language $\mathcal{L}^*$, with smallest element U_{s_0} and two Update Answer-Set at state s, M and M'. Then, M is preferred over M' iff some $i \leq s$ exists such that:*

- $\{r : r \in P_i, r \in Rej\,(M, s, \mathcal{P})\} \subset \{r : r \in P_i, r \in Rej\,(M', s, \mathcal{P})\}$
- $\{r : r \in P_j, r \in Rej\,(M, s, \mathcal{P})\} \subset \{r : r \in P_j, r \in Rej\,(M', s, \mathcal{P})\}$ *for all* $i < j \leq s$.

An update answer-set at state s, M, is strictly minimal *if no update Answer-Set at state s, M', is preferred over M.*

Clearly every strictly minimal update Answer-Set is minimal, but not vice versa.

Note that these definitions can directly be applied for the case of generalized extended logic programs, just by replacing $Rej\,(\_,\_,\_)$ with $Rej^*\,(\_,\_,\_)$.

Inheritance Programs of Buccafurri et al.

In [44] the authors propose a knowledge representation language, called DLP$^<$, which extends disjunctive logic programming (with strong negation) by inheritance. The addition of inheritance, they claim, enhances the knowledge modelling features of the language providing a natural representation of default reasoning with exceptions. They provide a declarative model-theoretic semantics of DLP$^<$, which is shown to generalize the Answer-Set Semantics of disjunctive logic programs. Since the disjunctive case is not dealt with in Dynamic Logic Programming, nor by the other approaches to updates, we present only the framework for the non-disjunctive case.

According to [44], a DLP$^<$*-program*, $P^<$, is a finite set $\{\langle o_1, P_1\rangle, \ldots, \langle o_n, P_n\rangle\}$ of object identifiers o_i $(1 \leq i \leq n)$ and associated ELPs P_i, together with a strict partial order "$<$" between object identifiers (pairs $\langle o_i, P_i\rangle$ are called *objects*).

According to their framework, conflict resolution between threatening rules, when determining properties of objects, is achieved in favor of rules which are *more specific* according to the hierarchy, in the sense that rule $r \in P_k$ is considered to represent more specific information than rule $r' \in P_l$ whenever $o_k < o_l$ holds $(1 \leq k, l \leq n$ and $k \neq l)$. In the following, $\rho(P^<)$ denotes the multiset of all rules appearing in the programs of $P^<$.

Definition 53 (Threatening Rules) *[44]Given two ground rules r_1 and r_2 we say that r_1* threatens *r_2 if:*

- $H(r_1) = -L$ *and* $H(r_2) = L$
- $obj\_of(r_1) < obj\_of(r_2)$.

Definition 54 (Overridden Rules) *[44] Given an interpretation I and two ground rules r_1 and r_2 such that r_1 threatens r_2 on L we say that r_1 overrides r_2 on L in I if:*

- $-L \in I$,
- $B(r_2)$ *is true in* I.

A (defeasible) rule $r \in \rho(P^<)$ is overridden in I if there exists $r_1 \in \rho(P^<)$ such that r_1 overrides r on L in I.

Definition 55 (Models and Minimal Models of $P^<$) *[44]An interpretation I is a* model *of $P^<$ iff every rule in $\rho(P^<)$ is either overridden or true in I. I is* minimal *iff it is the least model of all these rules.*

Definition 56 (Answer-Sets of $P^<$) *[44]Let $P^<$ be a* DLP$^<$*-program. Let $G_I(P^<)$ be the reduct of $P^<$ with respect to I obtained by:*

- *deleting any rule $r \in \rho(P^<)$ which is either overridden in I or defeated by I;*
- *deleting all default literals in the bodies of the remaining rules of $\rho(P^<)$.*

Then, I is an Answer-Set *of $P^<$ iff it is a minimal model of $G_I(P^<)$.*

Intuitively an Answer-Set of $P^<$ is obtained in a similar way as the models of the different update frameworks: given an interpretation, first we determine the a set of rules to be discarded and then we check if the interpretation is a model of the remaining rules. In [77], the authors have shown that if one only considers orders between objects that amount to a sequence of objects, then Inheritance Programs are equivalent to the update framework of Eiter et al. This will be elaborated upon in the following Subsection.

Comparisons

In this section we explore and elaborate upon the different logic program update mechanisms. Some of the results have been established in [77].

Since the update framework of Leite and Pereira employs a different language to encode update specifications, we will start by presenting a translation of extended update programs consisting of in- and out-rules into generalized extended logic programs. Subsequently, based on these generalized extended logic programs we present an alternative, nevertheless equivalent, semantical characterization of $\mathcal{P}$-Justified Updates. This will allow for a simpler comparison between the different approaches, in particular with DLP.

The translation of extended update programs into extended logic programs is as follows:

Definition 57 (Translation of UPs into GLPs) *Let P^{in_out} be an extended update program in the language $\mathcal{L}^*$. Its* translation into a generalized extended logic program *P is obtained from P^{in_out} by replacing each update rule (r) by the corresponding rule (r') where:*

- *If r is of the form* $in(p) \leftarrow in(q_1), ..., in(q_m), out(s_1), ..., out(s_n)$
  then r' is of the form $p \leftarrow q_1, ...q_m, not\ s_1, ..., not\ s_n$
- *If r is of the form* $out(p) \leftarrow in(q_1), ..., in(q_m), out(s_1), ..., out(s_n)$
  then r' is of the form $not\ p \leftarrow q_1, ...q_m, not\ s_1, ..., not\ s_n$

From now on, we will assume that every extended update program has been previously translated into a generalized extended logic program according to the previous mapping. The following theorems establishes an alternative characterizations of Extended $\mathcal{P}$-Justified Updates.

Theorem 43 (Extended $\mathcal{P}$-Justified Updates at state s) *Let $\mathcal{P} = \{ P_s : s \in \mathcal{T}\}$ be a* Sequence of Generalized Extended Logic Programs. *Let $s \in \mathcal{T}$. An extended interpretation M_s is an extended $\mathcal{P}$-*Justified Update *at state s, iff M_s is a (extended) stable model of:*

$$\rho(\mathcal{P})_s - Reject^*(\mathcal{P}, s, M_s) \tag{3.101}$$

where

$$\rho(\mathcal{P})_s = \bigcup_{i \leq s} P_i \tag{3.102}$$

$$Reject^*(\mathcal{P}, s, M_s) = \{r \in P_i \mid \exists r' \in P_j, i < j \leq s, r \bar{\bowtie} r' \wedge M_s \vDash B(r')\} \tag{3.103}$$

and $r \bar{\bowtie} r'$ iff $H(r) = not\ H(r')$ or $H(r) = -H(r')$.

Proof. *The proof immediately follows from the results in [49], namely in what concerns the correctness of the transformation, in which the mapping in Definition 47 was based, in capturing the semantics of programs with default negation in their heads with extended logic programs, where the new atoms A^p and A^n serve to encode the original objective literals A and $-A$. We will omit further details.* ∎

Now that every approach to updates can share a common language, we are ready to establish some bridges between them. We start with a theorem relating the approaches of Leite and Pereira with the extension of Eiter's approach presented in Definition 50:

Theorem 44 *Let $\mathcal{P} = \{ P_s : s \in \mathcal{T}\}$ be a* Sequence of Generalized Extended Logic Programs. *Let $s \in \mathcal{T}$. An interpretation M is a* Generalized Update Answer-Set at state s *if M is an extended $\mathcal{P}$-*Justified Update *at state s.*

Proof. *First of all, it is clear that for any generalized extended logic program P and one of its stable models M, if $r \in P$ is a rule such that $M \vDash B(r)$ and r' is a rule such that $H(r) = H(r')$, then M is also a stable model of $P \cup \{r\}$. Let $\Psi(\mathcal{P}, s, M_s) = \rho(\mathcal{P})_s - Reject^*(\mathcal{P}, s, M_s)$ and $\Pi(\mathcal{P}, s, M_s) = \bigcup_{s_i \leq s} \mathcal{P} - Rej^*(M_s, s, \mathcal{P})$. Then, by inspecting the definitions of $Reject^*(\mathcal{P}, s, M_s)$ and $Rej^*(M_s, s, \mathcal{P})$ we obtain that $\Psi(\mathcal{P}, s, M_s) - \Pi(\mathcal{P}, s, M_s) = R$ is a set of rules such that the following holds:*

$$\forall r' \in R, \exists r \in (\Psi(\mathcal{P}, s, M_s) \cap \Pi(\mathcal{P}, s, M_s)) : H(r') = H(r) \wedge H(r) \in M \wedge M \vDash B(r)$$

By repeatedly applying the property initially set forth, we obtain the result. ∎

In [77], the authors have established a correspondence between their update framework and Inheritance programs:

Theorem 45 *[77] Let $\mathcal{P} = \{ P_s : s \in \mathcal{T}\}$, $\mathcal{T} = \{1, ..., n\}$ be a* Sequence of Extended Logic Programs. *Let $P^< = \{\langle o_1, P_1\rangle, ..., \langle o_n, P_n\rangle\}$ with inheritance order $o_n < o_{n-1} < ... < o_1$. Then, an interpretation M is an* Update Answer-Set at state n *of $\mathcal{P}$ iff M is an* Answer-Set *of $P^<$.*

Note that inheritance programs have been defined for a larger class of programs, namely those with disjunctive heads, as well as for strict partial orders which are more expressive than simple sequences of objects. In a subsequent chapter we will extend Dynamic Logic Programming to allow for programs to be arranged according to acyclic directed graphs.

The previous theorems immediately provide us with the following corollary establishing a correspondence between Answer-Sets of inheritance programs and Justified Updates:

Corollary 46 *Let* $\mathcal{P} = \{ P_s : s \in \mathcal{T}\}$, $\mathcal{T} = \{1, ..., n\}$ *be a* Sequence of Extended Logic Programs. *Let* $P^< = \{\langle o_1, P_1 \rangle, ..., \langle o_n, P_n \rangle\}$ *with inheritance order* $o_n < o_{n-1} < ... < o_1$. *Then, an interpretation* M *is an* Answer-Set *of* $P^<$ *if* M *is an extended* $\mathcal{P}$-Justified Update *at state* n.

Now that we have established the comparisons between these three frameworks, we still need to compare these approaches with Dynamic Logic Programming.

We start with the following lemma:

Lemma 47 *Let* $\mathcal{P} = \{ P_s : s \in \mathcal{T}\}$, $\mathcal{T} = \{1, ..., n\}$ *be a* Sequence of Generalized Extended Logic Programs. *Let* $\mathcal{P}^{exp}$ *be the* Sequence of Extended Logic Programs *obtained from* $\mathcal{P}$ *by replacing each program* $P_s \in \mathcal{P}$ *by its expanded version* P_s^{exp}. *Then, an interpretation* M *is an extended* $\mathcal{P}$-Justified Update *at state* n *iff* M *is an extended* $\mathcal{P}^{exp}$-Justified Update *at state* n.

Proof. *According to Theorem 43, an extended interpretation* M *is an extended* $\mathcal{P}$-Justified Update *at state* n, *iff* M *is a (extended) stable model of:*

$$\rho(\mathcal{P})_n - Reject^*(\mathcal{P}, n, M)$$

or, according to the definition of stable models for generalized extended logic programs, iff

$$M = least\left((\rho(\mathcal{P})_n - Reject^*(\mathcal{P}, n, M))^{exp} \cup M^-\right)$$

M *is an extended* $\mathcal{P}^{exp}$-Justified Update *at state* n *iff* M *is a (extended) stable model of:*

$$\rho(\mathcal{P}^{exp})_n - Reject^*(\mathcal{P}^{exp}, n, M)$$

or, according to the definition of stable models for generalized extended logic programs, iff

$$M = least\left((\rho(\mathcal{P}^{exp})_n - Reject^*(\mathcal{P}^{exp}, n, M))^{exp} \cup M^-\right)$$

It is clear that

$$(\rho(\mathcal{P})_n - Reject^*(\mathcal{P}, n, M))^{exp} = \rho(\mathcal{P}^{exp})_n - Reject^*(\mathcal{P}^{exp}, n, M)$$

and also that:

$$(\rho(\mathcal{P}^{exp})_n - Reject^*(\mathcal{P}^{exp}, n, M))^{exp} = \rho(\mathcal{P}^{exp})_n - Reject^*(\mathcal{P}^{exp}, n, M)$$

it follows that M *is an extended* $\mathcal{P}$-Justified Update *at state* n *iff* M *is an extended* $\mathcal{P}^{exp}$-Justified Update *at state* n. ■

And we continue with a theorem stating that every extended stable model is an extended $\mathcal{P}$-*Justified Update*.

Theorem 48 *Let* $\mathcal{P} = \{ P_s : s \in \mathcal{T}\}$ *be a* Sequence of Extended Generalized Logic Programs. *Let* $s \in \mathcal{T}$. *Let* M_s *be an extended stable model of* $\mathcal{P}$ *at state* s. *Then* M_s *is an extended* $\mathcal{P}$-Justified Update *at state* s.

Proof. *Assume that* $\mathcal{P}$ *is in its expanded version. According to Definition 44, an interpretation* M_s *is an extended stable model of* $\mathcal{P}$ *at state* s *iff:*

$$M_s = least\left([\rho(\mathcal{P})_s - Reject(\mathcal{P}, s, M_s)] \cup Default(\rho(\mathcal{P})_s, M)\right) \qquad (3.104)$$

where

$$\rho(\mathcal{P})_s = \bigcup_{i \leq s} P_i$$

$$Reject(\mathcal{P}, s, M_s) = \{r \in P_i \mid \exists r' \in P_j, i < j \leq s, r \bowtie r' \wedge M_s \vDash B(r')\}$$

$$Default(\rho(\mathcal{P})_s, M) = \{not\, A \mid \nexists r \in \rho(\mathcal{P})_s : (H(r) = A) \wedge M_s \vDash B(r)\}$$

*According to Theorem 43, an interpretation M_s is an extended $\mathcal{P}$-*Justified Update *at state s iff it is a (extended) stable model of:*

$$\rho(\mathcal{P})_s - Reject^*(\mathcal{P}, s, M_s)$$

or, alternatively, iff:

$$M_s = least\left([\rho(\mathcal{P})_s - Reject^*(\mathcal{P}, s, M_s)] \cup M_s^-\right) \tag{3.105}$$

Note that the set of rules $\rho(\mathcal{P})_s - Reject(\mathcal{P}, s, M_s) \cup M_s^-$ is already expanded. Since for expanded programs we can replace the set $Reject^*(\mathcal{P}, s, M_s)$ with the set $Reject(\mathcal{P}, s, M_s)$, because the condition based on $\bar{\bowtie}$ can be reduced to that based on $\bowtie$ (for every rule r' that rejects a rule r such that $H(r) = -H(r')$, there is a rule r'' in the expanded version such that $H(r) = not\ H(r'')$ making r belong to the set of rejected rules), and since we clearly have that

$$Default(\rho(\mathcal{P})_s, M) \subseteq M_s^-$$

then, if M_s satisfies (3.104), then it also satisfies (3.105). ■

The converse of the previous theorem does not hold in general. Consider the example:

Example 24 *Take the two logic programs:*

$$P_1 = \{a \leftarrow\} \qquad P_2 = \{not\, a \leftarrow not\, a\}$$

The only stable model at state 2 is $\{a\}$. However, there are two justified updates namely $\{a\}$ and $\{\}$. If P_2^* was to be replaced with $\{-a \leftarrow not\, a\}$, so that it constitutes a valid input for the update Answer-Set semantics of Eiter et al., then, the sequence of programs P_1, P_2^* has a single stable model at state two, namely $\{a\}$ and two update Answer-Sets $\{a\}$ and $\{-a\}$.

Examples such as the previous one constitute one of the reasons why our own earlier semantics of updates based on Justified Updates evolved into the different semantics of Dynamic Logic Programming. It is widely accepted, when dealing with semantics of logic programs, that the addition of a tautological rule should not change the semantics of a given program. Should the update of some theory with a tautology change its semantics? Although the study of updates of non-monotonic theories is a field that is still in its early years, and a set of guiding postulates, as those existing for classical logic based updates [116], have not been set forth yet, we clearly believe that an update with a tautological rule should not change the semantics of a theory. In support of our claim we also call on all the work that has been established in the field of interpretation updates [157]. In particular, we claim that an update semantics, when dealing with the update of one program by another program, should coincide with the interpretation based approach if the initial program is purely extensional, i.e. if it encodes an interpretation. This result has been established for DLP in Theorem 18. The previous example, with its purely extensional initial program P_1, shows that such result does not hold for the Justified Update based semantics.

In [77], the authors point out other examples where some circularities are not removed, such as in the following one:

Example 25 *Take the two logic programs:*

$$P_1 = \left\{ \begin{array}{c} a \leftarrow b \\ b \leftarrow \end{array} \right\} \qquad P_2 = \{not\, b \leftarrow not\, a\}$$

For these programs, there are two stable models at state 2, *namely* $\{a, b\}$ *and* $\{\}$. *The Justified Update semantics coincides for this example.*

Eiter et al. point out that this example is somewhat similar to the previous one and that if one does not accept the model $\{\}$ in the first example, then one should also not accept the model $\{\}$ because the update with the rule $not\, b \leftarrow not\, a$ is somehow cyclic. We argue that such update is not cyclic nor tautological per se. Its possible cyclic or tautological properties can only be inferred if we look at the initial program as well. And, in this example, the rule $not\, b \leftarrow not\, a$ provides us with a new way of obtaining $not\, b$, namely by assuming atom a to be false by default, which, contrary to the previous example, has not been previously defined (since fact $b \leftarrow$ is rejected) and thus can in fact be assumed by default.

Note however that DLP still does not resolve all problems concerning the updates by tautological programs, namely when some form of contradiction is present, such as for example when we update the contradictory program $\{not\, a \leftarrow; \quad a \leftarrow\}$ with the tautological program $\{a \leftarrow a\}$. In this example, the interpretation $\{a\}$ is a stable model (and also a Justified Update and a Update Answer-set) since the tautological rule $a \leftarrow a$ rejects the initial rule $not\, a \leftarrow$. Searching for a semantics for updates based on causal rejection that is completely immune to tautological updates is still an open and non-trivial problem.

To conclude on this subject,we observe that, if desired, the notions of minimal and strictly minimal models can also be directly applied to DLP.

As a corollary of the previous theorem, we obtain the relationship between Dynamic Logic Programming and generalized Update Answer-Sets:

Corollary 49 *Let* $\mathcal{P} = \{ P_s : s \in \mathcal{T}\}$ *be a* Sequence of Extended Generalized Logic Programs. *Let* $s \in \mathcal{T}$. *Let* M_s *be an* extended stable model of $\mathcal{P}$ *at state* s. *Then* M_s *is an extended* Generalized Update Answer-Set at state s.

Note that these semantics for updates suggest the existence of another possible semantics for sequences of programs, using the definition of rejected rules of the update answer-set semantics and the definition of defaults of DLP. We call such semantics *U-Semantics*, defined by its set of *U-models* as follows:

Definition 58 (U-Models at state s**)** *Let* $\mathcal{P} = \{P_s : s \in \mathcal{T}\}$ *be an ordered sequence of generalized extended logic programs* P_s *in the language* $\mathcal{L}^*$, *with smallest element* U_{s_0}, *and* M *a generalized extended interpretation of* $\mathcal{L}^*$. M *is a* U-model at state s *iff:*

$$M = least\left(\left[\rho\left(\mathcal{P}\right)_s - Rej^*\left(M, s, \mathcal{P}\right)\right] \cup Default\left(\rho\left(\mathcal{P}\right)_s, M\right)\right) \tag{3.106}$$

where

$$\rho(\mathcal{P})_s = \bigcup_{i \leq s} P_i$$

$$Rej^*(M, s, \mathcal{P}) = \left\{ \begin{array}{r} r \in P_{s_1} \mid \exists r' \in P_{s_2} \setminus Rej^*(M, s, \mathcal{P}), s_1 < s_2 \leq s, \\ r \bar{\bowtie} r', M \vDash B(r') \cup B(r) \end{array} \right\}$$

$$Default(\rho(\mathcal{P})_s, M) = \{not\, A \mid \nexists r \in \rho(\mathcal{P})_s : (H(r) = A) \wedge M \vDash B(r)\}$$

and $r \bar{\bowtie} r'$ *iff* $H(r) = not\ H(r')$ *or* $H(r) = -H(r')$.

Note that, as before, we could use $\bowtie$ instead of $\bar{\bowtie}$ if we use the expanded versions of programs.

This semantics allows more models than DLP and less models that the update answer-set semantics. We state the following results, omitting the proof for it being rather trivial given the previous results:

Proposition 50 *Let* $\mathcal{P} = \{P_s : s \in \mathcal{T}\}$ *be a* Sequence of Extended Generalized Logic Programs. *Let* $s \in \mathcal{T}$. *Let* M_s *be an extended stable model of* $\mathcal{P}$ *at state* s. *Then* M_s *is an* U-model *at state* s.

Proposition 51 *Let* $\mathcal{P} = \{P_s : s \in \mathcal{T}\}$ *be a* Sequence of Extended Generalized Logic Programs. *Let* $s \in \mathcal{T}$. *Let* M_s *be an* U-model *at state* s. *Then* M_s *is an* Generalized Update Answer-Set at state s.

The relationships stated in the previous results can be summarized as follows:

Proposition 52 *Let* $\mathcal{P} = \{P_s : s \in \mathcal{T}\}$ *be a* Sequence of Extended Generalized Logic Programs. *Let* $s \in \mathcal{T}$. *Let* $DLP(\mathcal{P})_s$ *denote the set of extended stable models of* $\mathcal{P}$ *at state* s; $JU(\mathcal{P})_s$ *denote the set of extended* $\mathcal{P}$-Justified Update *at state* s; $AS(\mathcal{P})_s$ *denote the set of* Generalized Update Answer-Set at state s; *and* $U(\mathcal{P})_s$ *denote the set of* U-models *at state* s. *Then:*

$$DLP(\mathcal{P})_s \subseteq JU(\mathcal{P})_s \subseteq AS(\mathcal{P})_s$$
$$DLP(\mathcal{P})_s \subseteq U(\mathcal{P})_s \subseteq AS(\mathcal{P})_s$$

We now show some examples that illustrate the different results obtained according to the different semantics:

Example 26 *Let* $\mathcal{P}_a = P_{a1} \oplus P_{a2} \oplus P_{a3}$, $\mathcal{P}_b = P_{b1} \oplus P_{b2}$ *and* $\mathcal{P}_c = P_{c1} \oplus P_{c2}$ *be Dynamic Logic Programs where:*

$$P_{a1} = \{a \leftarrow\} \qquad P_{b1} = \{a \leftarrow\} \qquad P_{c1} = \{not\, a \leftarrow; \quad a \leftarrow\}$$
$$P_{a2} = \{not\, a \leftarrow\} \qquad P_{b2} = \{not\, a \leftarrow not\, a\} \qquad P_{c2} = \{a \leftarrow a\}$$
$$P_{a3} = \{a \leftarrow a\}$$

The following table summarizes the set of models obtained according to the several semantics:

	$DLP(\mathcal{P})_s$	$JU(\mathcal{P})_s$	$U(\mathcal{P})_s$	$AS(\mathcal{P})_s$
$\mathcal{P}_a$ *with* $s = a3$	$\{not\, a\}$	$\{not\, a\}$	$\{not\, a\}$ $\{a\}$	$\{not\, a\}$ $\{a\}$
$\mathcal{P}_b$ *with* $s = b2$	$\{a\}$	$\{not\, a\}$ $\{a\}$	$\{a\}$	$\{not\, a\}$ $\{a\}$
$\mathcal{P}_c$ *with* $s = c2$	$\{a\}$	$\{a\}$	$\{a\}$	$\{a\}$

This table shows how the update at state a3, with a tautology, changes the semantics of $\mathcal{P}_a$ (note that all the semantics agree that at state a2 the only model should be $M = \{not\, a\}$) for the cases of the Generalized Update Answer-Sets and U-semantics. The same happens in $\mathcal{P}_b$, this time for the cases of Generalized Update Answer-Sets and $\mathcal{P}$-Justified Updates. It is also important to note that DLP is immune to both these tautological updates. But none of these semantics are immune to all tautological updates, as shown by the third scenario ($\mathcal{P}_c$) where the contradiction existing at state c1 is somehow removed by the tautological update.

We finalize this Subsection by mentioning classes of programs for which some of the semantics coincide. Some of these conditions, were established in [77] for the class of extended logic programs and for generalized (normal) logic programs. We now generalize those results for the case of generalized extended logic programs, although the proof is established exactly in the same manner as for the other classes of programs, and add some new results. Part of such conditions are based on the notion of AND/OR graphs, that we now recall as presented in [77].

An AND/OR-graph is a pair $G = \langle N, C\rangle$, where N is a finite set of AND-nodes or OR-nodes, and $C \subseteq N \times \bigcup_{i=0}^{|N|} N^i$ is a set of connectors such that C is a function, i.e., for each $I \in N$ there is at most one tuple $\langle O_1, \ldots, O_k\rangle \in \bigcup_{i=0}^{|N|} N^i$ such that $\langle I, O_1, \ldots, O_k\rangle \in C$. We call I the *input node* and $O_1, \ldots, O_k$ the *output nodes* of $\langle I, O_1, \ldots, O_k\rangle \in C$. As well, $\langle I, O_1, \ldots, O_k\rangle$ itself is referred to as a k*-connector*.

The concept of a path, as defined in ordinary graphs, can be generalized to AND/OR-graphs as follows. Let $\langle R, O_1, \ldots, O_k\rangle$, $k \geq 0$, be the connector for a node R in G. A tree p is a *path rooted at R in G* if the following conditions hold:

1. if $k = 0$, then $p = \langle R\rangle$;

2. if $k > 0$ and R is an AND-node, then $p = \langle R, p_1, \ldots, p_k\rangle$, where $p_1, \ldots, p_k$ are paths rooted at $O_1, \ldots, O_k$ in G; and

3. if $k > 0$ and R is an OR-node, then $p = \langle R, p_i\rangle$, for some $1 \leq i \leq k$, where p_i is a path rooted at O_i in G.

Note that p might be an infinite tree. Furthermore, the *graph associated with a path* p, $G(p)$, is the directed graph whose nodes are the nodes of G occurring in p and whose edges contain, for every node R in the recursive definition of p, $R \to O_1, \ldots, R \to O_k$ if R is an AND-node, and $R \to O_i$ if R is an OR-node. Next, we will define how an AND/OR-graph can be assigned to a sequence of generalized extended logic programs $\mathcal{P} = \{\, P_s : s \in \mathcal{T}\}$, and how such a graph can be reduced with respect to an interpretation M.

Definition 59 *[77] Let $\mathcal{P} = \{\, P_s : s \in \mathcal{T}\}$, $\mathcal{T} = \{1, ..., n\}$ be a sequence of GELPs over a language $\mathcal{L}^*$ generated by $\mathcal{K}^*$. We associate with $\mathcal{P}$ an AND/OR-graph, $G_{\mathcal{P}} = \langle N, C\rangle$, in the following way:*

1. *the set N consists of AND-nodes r for every rule r in $\mathcal{P}$, and OR-nodes Z for every $Z \in H(r) \cup B(r)$ and every r' in $\mathcal{P}$;*

2. *the set C consists of $(k+l)$-connectors $\langle r, A_1, ..., A_k, not\, A'_1, ..., not\, A'_l\rangle$ for every rule r in $\mathcal{P}$ of the form $H(r) \leftarrow A_1, ..., A_k, not\, A'_1, ..., not\, A'_l$, $k, l \geq 0$, and of m-connectors $\langle Z, r_1, ..., , r_m\rangle$ for all rules $r_1, ..., , r_m$ in $\mathcal{P}$ such that $H(r_i) = Z$, where $Z \in \mathcal{L}^*$.*

Definition 60 *[77] Let $\mathcal{P} = \{ P_s : s \in \mathcal{T}\}$, $\mathcal{T} = \{1, ..., n\}$ be a sequence of GELPs over a language $\mathcal{L}^*$ generated by $\mathcal{K}^*$ and let M be a generalized interpretation. The* reduced AND/OR-graph of $\mathcal{P}$ with respect to M, $G^M_{\mathcal{P}}$, *is the graph resulting from $G_{\mathcal{P}}$ by:*

1. *removing all AND-nodes r and their connectors (as well as removing r from all connectors containing it as output node), if either $r \in Reject(\mathcal{P}_n, n, M)$ or $M \not\models B(r)$ holds; and*

2. *replacing, for every atom A, the connector of $not\, A$ by the 0-connector $\langle not\, A\rangle$, if A is associated with a 0-connector after Step (1) and no $r \in Reject(\mathcal{P}_n, n, M)$ exists such that $H(r) = A$.*

We now define two conditions that will be used to establish the classes of programs for which the semantics coincide:

Definition 61 (Root Condition) *Let $\mathcal{P} = \{ P_s : s \in \mathcal{T}\}$, $\mathcal{T} = \{1, ..., n\}$ be a sequence of GELPs over a language $\mathcal{L}^*$ generated by $\mathcal{K}^*$, s one of its states, and let M be an interpretation. Let $\mathcal{P}^{exp}$ be obtained from $\mathcal{P}$ by replacing each program $P_s \in \mathcal{P}$ by its expanded version P^{exp}_s. We say that $\mathcal{P}$ and M obey the* root condition *at state s iff, for every objective atom $L \in \mathcal{K}^* \setminus M^+$, one of the following conditions holds:*

1. *For every rule r in $\mathcal{P}^{exp}$ such that $H(r) = L$, $S \not\models B(r)$.*

2. *There exists a path p in $G^S_{\mathcal{P}^{exp}}$ rooted at $not\, L$, such that $G(p)$ is acyclic.*

Definition 62 (Chain Condition) *Let $\mathcal{P} = \{ P_s : s \in \mathcal{T}\}$, $\mathcal{T} = \{1, ..., n\}$ be a sequence of GELPs over a language $\mathcal{L}^*$ generated by $\mathcal{K}^*$, s one of its states, and let M be an interpretation. Let $\mathcal{P}^{exp}$ be obtained from $\mathcal{P}$ by replacing each program $P_s \in \mathcal{P}$ by its expanded version P^{exp}_s. We say that $\mathcal{P}$ and M obey the* chain condition *at state s iff for each pair r, r' of rules $r \in P_i$ and $r' \in P_j$ such that $1 \leq i < j < s$, $H(r) = not\, H(r')$ and $M \models B(r) \cup B(r')$, one of the following holds:*

1. *$r' \notin Rej^*(M, s, \mathcal{P})$*

2. *$\exists r'' \in P_{s+1} \cup ... \cup P_n : H(r'') = not\, H(r')$ and $B(r'') \subseteq B(r)$.*

We are now ready to establish the results concerning some classes of programs for which some semantics coincide. In the following theorems, we consider $\mathcal{P} = \{ P_s : s \in \mathcal{T}\}$, $\mathcal{T} = \{1, ..., n\}$ to be a sequence of GELPs over a language $\mathcal{L}^*$ generated by $\mathcal{K}^*$, s one of its states, and M an interpretation.

Theorem 53 *Let $\mathcal{P}$ and M obey the* chain condition *at state s. Then, M is a $\mathcal{P}$-*Justified Update *iff M is a* Generalized Update Answer-Set.

Theorem 54 *Let $\mathcal{P}$ and M obey the* chain condition *at state s. Then, M is an* Extended Stable Model *iff M is a* U-model.

Theorem 55 *Let $\mathcal{P}$ and M obey the* root condition *at state s. Then, M is a $\mathcal{P}$-*Justified Update *iff M is a* Extended Stable Model.

Theorem 56 *Let $\mathcal{P}$ and M obey the* root condition *at state s. Then, M is a* Generalized Update Answer-Set *iff M is a* U-model.

Corollary 57 *Let $\mathcal{P}$ and M obey the* root and chain conditions *at state s. Then M is a* Generalized Update Answer-Set *iff M is a* U-model *iff M is a* $\mathcal{P}$-Justified Update *iff M is a* Extended Stable Model.

The proofs concerning the *root condition* are straight forward adaptations of proofs existing in [77]. The proof concerning the *chain condition* is straight forward, given standard logic programming results, and is omitted.

3.5.2 Other Approaches

We next briefly mention two other approaches to updates that, unlike the previous ones, are not directly based on a notion of causal rejection.

Program Updates Through Abduction of Inoue and Sakama

In [212], the authors propose an integrated framework to deal with three forms of theory change, namely *view updates, theory updates* and *contradiction removal.* We are only concerned with their approach to theory update. Inoue and Sakama propose the use of abduction as the basic mechanism to find a solution. According to their view of abduction, they start with an abductive program $\langle P, \mathcal{A}\rangle$ and a ground objective literal G, where P is an extended logic program and $\mathcal{A}$ a set of objective literals from the language of P called the abducibles. Then, a pair (E, F) is an explanation (resp. anti-explanation) of observation G with respect to $\langle P, \mathcal{A}\rangle$ if:

1. $(P \cup E) \setminus F \models_{sm} G$ (resp. $(P \cup E) \setminus F \not\models_{sm} G$);
2. $(P \cup E) \setminus F$ is consistent;
3. $E \subseteq \mathcal{A} \setminus P$ and $F \subseteq \mathcal{A} \cap P$.

Within this abductive framework, to perform theory update of an initial knowledge base represented by the extended logic program P with the update specification represented by the extended logic program Q, the authors define the abductive program $\langle P \cup Q, P \setminus Q\rangle$. Then, P' is the resulting program iff $P' = (P \cup Q)\setminus F$ where $(\emptyset, F)$ is a minimal anti-explanation of the observation $G = false$ with respect to $\langle P \cup Q, P \setminus Q\rangle$. By definition we have that: P' must be consistent; $Q \subseteq P' \subseteq P \cup Q$; and there is no consistent program P'' such that $P' \subset P'' \subseteq P \cup Q$.

Essentially what Sakama and Inoue propose is that every rule in the initial program P is made defeasible, minimally eliminating them from $P \cup Q$ until the resulting program is consistent.

In our opinion there are two major drawbacks to this approach:

- the first drawback concerns the requirement for consistency of the update of a program P by a program Q. Contradiction is not an evil manifestation that should be removed at any cost. Rather it is a phenomenon that can have several causes and each of its types should be dealt with accordingly, as we've mentioned before (for an extensive study of paraconsistent logic programming, the reader is referred to [49, 51]). Requiring P' to be consistent renders the desirable property such that an empty update does not cause any change not valid for Inoue and Sakama's proposal. If, as for DLP, we use the symbol $\oplus$ to denote the update operation, we have that $SEM(P \oplus \emptyset) = SEM(P)$ does not hold in general, the simplest counterexample being $P = \{a \leftarrow; -a \leftarrow\}$. In fact, when Sakama and Inoue propose the use of their framework to remove inconsistency, it amounts to update the original theory with an empty program, i.e. although they claim to have a framework to achieve three different types of theory change, they cannot be achieved separately, i.e. one cannot perform program updates without simultaneously removing inconsistency.

- the second drawback of Sakama and Inoue's approach concerns the commitment implied by each update, when the rules are physically removed, rendering them useless even if future updates invalidate the basis for such removal. Consider the simple case where we have the following three programs:

$$P_1: \ a \leftarrow \qquad P_2: \ \begin{array}{l} -a \leftarrow b \\ b \leftarrow \end{array} \qquad P_3: \ -b \leftarrow$$

According to Inoue and Sakama, after updating P_1 with P_2 and subsequently with P_3, atom a does not follow from the semantics of the resulting program. This is so because rule $a \leftarrow$ was eliminated when P_1 was updated with P_2 and cannot be reinstated when P_3 is used to update the result. Example 5 in the Introduction of this Chapter is an instantiation of this example. According to Inoue and Sakama, after the power is back on, represented by the (in this case extended) logic program $\{-power\_failure \leftarrow\}$, the TV is still not on.

One should also point out that this framework for updates is not based on a notion of causal rejection. Not only the previous example where the initial program P is contradictory serves to illustrate this, but also the following example where neither P nor Q is contradictory:

$$P = \{a \leftarrow; -a \leftarrow b\} \qquad Q = \{b\}$$

According to Sakama and Inoue, there are two possible updates, if each one of the rules of P is removed, even though Q does not have any rules for a nor $-a$. Again this is related to the fact that Inoue and Sakama perform a single operation consisting of a mixture of updates with revision, two forms of theory change that are widely accepted as distinct. According to DLP, the result of updating P with Q should be semantically equivalent to the program consisting of all three rules, i.e. contradictory. Then, if one wishes so, some form of contradiction removal should be applied.

Program Updates Through Priorities of Zhang and Foo

In [233], Zhang and Foo propose a framework for solving the problem of updating a knowledge base represented by means of an extended logic program, by means of another such program. Their solution is based on prioritized logic programs which they have proposed earlier in [232]. The process for computing updates is a rather elaborate one and we will not present all the details. Rather we will informally explain how such updates are accomplished and discuss some of its characteristics.

Starting with two extended logic programs, P_0 and P_1 where, as usual, P_0 represents the initial knowledge base and P_1 the update specification, Zhang and Foo propose that we first determine the Answer-Sets of P_0. Subsequently, each of those Answer-Sets is individually updated by P_1 according to a transformation based on inertia rules. We remark that such transformation yields results such as the ones obtained for model updates (eg. [12, 157, 194, 197]) i.e., based on a notion of minimal change of the models. Accordingly, for each of the Answer-Sets of P_0, we obtain a set of models, each represented by $B(P_0, P_1)$. Then, based on each $B(P_0, P_1)$, a subset of the rules of P_0 is determined, $P_{(P_0,P_1)}$, such that $P_{(P_0,P_1)}$ is maximal and $B(P_0, P_1)$ is coherent with the program $P_{(P_0,P_1)} \cup P_1$ or, if $B(P_0, P_1)$ is inconsistent, then $P_{(P_0,P_1)}$ is any maximal subset of P_0 such that $P_{(P_0,P_1)} \cup P_1$ is well defined. Finally, Zhang and Foo define a prioritized logic program based on $P_{(P_0,P_1)} \cup P_1$, assigning higher priority to P_1, to finally determine the reducts of such program which are the possible resulting update programs. Note that this is a very informal and brief explanation of the process. For further details the reader is referred to [233].

The approach of Zhang and Foo is more in the spirit of the possible models approach of Winslett ([228]), where the models of the initial knowledge base are first determined before the updates are performed, and suffers from some drawbacks. First, and quite importantly, the result of updating one logic program by another logic program is a set of programs and not just one. This is particularly important when we want to perform a sequence of updates which renders an exponential growth in the number of knowledge bases to be considered. Also, in what concerns this issue, some cases exist where it is difficult to accept a set of programs instead of just one, as illustrated by the following example:

Example 27 *Consider the following logic programs:*

$$P_0 = \{p \leftarrow; r \leftarrow not\, q; q \leftarrow not\, r\}$$
$$P_1 = \{-p \leftarrow\}$$

According to Zhang and Foo, the result of updating P_0 with P_1 are the following two logic programs U' and U'':

$$U' = \{-p \leftarrow; r \leftarrow not\, q\}$$
$$U'' = \{-p \leftarrow; q \leftarrow not\, r\}$$

We cannot find any intuitively reasonable explanation for the result of updating P_0 with P_1 not to be the program U (or any update equivalent one):

$$U = \{-p \leftarrow; r \leftarrow not\, q; q \leftarrow not\, r\}$$

Furthermore, if we wish to perform another update specified by $P_2 = \{-r \leftarrow\}$, intuitively, we would expect the result of updating P_0 with P_1 and with P_2 to be a program such that its semantics would have atom q as a consequence. According to Zhang and Foo this is not the case because if we take U' as the result of updating P_0 with P_1 (and every possible result must be considered), when we update with P2 we cannot conclude atom q because the rule $q \leftarrow not\, r$ was rejected, for no apparent reason.

The previous example suggests that an empty update changes the initial program, even if it is not contradictory as happened with the semantics of Inoue and Sakama. Take the program $P_0 = \{r \leftarrow not\, q; q \leftarrow not\, r\}$, to which we apply an empty update program. The result of such an update is not P_0, nor an update equivalent one, but rather the set of programs composed of $P_0' = \{q \leftarrow not\, r\}$ and $P_0'' = \{r \leftarrow not\, q\}$.

In the previous example, even though some rules were rejected in one of the possible results, they are still present in the other option. But this does not always happen in the approach of Zang and Foo. Situations occur where rules are, unnecessarily, permanently rejected such as illustrated by the next example:

Example 28 *Consider the following logic programs:*

$$P_0 = \{r \leftarrow not\, q\}$$
$$P_1 = \{q \leftarrow not\, r\}$$

According to Zhang and Foo, the result of updating P_0 with P_1 is the following logic program U':

$$U' = \{q \leftarrow not\, r\}$$

Again, we cannot see any reasonable justification for the update of P_0 with P_1 not be the program U (or an update equivalent one):

$$U = \{r \leftarrow not\, q; q \leftarrow not\, r\}$$

And, unlike in the previous example, in this case there is no possible scenario where the rule $r \leftarrow not\, q$ still exists.

To conclude, we believe that the approach of Zhang and Foo is not a satisfactory solution to the problem of updating knowledge bases represented by logic programs, nor any other solution based on the models of the initial theory for that matter. We believe that the notion of updates based on causal rejection of rules, in general, is the only one providing acceptable results.

3.6 Summary and Open Issues

We defined a program transformation that takes two generalized logic programs P and U, and, produces the updated logic program $P \oplus U$ resulting from the update of program P by U. We provided a complete characterization of the semantics of program updates $P \oplus U$ and established their basic properties. Our approach generalizes the so called *revision programs* introduced in [157]. Namely, in the special case when the initial program is just a set of facts, our program update coincides with the justified revision of [157]. In the general case, when the initial program also contains rules, our program updates characterize precisely which of these rules remain valid by inertia, and which are rejected. We also showed how strong (or explicit or *"classical")* negation can be easily incorporated into the framework of program updates.

With the introduction of dynamic program updates, we have extended program updates to ordered sets of logic programs (or modules). When this order is interpreted as a time order, dynamic program updates describe the evolution of a logic program which undergoes a sequence of modifications. This opens up the possibility of incremental design and evolution of logic programs, leading to the paradigm of *dynamic logic programming.* We believe that dynamic programming significantly facilitates *modularization* of logic programming and, thus, modularization of non-monotonic reasoning as a whole.

We have explored some properties of DLP and presented some illustrative example. Such examples show that ordered sets of program modules need not necessarily be seen as just a temporal evolution of a logic program. Different modules can also represent different sets of priorities, or viewpoints of different agents. In the case of priorities, a dynamic program update specifies the exact meaning of the *"union"* of the modules, subject to the given priorities.

On a subsequent Chapter we will explore how such different encodings for the sequence of states can be combined to express, for example, the evolution in time of a set of programs related according to some priority hierarchy.

In what concerns those issues not explored in this work, we highlight:

Postulates for Updates: the basic postulates for updates in classical propositional logic, set forth in [116], do not apply when considering updates of non-monotonic theories. This was shown by the basic examples that served as the initial motivation for this work, and subsequently explored in [77]. It is in order to establish a set of postulates to be obeyed by any reasonable semantics for such non-monotonic theory updates, and against which such semantics can be tested and compared.

Combine Updates with Revision: there has been an extensive work on the subject of revision in non-monotonic theories (cf. [3, 10, 11, 33, 87, 88, 184, 202, 229, 230]). While revision deals with evolving representations of static worlds, updates deal with evolving worlds. One future direction for research is to study the combination of revision and updates so as to combine them into one single unified framework. This would allow to differentiate newly incoming information as being of an update nature from that of a revision nature, i.e. information concerning one particular state for which we already have some incomplete information.

Contradiction Removal: somehow related to the previous item is the subject of contradiction removal, which we have previously mentioned when we addressed the several possible ways contradiction may arise in a DLP setting. One other direction for future research is the definition of paraconsistent semantics for DLP to subsequently deal with, and eventually remove, such contradictions, namely by means of abduction.

Combine Updates with Preferences: several authors have been working on the subject of reasoning with preferences [38, 39]. Preferences and Updates are two distinct forms of reasoning and serve different purposes and goals. While preferences usually deal with incomplete knowledge modelled with default rules, Updates deal with dynamic worlds. Combining both forms of reasoning is certainly an interesting topic of research. Preliminary results in this direction can be found in [13].

Well Founded Semantics for Updates: three-valued semantics have been extensively studied and their usefulness for representing and reasoning with incomplete knowledge established. It is therefore important to define a well founded version for the semantics of DLP. In [130, 141–143], the notion of justified updates was also established for the three valued case. This provides a starting point for setting forth its DLP counterpart. In [17], the authors have made a first attempt of defining such semantics, at the transformational level. It is still not clear if such transformational based semantics yields the intuitively desirable results, for which a declarative characterization of such semantics is needed.

Other Semantics for Updates: immunity to tautologies has always been a desirable property for logic based systems. Finding a suitable semantics for logic program updates, based on the notion of causal rejection of rules and enjoying the intuitions we have explored, that is simultaneously immune to all tautological updates is a non-trivial open issue.

Chapter 4

Languages of Updates

Whereas DLP provides a framework and semantics to determine the meaning of sequences of logic programs, it does not provide a mechanism to construct such programs. Languages of updates accomplish this goal, and are the subject of this Chapter. We start with an overview of the language of updates LUPS [15] and its extension EPI [75]. Then we identify an intuitively incorrect behaviour of LUPS semantics and a possible, important, extension to its syntax. To address these issues, the Knowledge Update Language (KUL) is introduced and compared to its predecessors. Finally, we present some illustrative examples and show how KUL can be used to specify the effects of actions. Parts of this Chapter appeared in [9, 131].

4.1 Introduction

In the previous Chapter we have introduced Dynamic Logic Programming as a paradigm to express knowledge as sequences of states, each represented by a logic program. The meaning of such sequences of logic programs, at each state, was assigned by means of a model theoretic semantics based on the notion of its stable models.

Whereas DLP provides a meaning to sequences of logic programs, it says nothing about how to obtain them. Each logic program can represent newly incoming information, totally independent from the previous states, but can also depend on the previous state of affairs. To allow the specification of such logic programs whose construction can depend on the previous state, Alferes et al. introduced the language of updates LUPS [15]. The language LUPS is based on a notion of update commands that allow the specification (construction) of logic programs. Each command in LUPS, which can be issued in parallel with other LUPS commands, specifies an update action, basically encoding the assertion or retraction of a logic program rule. A collection of such commands, whose execution can be made dependent on the semantics of the current sequence of logic programs, specifies the next logic program to be added to such sequence.

Subsequently, Eiter et al. proposed to extend the LUPS language, introducing the language EPI [75]. EPI introduces the ability to access external observations and make the execution of commands to depend upon it. Furthermore the execution of EPI commands can be made dependent on the concurrent execution of other commands.

Although based on LUPS, EPI was mainly designed as a language to specify update policies in knowledge bases that evolve according to external observations.

In this Chapter we present a detailed overview of LUPS, together with a brief review of some of the main features of EPI. Subsequently we take a closer look at the semantics of LUPS where we identify an intuitively incorrect behaviour in what concerns a subset of its commands. The same problem occurs in EPI. We also identify an important extension to the syntax of LUPS. Then, we propose a Knowledge Update Language (KUL) that extends the syntax of LUPS and changes the semantics according to the desirable behaviour. Such desirable behaviour is partially expressed by means of a property that we prove valid for KUL, but not for LUPS and EPI. Finally, we explore some illustrative examples, namely showing how to encode action specifications in update languages.

4.2 Languages for Updates: Overview

4.2.1 LUPS

In [15], the authors argue that besides assigning a meaning to a sequence of logic programs, one also needs a language to specify how such sequence of programs is to be constructed i.e., besides declaratively specifying the states of a KB, it is advantageous to also declaratively specify the state transitions. And these state transitions should be allowed to depend on the states themselves. To this purpose, the language of updates *LUPS* [15] was introduced. Here we recall the language of updates *LUPS* closely following its original formulation in [15]. The object language of *LUPS* is that of generalized logic programs. A sentence U in *LUPS* is a set of simultaneous update commands (or actions) that, given a pre-existing sequence of logic programs $P_0 \oplus \cdots \oplus P_n$ (i.e. a dynamic logic program), whose semantics corresponds to our knowledge at a given state, produces a sequence with one more program, $P_0 \oplus \cdots \oplus P_n \oplus P_{n+1}$, corresponding to the knowledge that results from the previous sequence after performing all the simultaneous commands. A program in *LUPS* is a sequence of such sentences.

Given a program in *LUPS*, its semantics is defined by means of a dynamic logic program generated by the sequence of commands.

In this update framework, knowledge evolves from one knowledge state to another as a result of update commands stated in the object language. Without loss of generality it is assumed that the initial knowledge state is empty. Given the *current knowledge state*, its *successor knowledge state* is produced as a result of the occurrence of a set U of simultaneous *updates*. The knowledge state obtained by performing the sequence of updates $U_1, U_2, \ldots, U_n$ is denoted by $U_1 \otimes U_2 \otimes \cdots \otimes U_n$. So defined sequences of updates will be called *update programs*. In other words, an update program is a finite sequence $\mathcal{U} = \{U_s : s \in S\}$ of updates indexed by the set $S = \{1, 2, \ldots, n\}$. Each update is a set of update commands. Update commands (defined below) specify *assertions* or *retractions* to the current knowledge state. By the current knowledge state we mean the one resulting from the last update performed.

Knowledge can be queried at any state $t \leq n$, where n is the index of the current knowledge state. A query will be denoted by:

$$\textbf{holds } L_1, \ldots, L_k \textbf{ at } t?$$

and is true iff the conjunction of its literals holds at the state obtained after the tth update. If $t = n$, the state reference "**at** t" is skipped.

Update commands specify assertions or retractions to the current knowledge state. In *LUPS* a simple assertion is represented by the command:

$$\textbf{assert } L \leftarrow L_1, \ldots, L_k \textbf{ when } L_{k+1}, \ldots, L_m \tag{4.1}$$

Its meaning is that if $L_{k+1}, \ldots, L_m$ is true in the current state, then the rule $L \leftarrow L_1, \ldots, L_k$ is added to its successor state, and persists by inertia, until possibly retracted or overridden by some future update command.

In order to represent rules and facts that do not persist by inertia, i.e. that are one-state events, LUPS includes the modified form of assertion:

$$\textbf{assert event } L \leftarrow L_1, \ldots, L_k \textbf{ when } L_{k+1}, \ldots, L_m \tag{4.2}$$

The retraction of rules is performed with the two update commands:

$$\textbf{retract } L \leftarrow L_1, \ldots, L_k \textbf{ when } L_{k+1}, \ldots, L_m \tag{4.3}$$

$$\textbf{retract event } L \leftarrow L_1, \ldots, L_k \textbf{ when } L_{k+1}, \ldots, L_m \tag{4.4}$$

Its meaning is that, subject to precondition $L_{k+1}, \ldots, L_m$ (verified at the current state) rule $L \leftarrow L_1, \ldots, L_k$ is either retracted from its successor state onwards, or just temporarily retracted in the successor state (if governed by **event**).

Normally assertions represent newly incoming information. Although its effects remain by inertia (until contravened or retracted), the assert command itself does not persist. However, some update commands may desirably persist in the successive consecutive updates. This is especially the case of laws which, subject to some preconditions, are always valid, or of rules describing the effects of an action. In the former case, the update command must be added to all sets of updates, to guarantee that the rule remains indeed valid. In the latter case, the specification of the effects must be added to all sets of updates, to guarantee that, when the action takes place, its effects are enforced.

To specify such persistent update commands, *LUPS* introduces the following commands:

$$\textbf{always } L \leftarrow L_1, \ldots, L_k \textbf{ when } L_{k+1}, \ldots, L_m \tag{4.5}$$

$$\textbf{always event } L \leftarrow L_1, \ldots, L_k \textbf{ when } L_{k+1}, \ldots, L_m \tag{4.6}$$

$$\textbf{cancel } L \leftarrow L_1, \ldots, L_k \textbf{ when } L_{k+1}, \ldots, L_m \tag{4.7}$$

The first two statements mean that, in addition to any new set of arriving update commands, the persistent update command keep executing with them too. In the first case without, and in the second one with the **event** keyword. The third statement cancels execution of this persistent update, once the conditions for cancellation are met.

Definition 63 (LUPS) *An update program in LUPS is a finite sequence of updates, where an update is a set of commands of the form (4.1) to (4.7).*

The semantics of *LUPS* is defined by incrementally translating update programs into sequences of generalized logic programs and by considering the semantics of the *DLP* formed by them.

Let $\mathcal{U} = U_1 \otimes \ldots \otimes U_n$ be a *LUPS* programs. At every state t the corresponding *DLP*, $\Upsilon_t(\mathcal{U}) = \mathcal{P}_t$, is determined.

The translation of a *LUPS* program into a dynamic program is made by induction, starting from the empty program P_0, and for each update U_t, given the already built dynamic program $P_0 \oplus \cdots \oplus P_{t-1}$, determining the resulting program $P_0 \oplus \cdots \oplus P_{t-1} \oplus P_t$. To cope with persistent update commands, associated with every dynamic program in the inductive construction, a set containing all currently active persistent commands is considered, i.e. all those commands that were not cancelled until that point in the construction, from the time they were introduced. To be able to retract rules, a unique identification of each such rule is needed. This is achieved by augmenting the language of the resulting dynamic program with a new propositional variable "$N(R)$" for every rule R appearing in the original *LUPS* program.

Definition 64 (Translation into dynamic logic programs) *Let $\mathcal{U} = U_1 \otimes \cdots \otimes U_n$ be an update program. The corresponding dynamic logic program $\Upsilon(\mathcal{U}) = \mathcal{P} = P_0 \oplus \cdots \oplus P_n$ is obtained by the following inductive construction, using at each step t an auxiliary set of persistent commands PC_t:*

Base step: $P_0 = \{\}$ with $PC_0 = \{\}$.

Inductive step: Let $\Upsilon_{t-1}(\mathcal{U}) = \mathcal{P}_{t-1} = P_0 \oplus \cdots \oplus P_{t-1}$ with the set of persistent commands PC_{t-1} be the translation of $\mathcal{U}_{t-1} = U_1 \otimes \cdots \otimes U_{t-1}$. The translation of $\mathcal{U}_t = U_1 \otimes \cdots \otimes U_t$ is $\Upsilon_t(\mathcal{U}) = \mathcal{P}_t = P_0 \oplus \cdots \oplus P_{t-1} \oplus P_t$ with the set of persistent commands PC_t, where:

$$
\begin{aligned}
PC_t = {} & PC_{t-1} \cup \{\textbf{assert } R \textbf{ when } \phi : \textbf{always } R \textbf{ when } \phi \in U_t\} \cup \\
& \cup \{\textbf{assert event } R \textbf{ when } \phi : \textbf{always event } R \textbf{ when } \phi \in U_t\} \cup \\
& - \left\{\textbf{assert [event] } R \textbf{ when } \phi : \textbf{cancel } R \textbf{ when } \psi \in U_t \wedge \bigoplus \mathcal{P}_{t-1} \models_{sm} \psi\right\} - \\
& - \left\{\textbf{assert [event] } R \textbf{ when } \phi : \textbf{retract } R \textbf{ when } \psi \in U_t \wedge \bigoplus \mathcal{P}_{t-1} \models_{sm} \psi\right\} -
\end{aligned}
$$

$$NU_t = U_t \cup PC_t$$

$$
\begin{aligned}
P_t = {} & \left\{N(R) \leftarrow : \textbf{assert [event] } R \textbf{ when } \phi \in NU_t \wedge \bigoplus \mathcal{P}_{t-1} \models_{sm} \phi\right\} \cup \\
& \cup \left\{H(R) \leftarrow B(R), N(R) : \textbf{assert [event] } R \textbf{ when } \phi \in NU_t \wedge \bigoplus \mathcal{P}_{t-1} \models_{sm} \phi\right\} \cup \\
& \cup \left\{not\, N(R) \leftarrow : \textbf{retract [event] } R \textbf{ when } \phi \in NU_t \wedge \bigoplus \mathcal{P}_{t-1} \models_{sm} \phi\right\} \cup \\
& \cup \left\{not\, N(R) \leftarrow : \textbf{assert event } R \textbf{ when } \phi \in NU_{t-1} \wedge \bigoplus \mathcal{P}_{t-2} \models_{sm} \phi\right\} \cup \\
& \cup \left\{N(R) \leftarrow : \textbf{retract event } R \textbf{ when } \phi \in NU_{t-1} \wedge \bigoplus \mathcal{P}_{t-2} \models_{sm} \phi, N(R)\right\}
\end{aligned}
$$

Definition 65 (LUPS Semantics) *Let $\mathcal{U}$ be an update program. A query*

$$\textbf{holds } L_1, \ldots, L_n \textbf{ at } t$$

is true in $\mathcal{U}$ iff $\bigoplus_t \Upsilon(\mathcal{U}) \models_{sm} L_1, \ldots, L_n$.

4.2.2 EPI

Eiter et al. introduced the language EPI [75] which propose to extend LUPS with two main features:

External Observations: As Eiter et al. point out, LUPS was not conceived for handling a yet unknown update which may arrive as the environment evolves, therefore lacking the possibility to allow the specification of how an agent should react upon the arrival of such an update. The language EPI facilitates access to external observations, allowing commands expressing sentences such as "retract rule R if rule R' is observed" which would be encoded by a command of the form:

$$\textbf{assert } R \textbf{ when } \mathbf{E}:R'$$

This extension enables the flexible handling of external observations such as simply recording changes in the environment, skipping uninteresting updates, or applying default actions.

Concurrency Dependencies EPI allows the specification of commands whose execution depends on the concurrent execution of other commands. For example, we may specify that some rule R should only be asserted if some rule R' is simultaneously retracted.

We will not present the technical details of EPI, for which the reader is referred to [75]. To our purposes we just need to keep the intuition behind these two features which will be adopted in a subsequent Chapter. Nevertheless, we finish this Section with some remarks on EPI.

In EPI, unlike in LUPS where the knowledge base evolves according to a sequence of concurrent update commands, there is a fixed update policy, specified by a set of update commands, which is evaluated according to a sequence of external observations to determine, at each state transition, which of the update commands specified by the update policy should be executed.

Although Eiter et al. claim that EPI is an extension of LUPS, it does not appear to be so. This shift in paradigm from a sequence of updates in LUPS to a sequence of external observations that trigger updates in EPI make them rather divergent in essence. For example, in LUPS, a persistent command of the form

$$\textbf{always } L \leftarrow L_1, \ldots, L_k \textbf{ when } L_{k+1}, \ldots, L_m$$

until cancelled, is to be evaluated at every state transition and, at every transition such that $L_{k+1}, \ldots, L_m$ holds, the rule $L \leftarrow L_1, \ldots, L_k$ is asserted. In EPI, if the same persistent commands belongs to the update policy, after the first state such that $L_{k+1}, \ldots, L_m$ holds, the rule $L \leftarrow L_1, \ldots, L_k$ will be asserted at *every* future state transition, even if $L_{k+1}, \ldots, L_m$ does not hold anymore. The authors do not present any examples showing the usefulness of this treatment of persistent commands, and we cannot find any reason that supports this semantics.

In what concerns commands whose execution depends on the concurrent execution of other commands, if we have the following command

$$\textbf{assert } R \textbf{ when } (\textbf{assert } R_1)$$

it seems reasonable to expect that rule R is asserted whenever rule R_1 is asserted. In EPI, if we have an update policy consisting of the previous command together with the following command

$$\textbf{always } R_1$$

then, even though rule R_1 was asserted due to the second command, rule R would not be asserted. This is so because the semantics of EPI does not treat the **always** command as an **assert** command that besides asserting the specified rule also persists to the subsequent states, but rather as a different unrelated command.

4.3 A New Semantics for Non-inertial Commands

In *LUPS*, the authors introduced a class of commands whose immediate effect should only hold in the successor state and should not persist by inertia in subsequent states. This kind of non-inertial commands are indicated by the keyword **event** such as the statement:

assert event *Rule* **when** *Condition*

According to the intuitive reading above, if we want to update an initial KB, P_1, with two consecutive updates U_2 and U_3, such that U_2 only contains such non-inertial commands, and U_3 is empty, it seems reasonable to expect that, after the second update, U_3, what holds true is exactly equal to what held true before the first update, i.e. what holds true at P_1. Unfortunately this is not the case in *LUPS*, as illustrated by the following example:

Example 29 *Consider the simple case where* $P_1 = \{a \leftarrow\}$*, possibly obtained by a past update command such as* **assert** $a \leftarrow$*, and the following sequence of updates:*

$$U_2 = \{\textbf{assert event } a \leftarrow\}$$
$$U_3 = \{\}$$

At state 3, i.e. after the update U_3*, according to the semantics of* LUPS *we have* $M_3 = \{\}$ *as the only stable model, i.e.* a *is not a consequence of the knowledge base at state 3.*

In this example, $M_3 = \{\}$ is the only stable model because the command **assert event** $a \leftarrow$ asserts the rule $a \leftarrow$ at state 2, but then causes the removal of all rules (past and present) of the form $a \leftarrow$, i.e. both the rule specified by U_2 and the rule of P_1 are removed. We argue that $M_3' = \{a\}$ should be the only stable model at state 3, because the command **assert event** $a \leftarrow$ should not affect (remove at state 3) the rule $a \leftarrow$ that was previously asserted at state 1, i.e. the rule in P_1. Let us look at another example:

Example 30 *Consider a slight modification in the previous example, such that the initial program is, now,* $P_1^* = \{a \leftarrow not\ \bot\}$ *(where, as usual,* $\bot$ *is a reserved proposition with the property of being false in every stable model i.e., not* $\bot$ *belongs to every stable model). If the same update sequence is performed, after the update* U_3 *we have* $M_3^* = \{a\}$ *as the only stable model.*

As we have seen, updates are somewhat syntactical in nature, but in this example, this syntactical difference in behaviour should not exist. We argue that both examples should have the same outcome, i.e. they should both have $M = \{a\}$ as the only stable model at state 3. To avoid such problem, we argue that an event command should be exerted on the single asserted (or retracted) instance of a rule and not on all other syntactically equal rules.

The main contribution of this Chapter is a proposal for a change in the semantics of *LUPS* to correct this undesirable behaviour.

The second contribution of this Chapter resides in the extension of the *LUPS* syntax with the introduction of a persistent retract command, and with a modification to the semantics of the retraction command of LUPS. We start with the motivation for the change in semantics for the retraction command of LUPS. In LUPS a retraction command, if executed, not only retracts the specified rule from the object level knowledge base, but also cancels (removes) any persistent assertion command for such rule. We do not believe that such reading of retractions is intuitive nor helpful in practical examples. If not, consider the following simple case:

Example 31 *Consider a scenario where there is one available action (α) which causes the assertion of rule (rule). This would be encoded by the statement*

$$\textbf{always}\ rule\ \textbf{when}\ \alpha$$

Let us suppose that we have previously performed action α and we want to retract rule from the knowledge base. The intuitive command to be performed would be **retract** *rule. But according to the semantics of LUPS, the execution of* **retract** *rule would cause the effective retraction of rule, but as a side effect would also cause the cancellation of the statement* **always** *rule* **when** *α, i.e. action α would no longer be available.*

We argue that the semantics of the retraction command should only retract the specified rule, leaving intact any existing persistent commands for the same rule. In this Chapter, we change the semantics accordingly.

In *LUPS*, besides the assertion and retraction commands, denoted by the keywords **assert** and **retract** respectively, that may only contribute to the state transition for which they were specified, there is a command, denoted by the keyword **always**, which can be seen as a permanent assert command, i.e. until it is cancelled, it will cause the assertion of a specific rule every time the specified condition holds. We argue that such persistent command should also exist for the retraction of rules. To illustrate our claim, let us consider the following example from [15]:

Example 32 *Consider the following scenario: -once Republicans take over both Congress and the Presidency they establish a law stating that abortions are punishable by jail; -once Democrats take over both Congress and the Presidency they abolish such a law; -in the meantime, there are no changes in the law because always either the President or the Congress vetoes such changes. The specification in* LUPS, *as presented in [15], is*[1]*:*

Persistent update commands:

$$\textbf{always}\ jail(X) \leftarrow abortion(X)\ \textbf{when}\ repC, repP \tag{4.8}$$

$$\textbf{always}\ not\, jail(X) \leftarrow abortion(X)\ \textbf{when}\ not\, repC, not\, repP \tag{4.9}$$

The authors further state that in this example, alternatively, instead of the second clause they could have used a retract statement:

$$\textbf{retract}\ jail(X) \leftarrow abortion(X)\ \textbf{when}\ not\, repC, not\, repP \tag{4.10}$$

noting that, in this example, since there is no other rule implying jail, retracting the rule is safely equivalent to retracting its conclusion.

We argue that neither of the proposed solutions, to represent the abolition of the abortion law when the Democrats take over (commands (4.9) and (4.10)), properly represents the intuition stated in the scenario.

[1]Where the rules with variables simply stand, as usual, for all the ground rules that result from replacing the variables by all the ground terms in the language.

The argument against the use of command (4.9) is implicitly stated by the authors of [15] when they say that "*since there is no other rule implying jail, retracting the rule is safely equivalent to retracting its conclusion*". In fact, if there were other rules implying jail, which is fair to expect in a realistic scenario, such as for example a rule stating that assassinations are punishable by jail, then some undesirable effects would occur. Suppose such a rule was represented by an update command, at the initial state, of the form:

$$\textbf{assert}\ jail(X) \leftarrow assassination(X) \tag{4.11}$$

If this command had been previously issued, then, after the Democrats take over both Congress and the Presidency, someone ($mary$) that both assassins someone and performs an abortion would *not* be punished by jail. This is so because the rule asserted by command (4.9) would reject, according to the DLP semantics, the previously asserted rule specified by command (4.11). The resulting knowledge base would have $not\, jail(mary)$ as a consequence.

The argument against the use of command (4.10) resides in the fact that, to effectively represent the intended meaning, this command would have to belong to every update i.e. it would have to be explicitly added to the specification of *every* state transition. Not only this does not add to the simplicity of the language but, also, the fact that the representation of the effect of Republicans taking over requires a single update command, and that the representation of the effect of Democrats taking over requires several update commands, one at each update, is somehow unintuitive. To this add the fact that the execution of one of such retraction commands would also cancel the persistent assertion command representing the case when Republicans take over i.e. after Democrats control the government, when Republicans win both Congress and the Presidency the abortion law would not be reinstated because the corresponding persistent command had been removed by means of the retraction command, as explained above.

The introduction of the **always** command in [15] was justified with the need to avoid consecutive repetitions of the **assert** command. We believe that such persistent command should also exist for the retraction of rules. A command that, until cancelled, retracts a specific rule from the KB every time the specified condition holds. In this Chapter, we introduce such command.

Throughout, to differentiate the original *LUPS* language and the extended and modified version here proposed, we refer to the latter as *KUL (Knowledge Update Language)*.

The remainder is structured as follows: First, in Sect.4.3.1, we introduce the syntax of the extended language *KUL*. In Sect.4.3.2 we propose a semantics for this extended language that corrects the above mentioned problem. In Sect.4.3.3 we illustrate with two examples. In Sect. 4.3.4 we compare both semantics by means of a desirable property.

4.3.1 *KUL* - Syntax

In this Section we formalize the language of *KUL*. We will keep all the commands of *LUPS*, with a slight modification in the syntax of two of such commands, which will be explained below, and introduce the above mentioned persistent retract command and its corresponding cancellation command.

The language of *KUL* will contain the basic non-persistent commands for the assertion and retraction of rules, denoted by the keywords **assert** and **retract**. They are of the form:

$$\textbf{assert } L \leftarrow L_1, \ldots, L_k \textbf{ when } L_{k+1}, \ldots, L_m \tag{4.12}$$
$$\textbf{retract } L \leftarrow L_1, \ldots, L_k \textbf{ when } L_{k+1}, \ldots, L_m \tag{4.13}$$

Both these commands can be made persistent, i.e. until cancelled they are added to all subsequent updates. We will identify such persistent commands by prefixing the non-persistent commands with the keyword **always**. They are thus of the form:

$$\textbf{always assert } L \leftarrow L_1, \ldots, L_k \textbf{ when } L_{k+1}, \ldots, L_m \tag{4.14}$$
$$\textbf{always retract } L \leftarrow L_1, \ldots, L_k \textbf{ when } L_{k+1}, \ldots, L_m \tag{4.15}$$

Note here the first modification in the syntax of a *LUPS* command. In *LUPS*, command (4.14) does not have the keyword **assert**, being identified by the keyword **always** alone. Since we are now introducing the persistent retraction command, this new notation becomes more symmetrical and therefore more intuitive.

All the previous commands are inertial. To obtain the corresponding non-inertial commands one simply adds the keyword **event** to obtain the following commands:

$$\textbf{assert event } L \leftarrow L_1, \ldots, L_k \textbf{ when } L_{k+1}, \ldots, L_m \tag{4.16}$$
$$\textbf{retract event } L \leftarrow L_1, \ldots, L_k \textbf{ when } L_{k+1}, \ldots, L_m \tag{4.17}$$
$$\textbf{always assert event } L \leftarrow L_1, \ldots, L_k \textbf{ when } L_{k+1}, \ldots, L_m \tag{4.18}$$
$$\textbf{always retract event } L \leftarrow L_1, \ldots, L_k \textbf{ when } L_{k+1}, \ldots, L_m \tag{4.19}$$

Just as in *LUPS* there is a cancellation command for the persistent command **always**, denoted by the keyword **cancel**, so there will be one in *KUL* but now denoted by the keyword **cancel assert**, to simplify the introduction of a cancellation command for the persistent retraction command, which will be denoted by the keyword **cancel retract**. These two commands are:

$$\textbf{cancel assert } L \leftarrow L_1, \ldots, L_k \textbf{ when } L_{k+1}, \ldots, L_m \tag{4.20}$$
$$\textbf{cancel retract } L \leftarrow L_1, \ldots, L_k \textbf{ when } L_{k+1}, \ldots, L_m \tag{4.21}$$

The syntax of the update commands of *KUL* is, formally:

Definition 66 (*KUL* - Update Commands) *A* KUL *update command, or* command *for short, is a propositional expression of any of the forms*[2]

$$[\textbf{always }]\,\textbf{assert}\,[\textbf{ event}]\ R \textbf{ when } \phi \tag{4.22}$$
$$[\textbf{always }]\,\textbf{retract}\,[\textbf{ event}]\ R \textbf{ when } \phi \tag{4.23}$$
$$\textbf{cancel assert } R \textbf{ when } \phi \tag{4.24}$$
$$\textbf{cancel retract } R \textbf{ when } \phi \tag{4.25}$$

where R is a rule of the form $L \leftarrow L_1, \ldots, L_k$ and ϕ is a (possibly empty) conjunction of literals, $L_{k+1}, \ldots, L_m$, where L and each L_i are literals. If ϕ is empty, we simply omit the **when** *keyword. We refer to those commands* without *(resp.* with*) the keyword* **event** *as* inertial *(resp.* non-inertial*) commands. We refer to those commands* with *(resp.* without*) the keyword* **always** *as* persistent *(resp.* non-persistent*) commands.*

[2]Where [**a**] will be used for notational convenience denoting either the presence or absence of **a**.

The following table summarizes the correspondence between the syntax of *LUPS* and that of *KUL*:

LUPS		*KUL*
assert [event]	$\leftrightarrow$	**assert** [event]
retract [event]	$\leftrightarrow$	**retract** [event] + **cancel assert**
always [event]	$\leftrightarrow$	**always assert** [event]
non existing		**always retract** [event]
cancel	$\leftrightarrow$	**cancel assert**
non existing		**cancel retract**

An update program in *KUL* is defined as follows:

Definition 67 (*KUL* - Update Program) *An update program in* KUL *is a finite sequence of updates, where an update is a set of commands of the form (4.22) to (4.25).*

4.3.2 *KUL* - Semantics

The semantics of *KUL* is defined by incrementally translating update programs into sequences of generalized logic programs and by considering the semantics of the *DLP* formed by them.

Let $\mathcal{U} = U_1 \otimes ... \otimes U_n$ be a *KUL* update program. At every state t we determine the corresponding *DLP*, $\Upsilon_t(\mathcal{U}) = \mathcal{P}_t$.

The translation of a *KUL* program into a dynamic program is similar to the one presented for *LUPS*. It is made by induction, starting from the empty program P_0 and, for each update U_t, given the already built dynamic program $P_0 \oplus \cdots \oplus P_{t-1}$, determining the resulting program $P_0 \oplus \cdots \oplus P_{t-1} \oplus P_t$. To cope with persistent update commands, as for the *LUPS* semantics, we also consider a set containing all currently active persistent commands, although its definition must be extended to deal with the newly introduced persistent retraction commands. As in *LUPS*, the retraction of rules imposes its unique identification. Therefore, the language of the resulting dynamic logic program must be extended with a new propositional variable "$N(R)$" for every rule R appearing in the original *LUPS* program. To properly handle non-inertial commands, we also need to uniquely associate those rules appearing in non-inertial commands with the states they belong to. To this end, the language of the resulting dynamic logic program must also be extended with a new propositional variable "$Ev(R,S)$" for every rule R appearing in a non-inertial command in the original *LUPS* program, and every state S.

We now present the translation for *KUL*:

Definition 68 (Translation into dynamic logic programs) *Let* $\mathcal{U} = U_1 \otimes \cdots \otimes U_n$ *be a* KUL *update program. The corresponding dynamic logic program* $\Upsilon^*(\mathcal{U}) = \mathcal{P} = \mathcal{P}_n = P_0 \oplus \cdots \oplus P_n$ *is obtained by the following inductive construction, using at each step* t *an auxiliary set of persistent commands* PC_t*:*

Base step: $P_0 = \{\}$ with $PC_0 = \{\}$.

Inductive step: Let $\Upsilon^*_{t-1}(\mathcal{U}) = \mathcal{P}_{t-1} = P_0 \oplus \cdots \oplus P_{t-1}$ with the set of persistent commands PC_{t-1} be the translation of $\mathcal{U}_{t-1} = U_1 \otimes \cdots \otimes U_{t-1}$. The translation of

$\mathcal{U}_t = U_1 \otimes \cdots \otimes U_t$ is $\Upsilon_t^*(\mathcal{U}) = \mathcal{P}_t = P_0 \oplus \cdots \oplus P_{t-1} \oplus P_t$ with the set of persistent commands PC_t, where:

$$\begin{aligned} PC_t = PC_{t-1} &\cup \{\textbf{assert } R \textbf{ when } \phi : \textbf{always assert } R \textbf{ when } \phi \in U_t\} \cup \\ &\cup \{\textbf{retract } R \textbf{ when } \phi : \textbf{always retract } R \textbf{ when } \phi \in U_t\} \cup \\ &\cup \{\textbf{assert event } R \textbf{ when } \phi : \textbf{always assert event } R \textbf{ when } \phi \in U_t\} \cup \\ &\cup \{\textbf{retract event } R \textbf{ when } \phi : \textbf{always retract event } R \textbf{ when } \phi \in U_t\} \cup \\ &- \left\{\textbf{assert [event] } R \textbf{ when } \phi : \textbf{cancel assert } R \textbf{ when } \psi \in U_t \wedge \bigoplus \mathcal{P}_{t-1} \models_{sm} \psi\right\} - \\ &- \left\{\textbf{retract [event] } R \textbf{ when } \phi : \textbf{cancel retract } R \textbf{ when } \psi \in U_t \wedge \bigoplus \mathcal{P}_{t-1} \models_{sm} \psi\right\} \end{aligned}$$

$$NU_t = U_t \cup PC_t$$

$$\begin{aligned} P_t = &\left\{not\, N(R) \leftarrow : \textbf{retract } R \textbf{ when } \phi \in NU_t \wedge \bigoplus \mathcal{P}_{t-1} \models_{sm} \phi\right\} \cup \\ &\cup \left\{N(R) \leftarrow; H(R) \leftarrow B(R), N(R) : \textbf{assert } R \textbf{ when } \phi \in NU_t \wedge \bigoplus \mathcal{P}_{t-1} \models_{sm} \phi\right\} \cup \\ &\cup \left\{H(R) \leftarrow B(R), Ev(R,t) : \textbf{assert event } R \textbf{ when } \phi \in NU_t \wedge \bigoplus \mathcal{P}_{t-1} \models_{sm} \phi\right\} \cup \\ &\cup \left\{not\, N(R) \leftarrow Ev(R,t) : \textbf{retract event } R \textbf{ when } \phi \in NU_t \wedge \bigoplus \mathcal{P}_{t-1} \models_{sm} \phi\right\} \cup \\ &\cup \{not\, Ev(R, t-1) \leftarrow; Ev(R,t) \leftarrow\} \end{aligned}$$

Note that the body of every rule R must be extended either with the predicate $N(R)$ or with the predicate $Ev(R,t)$. The differences between this transformation and the original $LUPS$ transformation are the following: - the modification in the definition of the set of active persistent commands, PC_t, to deal with the newly introduced persistent retraction command and the corresponding cancellation command; - the modification in the definition of the generalized logic program at state t, P_t, to properly deal with non-inertial commands. This is achieved by treating inertial and non-inertial rules in a separate manner: the former are dealt with as in LUPS while the latter are extended with the predicate $Ev(R,t)$ which is only made true for the duration of one state. This is achieved simply by including the rules $not\, Ev(R, t-1) \leftarrow$ and $Ev(R,t) \leftarrow$ in the generalized logic program of every state.

The semantics of KUL is, as expected:

Definition 69 (*KUL* Semantics) *Let $\mathcal{U} = U_1 \otimes ... \otimes U_n$ be a* KUL *program. A query* **holds** $L_1, \ldots, L_k$ **at** t? *is true in $\mathcal{U}$ iff $\bigoplus \Upsilon_t^*(\mathcal{U}) \models_{sm} L_1, \ldots, L_k$, or, equivalently, iff $\bigoplus \mathcal{P}_t \models_{sm} L_1, \ldots, L_k$. By $SM(\mathcal{U})$ we mean the set of all stable models of $\Upsilon^*(\mathcal{U})$ at state n, modulo the newly introduced atoms $N(R)$ and $Ev(R,S)$, and their corresponding default literals.*

KUL embeds Dynamic Logic Programming as stated in the following Theorem:

Theorem 58 *Let $\mathcal{P} = P_1 \oplus ... \oplus P_s$ be a DLP. Let $\mathcal{U} = U_1 \otimes ... \otimes U_s$ such that*

$$U_i = \{\textbf{assert } r : r \in P_i\}$$

for every $1 \leq i \leq s$. Let ϕ be a conjunction of literals of the underlying object language of $\mathcal{P}$. Then, $\bigoplus_i \mathcal{P} \models_{sm} \phi$ iff **holds** ϕ **at** i? *is true in $\mathcal{U}$. Furthermore, $SM(\Upsilon_i^*(\mathcal{U})) = SM(P_1 \oplus ... \oplus P_i)$ when restricted to the underlying object language of $\mathcal{P}$.*

Proof. *Let $\mathcal{P}$ and $\mathcal{U}$ be as defined above. Then, $\Upsilon_i^*(\mathcal{U}) = P_0' \oplus P_1' \oplus \cdots \oplus P_i'$ is such that $(1 \leq n \leq i)$:*

$$P_0' = \{\}$$
$$P_n' = \{N(r) \leftarrow; H(r) \leftarrow B(r), N(r) : r \in P_n\} \cup \{not\, Ev(R, t-1) \leftarrow; Ev(R, t) \leftarrow\}$$

since the literals not $Ev(R, t-1)$ and $Ev(R, t)$ cannot belong to ϕ, nor those of the form $N(R)$, and there are no rules for not $N(R)$, and since P_0' can be simply eliminated for being empty, $SM\,(\Upsilon_i^*(\mathcal{U})) = SM\,(P_1'' \oplus \cdots \oplus P_i'')$ where

$$P_n'' = \{H(r) \leftarrow B(r) : r \in P_n\}$$

Note that $P_n'' = P_n$. It follows that $\bigoplus_i \mathcal{P} \models_{sm} \phi$ iff $\bigoplus \Upsilon_i^*(\mathcal{U})' \models_{sm} \phi$ iff $P_1'' \oplus \cdots \oplus P_i'' \models_{sm} \phi$. ■

Corollary 59 *KUL generalizes interpretation updates [157].*

Corollary 60 *KUL generalizes logic programs under the stable model semantics.*

4.3.3 Illustrative Examples

There follows an example to illustrate the different behaviour between *LUPS* and *KUL*:

Example 33 *Consider a public building with several floors. Initially, the security policy of the building states that any person (P) is allowed into any of its floors (F) if and only if they have a special permit for that floor. This can be represented by the update U_1:*

$$\begin{array}{ll} U_1: & \textbf{assert}\,(allowed(P,F) \leftarrow permission(P,F)) \\ & \textbf{assert}\,(not\, allowed(P,F) \leftarrow not\, permission(P,F)) \end{array}$$

Later on, the administration decided to open up a public relations office, to be situated in the ground floor. They had to update the security policy which, from then on, would allow any person in the ground floor provided they have some form of identification. Let us suppose this happened in the second day (state), and is represented by the update U_2:

$$U_2: \ \textbf{assert}\,(allowed(P, ground) \leftarrow id(P))$$

Further down the line (on the third day), the administration decided to declare an open day, once every now and then, when everyone, for the duration of a single day, was allowed to visit the entire building, provided they have some form of Id. This is represented by the update U_3:

$$U_3: \ \textbf{always assert event}\ (allowed(P,F) \leftarrow id(P))\ \textbf{when}\ open\_day$$

Suppose that both Mary and John have Ids and Mary has a permission for the second floor, represented by the facts permission(mary, second), id(john) and id(mary), in the KB. At day five there is an open day represented by the update at state 4:

$$U_4: \ \textbf{assert event}\ (open\_day \leftarrow)$$

According to the KUL *semantics, at state 4 Mary is allowed in the ground and second floors, and John is only allowed in the ground floor; at state 5 both Mary and John are allowed in all floors of the building; at state 6 and thereafter everything is back as it was at state 4, with Mary being allowed in the ground and second floors, and John only being allowed in the ground floor, as expected. If this problem was to be tackled with the semantics of* LUPS, *everything would be the same until (and including) state 5 but, at state 6, John and Mary (and anybody else) would no longer be allowed in the ground floor, which seems to be rather unintuitive. This is so because not only the rule asserted by the* **always assert event** *command in* U_3 *is removed, but so is the rule asserted by* U_2*, simply because it has the same syntax.*

We now show how Example 32 would be encoded in *KUL*:

Example 34 *Consider the scenario of Example 32. The specification in* KUL *would be:*

Persistent update commands:

$$\textbf{always assert } jail(X) \leftarrow abortion(X) \textbf{ when } repC, repP$$
$$\textbf{always retract } jail(X) \leftarrow abortion(X) \textbf{ when } not\, repC, not\, repP$$

If, as before, at the initial state we also have the following update command:

$$\textbf{assert } jail(X) \leftarrow assassination(X)$$

Then, after the Democrats take over both Congress and the Presidency, if Mary both assassins someone and performs an abortion, she will now be punished by jail, as intended. Furthermore, if afterwards the Republicans retake the government, the rule $jail(X) \leftarrow abortion(X)$ *is reinstated because the persistent assertion update command has been left intact when the Democrats took over.*

4.3.4 Comparison

In this section we compare *LUPS* and *KUL* by means of a property that partially characterizes the desired behaviour of the semantics with respect to non-inertial events.

Before we express this property, we start with the definition of *update program equivalence* for update programs, according to which two update programs are *update program equivalent* iff their semantics coincides after an arbitrary number of updates with arbitrary update programs. Formally:

Definition 70 (Update Program Equivalence) *Let* $\mathcal{U}_1$ *and* $\mathcal{U}_2$ *be two update programs. We say that* $\mathcal{U}_1$ *and* $\mathcal{U}_2$ *are* update program equivalent, *denoted by* $\mathcal{U}_1 \stackrel{\otimes}{\equiv} \mathcal{U}_2$*, iff for every update program* $\mathcal{Q}$*,* $\mathcal{U}_1 \otimes \mathcal{Q}$ *is semantically equivalent to* $\mathcal{U}_2 \otimes \mathcal{Q}$*, i.e.*[3]*:*

$$SM\,(\mathcal{U}_1 \otimes \mathcal{Q}) = SM\,(\mathcal{U}_2 \otimes \mathcal{Q})$$

where if $\mathcal{R} = R_{r_1} \otimes ... \otimes R_{r_n}$ *and* $\mathcal{S} = S_{s_1} \otimes ... \otimes S_{s_m}$ *are two update programs, by* $\mathcal{R} \otimes \mathcal{S}$ *we mean the update program* $R_{r_1} \otimes ... \otimes R_{r_n} \otimes S_{s_1} \otimes ... \otimes S_{s_m}$*.*

With this property, we can now come back to our main claim. In particular, we claim that if we have a sequence of updates such that only non-inertial commands are executed, the knowledge state before the execution of such sequence of commands and the knowledge state after the execution of all such commands should be *update program equivalent.* Intuitively we want the long term (more than one state) effect of

[3]Modulo the newly introduced atoms $Ev(R, S)$ and $N(R)$.

non-inertial commands to reside in their interaction with inertial commands, be they persistent or not. In particular, rules asserted or retracted by non-inertial commands should only change the semantics at the subsequent state by allowing and/or preventing the execution of other commands, at that subsequent state, which may be inertial and therefore change the semantics for more than just one state transition. In particular, if there is a sequence of updates without any inertial command to be executed, followed by a state transition specified by an empty update, after its execution the knowledge state should be *equivalent* to the initial one. In other words, the effect of non-inertial commands should be, in fact, non inertial. The referred empty update is necessary because the immediate effect of every non-inertial command holds for one state, i.e. we need an extra state transition for such effect to be removed.

This is formally defined as follows:

Definition 71 (Stability with respect to non-inertial commands) *An update language is* stable with respect to non-inertial commands *iff for every update programs* $\mathcal{U}_1$ *and* $\mathcal{U}_2$ *such that* $\mathcal{U}_1$ *consists of updates with non-persistent commands only, and* $\mathcal{U}_2$ *consists of updates with non-persistent, non-inertial commands only,*

$$\mathcal{U}_1 \otimes U_\emptyset \overset{\otimes}{\equiv} \mathcal{U}_1 \otimes \mathcal{U}_2 \otimes U_\emptyset$$

where $U_\emptyset$ *denotes an empty update.*

The restriction imposed on the updates of $\mathcal{U}_1$ to contain just non-persistent commands, i.e. without the keyword **always**, is justified by the fact that if such persistent commands were present, they could be executed at subsequent states, together with the updates of $\mathcal{U}_2$ and thus, invalidating our goal to have, at the state transitions corresponding to the updates of $\mathcal{U}_2$, only non-inertial commands being executed. Recall that an inertial command is valid at all subsequent states until cancelled. Note that to express our intuition, all we need is to guarantee that at the state transitions corresponding to the updates of $\mathcal{U}_2$ we only execute non-inertial commands. In fact, this would also be achieved if we would allow $\mathcal{U}_1$ to contain persistent non-inertial commands so as long as we ensure that at the state transition corresponding to $U_\emptyset$ no commands are executed, but we will keep to this simpler formulation.

Proposition 61 LUPS *[15] is not stable with respect to non-inertial commands.*

Example 29 above shows that *LUPS* is not stable with respect to non-inertial commands. It is worth noting that the recently proposed language of updates *EPI* [75], being based on the semantics of *LUPS*, is also not stable with respect to non-inertial commands, although some adaptations must be made to make the property applicable to EPI because of the fixed update policy it employs, i.e., instead of a sequence of updates one must consider an initial update policy with those non-inertial commands that are sequentially activated by external observations. The same example, adapted to *EPI*, also shows that *EPI* is not stable with respect to non-inertial commands.

Theorem 62 KUL *is stable with respect to non-inertial commands.*

Before we prove the Theorem, we prove the following Lemma:

Lemma 63 *Let $\mathcal{U} = U_1 \otimes \cdots \otimes U_n$ be a* KUL *update program. Let $\mathcal{P}_i = P_0 \oplus \cdots \oplus P_i$ be the dynamic logic program at state i obtained according to Definition 68. Then, for every stable model M of $\mathcal{P}_i$ it hods that*

$$Ev(R, i-j) \notin M, \forall 1 < j \leq i$$
$$Ev(R, i) \in M$$

Proof. *From the construction of $\mathcal{P}_i$. Since each P_t in the sequence $P_1 \oplus \cdots \oplus P_i$ contains the rules*

$$\{not\,Ev(R, t-1) \leftarrow; Ev(R, t) \leftarrow\}$$

it follows that every $Ev(R,t) \leftarrow$ rule in P_t is rejected by the rule $not\,Ev(R,t) \leftarrow$ in P_{t+1}. Since these are the only rules for $Ev(R,t)$, it follows that any stable model at state i must contain $Ev(R,i)$ and not contain $Ev(R, i-j), \forall 1 < j \leq i$. ■

Proof of Theorem 62. *Let $\mathcal{U} = U_1 \otimes \cdots \otimes U_n$ and $\mathcal{U}' = U'_1 \otimes \cdots \otimes U'_m$ be two* KUL *update programs such that $\mathcal{U}$ consists of updates with non-persistent commands only, and $\mathcal{U}'$ consists of updates with non-persistent, non-inertial commands only. Let $\emptyset$ be an empty update. Let $\mathcal{P}_{n+1} = P_0 \oplus \cdots \oplus P_n \oplus P_{n+1}$ be the dynamic logic program at state $n+1$ and PC_{n+1} the set of persistent commands at state $n+1$ obtained, from $\mathcal{U} \otimes \emptyset_{n+1}$ according to Definition 68. Clearly PC_{n+1} is empty since $\mathcal{U}$ consists of updates with non-persistent commands only. Furthermore we have that $P_{n+1} = \{not\,Ev(R,n) \leftarrow; Ev(R, n+1) \leftarrow\}$. Let $\mathcal{P}'_{n+m+1} = P_0 \oplus \cdots \oplus P_n \oplus P'_{n+1} \oplus \cdots \oplus P'_{n+m} \oplus P'_{n+m+1}$ be the dynamic logic program at state $n+m+1$ and PC_{n+m+1} the set of persistent commands at state $n+m+1$ obtained, from $\mathcal{U} \otimes \mathcal{U}' \otimes \emptyset_{n+m+1}$ according to Definition 68. Clearly PC_{n+m+1} is also empty. We have that $P_{n+m+1} = \{not\,Ev(R, n+m) \leftarrow; Ev(R, n+m+1) \leftarrow\}$. Furthermore, since $\mathcal{U}'$ consists of updates with non-inertial commands only, we have that every rule r in program P'_i, $n+1 \leq i \leq n+m$, such that $H(r) \notin \{N(R), not\,N(R), Ev(R,N), not\,Ev(R,N)\}$ is such that $Ev(r,i) \subseteq B(r)$, i.e. the body of every rule in P'_i, excluding those for the new atoms $N(R)$ and $Ev(R,N)$ (and their corresponding default literals), contains the atom $Ev(r,i)$ in its body. Since at state $n+m+1$ all those atoms $Ev(r,i)$ are false, and will always be false by the Lemma above, we can safely remove all those rules. Clearly the resulting DLP is update equivalent to $\mathcal{P}_{n+1}$ (Modulo the newly introduced atoms $Ev(R,S)$ and $N(R)$ and their corresponding default literals). Since $\mathcal{P}'_{n+m+1}$ is update equivalent to $\mathcal{P}_{n+1}$ and both sets of persistent commands are empty, it can easily be proved that $\mathcal{U} \otimes \emptyset_{n+1} \overset{\otimes}{\equiv} \mathcal{U} \otimes \mathcal{U}' \otimes \emptyset_{n+m+1}$.* ■

4.4 Reasoning About Actions

Definition 72 (Action) *Let $\mathcal{L}_\alpha = \{\alpha_1, \ldots, \alpha_m\}$ be a set of atoms from $\mathcal{K}$ where each $\alpha \in \mathcal{L}_\alpha$ represents an action. We call the elements of $\mathcal{L}_\alpha$* actions. *Typically, for every* action *there will be one (or more) update statements of the forms (4.22) and (4.23), where the action α appears in the environment observations.*

For example, in

always assert event $(L \leftarrow L_1, \ldots, L_k)$ **when** $L_{k+1}, \ldots, L_m, \alpha$

we have, intuitively, that α is an action whose preconditions are $L_{k+1}, \ldots, L_m$ and whose effect is an update that, according to its type, can model different kinds of actions, all in one unified framework. Examples of kinds of actions are:

- actions of the form

$$\alpha \textbf{ causes } F \textbf{ if } F_1, \ldots, F_k$$

  where $F, F_1, \ldots, F_k$ are fluents (such as in the language $\mathcal{A}$ of [96]) translates into the update command

$$\textbf{always assert}\,(F)\ \textbf{when}\ F_1, \ldots, F_k, \alpha$$

- actions whose epistemic effect is a rule update of the form

$$\alpha \textbf{ updates with } L \leftarrow L_1, \ldots, L_k \textbf{ if } L_{k+1}, \ldots, L_m$$

  translates into the update command

$$\textbf{always assert}\,(L \leftarrow L_1, \ldots, L_k)\ \textbf{when}\ L_{k+1}, \ldots, L_m, \alpha$$

- actions that, when performed in parallel, have different outcomes, of the form

$$\alpha_a \vee \alpha_b \textbf{ cause } L_1 \textbf{ if } L_{k+1}, \ldots, L_m$$
$$\alpha_a \wedge \alpha_b \textbf{ cause } L_2 \textbf{ if } L_{k+1}, \ldots, L_m$$

  translates into the three update commands:

$$\textbf{always assert}\,(L_1)\ \textbf{when}\ L_{k+1}, \ldots, L_m, \alpha_a, \mathit{not}\,\alpha_b$$
$$\textbf{always assert}\,(L_1)\ \textbf{when}\ L_{k+1}, \ldots, L_m, L_{k+1}, \ldots, L_m, \mathit{not}\,\alpha_a, \alpha_b$$
$$\textbf{always assert}\,(L_2)\ \textbf{when}\ L_{k+1}, \ldots, L_m, \alpha_a, \alpha_b$$

- actions with non-deterministic effects of the form

$$\alpha \textbf{ causes } L_1 \vee L_2 \textbf{ if } L_{k+1}, \ldots, L_m$$

  translates into the update commands (where β_a, β_b are new auxiliary predicates and I is a unique identifier of an occurrence of α):

$$\textbf{always assert}\,(L_1 \leftarrow \beta_a\,(I))\ \textbf{when}\ L_{k+1}, \ldots, L_m, \alpha\,(I)$$
$$\textbf{always assert}\,(L_2 \leftarrow \beta_b\,(I))\ \textbf{when}\ L_{k+1}, \ldots, L_m, \alpha\,(I)$$
$$\textbf{always assert}\,(\beta_a\,(I) \leftarrow \mathit{not}\,\beta_b\,(I))\ \textbf{when}\ L_{k+1}, \ldots, L_m, \alpha\,(I)$$
$$\textbf{always assert}\,(\beta_b\,(I) \leftarrow \mathit{not}\,\beta_a\,(I))\ \textbf{when}\ L_{k+1}, \ldots, L_m, \alpha\,(I)$$

  In this representation of the non-deterministic effects of an action α, we create two auxiliary actions (β_a, β_b) with deterministic effects, and make the effect of α be the non-deterministic choice between actions β_a or β_b.

We now show some examples:

Example 35 *[28]Mary is lifting a bowl of soup from the kitchen table, while John is opening the door to the dining room. Two represent this story we consider two fluents (atoms) $lifted$ and opened, together with two actions $lift$ and open. The effects of the actions can be described by the commands:*

$$\textbf{always assert}\,(\mathit{lifted})\ \textbf{when}\ \mathit{lift}$$
$$\textbf{always assert}\,(\mathit{opened})\ \textbf{when}\ \mathit{open}$$

The initial situation, where both the door is closed and the bowl is on the table could be specified by the initial update:

$$\textbf{assert}\ (not\, lifted)$$
$$\textbf{assert}\ (not\, opened)$$

Note that since all atoms are initially false by default, these two commands are not strictly necessary. After executing both actions open and lift, represented by the non-inertial assertions, at state s:

$$\textbf{assert event}\ (lift)$$
$$\textbf{assert event}\ (open)$$

we have that both lifted and opened are true, i.e. the following query is true:

$$\textbf{holds}\ lifted, opened\ \textbf{at}\ s+1?$$

In the previous example the effects of actions are completely independent. The next example describes a more complex scenario where effects of actions are mutually dependent:

Example 36 *(adapted from [97]) Whenever the bowl is filled with water, Mary needs to lift it with both hands not to spill the water which would happen if she would try to lift it with only one hand. To drink the water, Mary has to first lift the bowl filled with the liquid, and hold it lifted while drinking. Mary is happy if she is not thirsty and there is no water spilled. To represent this scenario we consider the fluents: $filled$, $lifted$, $happy$, $thirsty$ and $spilled$, together with the actions: $fill$, $drink$, $lift\_r$, $lift\_l$ and $hold$. The entire scenario could be specified by the following KUL commands:*

$$\begin{array}{l}
\textbf{assert}\ (happy \leftarrow not\, thirsty, not\, spilled)\\
\textbf{always assert}\ (filled)\ \textbf{when}\ fill, not\, lifted\\
\textbf{always assert}\ (lifted)\ \textbf{when}\ lift_r, lift_l\\
\textbf{always assert}\ (spilled)\ \textbf{when}\ filled, not\, lift_r, lift_l\\
\textbf{always assert}\ (spilled)\ \textbf{when}\ filled, not\, lift_l, lift_r\\
\textbf{always assert}\ (not\, filled)\ \textbf{when}\ filled, not\, lift_r, lift_l\\
\textbf{always assert}\ (not\, filled)\ \textbf{when}\ filled, not\, lift_l, lift_r\\
\textbf{always assert}\ (not\, lifted)\ \textbf{when}\ lifted, not\, hold\\
\textbf{always assert}\ (lifted)\ \textbf{when}\ lifted, hold\\
\textbf{always assert}\ (not\, thirsty)\ \textbf{when}\ filled, lifted, hold, drink\\
\textbf{always assert}\ (not\, filled)\ \textbf{when}\ filled, lifted, hold, drink
\end{array}$$

Let us further consider the initial situation where Mary is thirsty, the bowl is empty on the table and there is no water spilled, represented by the following updates:

$$\textbf{assert}\ (thirsty)$$
$$\textbf{assert}\ (not\, lifted)$$
$$\textbf{assert}\ (not\, filled)$$
$$\textbf{assert}\ (not\, spilled)$$

We can now check the outcome of several sequences of actions, starting from this initial situation.

- *Consider the following sequence of updates:*

$$U_2 = \{\textbf{assert event}\,(fill)\}$$
$$U_3 = \left\{ \begin{array}{c} \textbf{assert event}\,(lift\_r) \\ \textbf{assert event}\,(lift\_l) \end{array} \right\}$$
$$U_4 = \left\{ \begin{array}{c} \textbf{assert event}\,(drink) \\ \textbf{assert event}\,(hold) \end{array} \right\}$$

as the result of these updates we would obtain the following answers to the following queries:

holds *happy* **at** 3?	*is false*
holds *happy* **at** 4?	*is false*
holds *happy* **at** 5?	*is true*

- *Consider the following sequence of updates:*

$$U_2 = \left\{ \begin{array}{c} \textbf{assert event}\,(lift\_r) \\ \textbf{assert event}\,(lift\_l) \end{array} \right\}$$
$$U_3 = \left\{ \begin{array}{c} \textbf{assert event}\,(fill) \\ \textbf{assert event}\,(hold) \end{array} \right\}$$
$$U_4 = \left\{ \begin{array}{c} \textbf{assert event}\,(drink) \\ \textbf{assert event}\,(hold) \end{array} \right\}$$

as the result of these updates we would obtain the following answers to the following queries:

holds *happy* **at** 3?	*is false*
holds *happy* **at** 4?	*is false*
holds *happy* **at** 5?	*is false*
holds *filled* **at** 4?	*is false*
holds *lifted* **at** 3?	*is true*
holds *thirsty* **at** 5?	*is true*

i.e. since the bowl must be filled before it has been lifted, lifting it before filling it does not cause it to be filled and therefore the action drink does not cause Mary not to be thirsty.

- *Consider the following sequence of updates:*

$$U_2 = \{\textbf{assert event}\,(fill)\}$$
$$U_3 = \left\{ \begin{array}{c} \textbf{assert event}\,(lift\_r) \\ \textbf{assert event}\,(lift\_l) \end{array} \right\}$$
$$U_4 = \{\}$$
$$U_5 = \{\textbf{assert event}\,(drink)\}$$

as the result of these updates we would obtain the following answers to the following queries:

holds *happy* **at** 4?	*is false*
holds *happy* **at** 5?	*is false*
holds *happy* **at** 6?	*is false*
holds *lifted* **at** 4?	*is true*
holds *lifted* **at** 5?	*is false*
holds *thirsty* **at** 6?	*is true*

i.e. even though Mary correctly lifted the bowl by performing both $lift\_l$ *and* $lift\_r$ *actions at state 3, she did not hold it and, at state 5 when she performs the action* $drink$*, the bowl is no longer* $lifted$ *and Mary cannot satisfy her thirst.*

- *Consider the following sequence of updates:*

$$U_2 = \{\textbf{assert event}\,(fill)\}$$
$$U_3 = \{\textbf{assert event}\,(lift\_r)\}$$
$$U_4 = \{\textbf{assert event}\,(lift\_l)\}$$
$$U_5 = \{\textbf{assert event}\,(fill)\}$$
$$U_6 = \left\{ \begin{array}{c} \textbf{assert event}\,(lift\_r) \\ \textbf{assert event}\,(lift\_l) \end{array} \right\}$$
$$U_7 = \left\{ \begin{array}{c} \textbf{assert event}\,(drink) \\ \textbf{assert event}\,(hold) \end{array} \right\}$$

as the result of these updates we would obtain the following answers to the following queries:

holds *happy* **at** 6?	*is false*
holds *happy* **at** 7?	*is false*
holds *happy* **at** 8?	*is false*
holds *not thirsty* **at** 8?	*is true*
holds *not spilled* **at** 4?	*is false*
holds *not spilled* **at** 8?	*is false*

i.e. even though Mary finally managed to drink the water, she spilled some when she performed action $lift\_r$ *alone and cannot be happy.*

We finalize by showing how the traditional Yale Shooting Problem can be represented in *KUL*:

Example 37 *[105]The scenario involves three actions namely load, wait and shoot, and two fluents namely alive and loaded. There is a gun to be shot and a turkey to be shot at. Loading causes the gun to be loaded. Shooting the loaded gun has the effect that the turkey is no longer alive afterwards. Waiting has no effects. Let us suppose that initially the gun is unloaded and, of course, the turkey is alive. The effects of the three actions would be encoded by the following update commands:*

$$\textbf{always assert}\,(loaded)\ \ \textbf{when}\ load$$
$$\textbf{always assert}\,(not\,loaded)\ \ \textbf{when}\ loaded, shoot$$
$$\textbf{always assert}\,(not\,alive)\ \ \textbf{when}\ loaded, shoot$$

Where, for action wait there is no command since it has no effect other than inertia. To these statements we need to assert the initial situation[4]*:*

$$\textbf{assert}\,(alive)$$
$$\textbf{assert}\,(not\,loaded)$$

[4]Note that the second command is irrelevant since initially all atoms are assumed false by default.

Let these five commands constitute the initial update, U_1. If we have the following sequence of events: at state 2 load the gun; at state 3 wait, shoot at state 4 and wait for another state. These actions would be translated into the following four updates:

$$U_2 = \{\textbf{assert event}\,(load)\}$$
$$U_3 = \{\textbf{assert event}\,(wait)\}$$
$$U_4 = \{\textbf{assert event}\,(shoot)\}$$
$$U_5 = \{\textbf{assert event}\,(wait)\}$$

as the result of these updates we would obtain the following answers to the following queries:

holds *alive, not loaded* **at** 1?	*is true*
holds *alive, not loaded* **at** 2?	*is true*
holds *alive, loaded* **at** 3?	*is true*
holds *alive, loaded* **at** 4?	*is true*
holds *not alive, not loaded* **at** 5?	*is true*

We end this section with some brief remarks on the relationship between action languages and update languages.

As we have seen by the previous examples, it is possible, in some cases, to establish a correspondence between actions languages such as the languages $\mathcal{A}$ of [96] and $\mathcal{C}$ of [101], and update languages such as LUPS and KUL. The previous examples show how some typical examples in the actions domain can be encoded. But these examples, by themselves, do not provide sound bridges relating both domains. Since update languages were specifically designed to allow assertions and retraction of rules to allow for a knowledge base to evolve, action languages by only allowing the effects of actions to be fluents restrict themselves to purely extensional updates. From this purely syntactical point of view LUPS and KUL are more expressive. Action languages such as $\mathcal{C}$, on the other hand, were designed to express the notion of causality which is semantically different from the underlying notion of inertia found in the DLP semantics. It is thus natural to observe differences in the semantics between action languages and update languages. A detailed study of the bridges between both is certainly one of the main topics for future research, but clearly outside the scope of this work.

4.5 Conclusions and Open Issues

Along this Chapter we have overviewed the language of updates LUPS and briefly mentioned the main features of the update specification language EPI. We have identified an incorrect behaviour of the semantics of LUPS as well as an important extension to its set of commands. To address these issues we have introduced the Knowledge Update Language (KUL). We have compared KUL with LUPS by means of a desirable property that holds in the former but not in the later. It is worth stressing that all the applications examples, for LUPS, shown in the literature [16–18, 20] yield the same results when converted to KUL. On the other hand, the examples presented in Section 4.3.3 either cannot be expressed in LUPS or yield a different result.

We have also explored the applicability of KUL in the domain of actions by showing how some typical examples can be encoded.

The Knowledge Update Language is the starting point for the introduction of several features in the next Chapter.

Chapter 5

Knowledge and Behaviour Update Language

In this Chapter we extend the language of updates KUL *with several features, the most important being the possibility to allow the knowledge base to evolve not only due to external updates but also due to self updates. According to this extended framework, a knowledge base is composed not only of a DLP (representing the object level knowledge) but also of an update specification that partially encodes its future evolution, i.e. its behaviour. in this Chapter, we introduce the* Knowledge and Behaviour Update Language *(*KABUL*) to allow the specification of updates to both the object level knowledge base and the self-updates that encode the behaviour of the knowledge base.*

5.1 Introduction

In the previous chapter we have overviewed the language of updates *LUPS* and the related language of update specifications EPI. We have also proposed a new semantics correcting an undesirable behaviour with non-inertial commands, and extended the syntax with a new persistent retraction command and its corresponding cancellation command, introducing the language *KUL*. We have also shown how *KUL* can be used to specify the effects of actions by means of persistent commands.

This notion of allowing (persistent) commands to specify more than one state transition leads us to introduce of the concept of *Evolving Knowledge Bases*, i.e. transform an otherwise static knowledge base which is only capable of responding to outside stimuli to a dynamic one where update commands are made part of the knowledge base, making its evolution possible according to its own behaviour specification, possibly without any external updates.

An *Evolving Knowledge Base* is a knowledge base which can change due to external update commands, but which also contains an internal specification encoding its behaviour. According to this notion, an evolving knowledge base at some state s, consists of a tuple $\langle \mathcal{P}_s, SU_s \rangle$ where $\mathcal{P}_s = P_1 \oplus ... \oplus P_s$ is a dynamic logic program, and SU_s is the self update, i.e. a specification that partially encodes its future evolution. At each state transition, the knowledge base receives a set of external updates (EU_{s+1})

and perceives a set of external observations (EO_{s+1}). The self and external update are combined, evaluated against the dynamic logic program and external observations, to determine the next state of the evolving knowledge base $\langle \mathcal{P}_{s+1}, SU_{s+1} \rangle$:

$$\langle \mathcal{P}_s, SU_s \rangle \overset{\langle EU_{s+1}, EO_{s+1} \rangle}{\longrightarrow} \langle \mathcal{P}_{s+1}, SU_{s+1} \rangle$$

To specify such knowledge bases, we need an update language capable of not only specifying the assertions and retractions of the object level rules in the DLP, but also capable of updating the behaviour specified by the self update. One way to extend the existing languages of updates in order to express such statements, is to allow the update commands not only to specify the set of logic program rules that belong to the KB produced by the "current" state transition, but to also specify a set of commands that belong to the self update that will govern the next state transition, i.e. we need commands to assert and retract **assert** and **retract** commands, and we need to assert and retract these, in turn, i.e., we need nested (or embedded) commands.

Given that $\mathcal{P}_s$ encodes the object level knowledge and SU_s encodes the behaviour, we need to define a language capable of updating them both. To this purpose, we introduce the *Knowledge And Behaviour Update Language* (*KABUL*) as a language to specify *Evolving Knowledge Bases.*

Before we continue, allow us to draw attention to the existence of some desired update statements which are not representable, in a concise and simple way, in KUL. Among such are these:

- it is not possible to directly specify updates that depend on a sequence of conditions: since the commands of *KUL* (and *LUPS*) only allow for a conjunction of literals in their conditions which are to be evaluated at one state to, eventually, assert or retract a rule at the next state, it is not possible to directly specify an update statement such as "assert a rule R if some condition $Cond1$ is true after some condition $Cond2$ was true".

- it is not possible to directly specify delayed effects of actions, i.e. actions that, if executed at some state n, cause an effect at state $n + s$ such as for example a circuit with several consecutive delay gates where an input signal takes several state transitions to reach the output. This example will be explored below.

- *KUL* (and *LUPS*) allows, by means of its persistent commands, the specification of updates that will occur in the future (subsequent states). But the specification of such update statements that are valid for more than one state transition is quite limited. A language of updates should allow more flexibility in the specification of future updates, not captured by the persistent commands. For example, one should be able to specify, at some arbitrary state s, that n states from now some rule R should be retracted if some condition holds. In *KUL* (and *LUPS*) it is only possible to directly specify that, from now on, a rule R should (always) be retracted if some condition holds or, alternatively, wait for state $s+n$ to issue the update statement.

- it is not possible to directly specify an update that should be executed only once, at the first state transition on which its conditions are verified, and then cease to persist.

- in *KUL* (and *LUPS*), it is not possible to specify an update that depends on the concurrent execution of other commands. Note however that such conditions are possible in EPI, although the assigned semantics, as we have mentioned before, is not intuitive in the case where an update depends on the assertion of some rule and that rule is asserted by means of a persistent command.

- in *KUL* (and *LUPS*) it is not possible to specify an update that depends on the "*memorial*" presence (or absence) of a specific rule in the object knowledge base. One may want to make the assertion of a rule depend on it being absent from the knowledge base. Such an extension was suggested in [75] but not materialized there.

- when reasoning about actions in *KUL* (and *LUPS*), there is always the need for an intermediate state transition for the atom representing the action to be asserted, before its effects are verified. This causes irreparable damage in situations where we use *KUL* (and *LUPS*) as a language to specify the effects of actions together with its normal use for rule updates, as illustrated by the following example: suppose we have an action α whose specification is:

  $$\alpha \textbf{ causes } b \textbf{ if } c.$$

  specified by the command:

  $$\textbf{always assert } (b) \textbf{ when } c, \alpha$$

  Suppose that, at state s, we update the knowledge base with U_{s+1} only containing the non-inertial command:

  $$\textbf{assert event } (c)$$

  We expect c to be true at state $s+1$. If, at such state $s+1$ we perform the action α, since c is true at $s+1$ we would expect b to be true at the subsequent state $s+2$. The execution of such action would be encoded as an update U_{s+2} with the command:

  $$\textbf{assert event } (\alpha)$$

  But b is not true at state $s+2$. This is so because it takes one state transition for atom α to be asserted in the knowledge base. By that time, when α is true and the persistent command representing the specification of action α could be tested for its remaining conditions, c is no longer true and b never becomes true. Note that this is not an intrinsic problem with the *KUL* (and *LUPS*) language, but rather an unsatisfactory behaviour when used to reason about a combination of actions and other updates, something for which it was not originally designed.

- in *KUL* (and *LUPS*), it is not possible to directly specify the inhibition of a command. If we have a persistent command that we wish to inhibit at one particular state transition, it is only possible to cancel it, permanently removing it, and then to reassert it. This requires exact knowledge of all the commands that were previously issued. It would be desirable to specify the temporary inhibition of the update specified by one such commands without having to remove them. For example, one may wish to say that rule R should not be asserted at this state transition, without having to cancel every command that may assert it and then reassert them back.

When we say that it is not possible to directly specify some statement in KUL (and LUPS), we do not mean that it is strictly not possible. Since KUL (and LUPS) both generalize logic programs under the stable model semantics, everything that can be specified in the later can also be specified in the former. But we do not want to follow such a strong view on possibility of expression. Rather we are concerned with the high-level power of the language to allow simple and concise representations of the kind of statements we wish to express in the context of updates of knowledge bases. When defining such a high-level language we are usually faced with an option between two design stances: according to one of them we can identify a core set of commands, define its semantics, and on top of them build libraries of macros to be used when writing specifications of more complex problems; according to the other option we add to the language, as main entities, all those necessary commands. In this work we have opted to identify a set of commands that allow us to concisely represent what we desire, extending the core language KUL appropriately. We believe that the size of the language, in terms of the number of its constructs, is not overly large and allows for simple representations without the need for other macros. Nevertheless we do not make a strong claim that they constitute the minimal set required to achieve their purpose, but rather that they constitute a manageable set to achieve some degree of practicality.

In this section we set forth a language of updates, based on the commands and semantics of KUL, extended with several features, some of which inspired by the language EPI.

Before we continue, we will establish some slightly different conventions than those introduced before. In KUL (and $LUPS$), a command was an expression of, for example, the form:

$$\textbf{assert event}\ (R)\ \textbf{when}\ L_{k+1}, \ldots, L_m$$

From now on, to make the representations more concise, we replace the keyword **when** with the arrow ($\Leftarrow$). Also, we will be referring to the expression

$$\textbf{assert\_event}\ (R) \Leftarrow L_{k+1}, \ldots, L_m$$

as a *statement*. The part of a statement that is to the left of the ($\Leftarrow$) , will be called a command. For example,

$$\textbf{assert\_event}\ (R) \qquad \textbf{retract\_event}(R) \qquad \textbf{always\_assert}(R)$$

are *commands* and:

$$\begin{array}{r}\textbf{assert\_event}\ (R) \Leftarrow L_{k+1}, \ldots, L_m\\ \textbf{retract\_event}(R) \Leftarrow L_{k+1}, \ldots, L_m\\ \textbf{always\_assert}(R) \Leftarrow L_{k+1}, \ldots, L_m\end{array}$$

are *statements*.

There follows a brief summary of each of the improvements together with the underlying motivations. Further motivation and more detailed explanations will be presented throughout this section, when the formal definitions are established. The innovations set forth in this chapter fall into three distinct categories: framework, commands, and conditions.

Framework: The LUPS framework was originally described as a means to describe the logical consequences of a sequence of update statements. Accordingly, if we have an initial knowledge base encoded as a generalized logic program, which without loss of generality can be considered empty (everything is false by default), and apply to it a sequence of updates (sets of statements), the LUPS framework translates such a sequence of updates into a sequence of logic programs to be interpreted as a DLP. The semantics of LUPS is defined as being the semantics of such DLP. Such translation inductively constructs the sequence of logic programs using an auxiliary set of "active" persistent statements. If, after a sequence of such updates, we want to perform another update, the DLP alone, obtained by the previous transformation, is not enough to determine the result of performing another update. We still need such a set of "active" persistent statements.

If we take a closer look at the transformation of sequences of updates into sequences of logic programs, we can observe that the inductive definition can be easily seen as a constructive definition if, instead, we associate with each state not only the corresponding logic program but also the set of "active" persistent statements, i.e. if we promote such a set of persistent statements to be an integral part of each knowledge state. With this new way of looking at knowledge states, whereby with each state we associate a pair $\langle \mathcal{P}_s, PC_s \rangle$, where $\mathcal{P}_s = P_0 \oplus ... \oplus P_s$ is a dynamic logic program (also referred to as the object level KB) and PC_s is the set of "active" persistent statements at state s, we can discard all past update commands since $\langle \mathcal{P}_s, PC_s \rangle$ contains all necessary information to determine future knowledge states after subsequent updates. Note however that there is not a major paradigm shift. In fact, the inductive definition of the mentioned transformation can be directly adapted to this new perspective. From a higher level stand point, and having in mind the application of such a language of updates in the context of agent systems, it seems more appropriate to have one such agent's knowledge state be defined by the object level KB together with the update statements that have not been exhausted (can still produce knowledge changes), than to have the historical sequence of updates that led it to its present state. This is because the agent actually performs the updates, changing its mental state, sometimes having to make commitments when doing so. The constituents of the pair $\langle \mathcal{P}_s, PC_s \rangle$ can be seen as the historical evolution that represents the current state of knowledge, represented by the DLP $\mathcal{P}_s$, together with the specification for the future evolutions represented by PC_s, i.e. a duality between past and future where the past is not hypothetical but rather a concrete well defined body of knowledge.

As we've seen before, the persistent commands are to be (conditionally) executed not only to produce the state transition at which they were issued, but are also present at all subsequent state transitions until they are cancelled. In other words, **always** commands may specify (limited) sequences of state transitions.

If one agrees with the premises that a language for updates should allow for commands whose effect spans for more than one state transition, then it is reasonable to believe that *KUL* (and *LUPS*) is not expressive enough for such a purpose, in the sense that some desirable statements, specifying some updates that span for more than one state transition, cannot be directly expressed. For example, a statement such as "*update the KB with a certain rule when a certain condition holds after another certain condition held*", cannot be directly expressed in *KUL* (and *LUPS*). Such statement would have the form, in a *LUPS like* language, as

$$\textbf{always}\,(\textbf{always}\,(R)\ \textbf{when}\ L_{k+1}, \ldots, L_m)\ \textbf{when}\ L_{m+1}, \ldots, L_n$$

In general, *KUL* (and *LUPS*) does not allow the specification of updates whose execution depends on conditions on more than one state. Such statements would allow for the specification of delayed effects of actions, i.e. statements of the form "*a certain action at some state n causes a certain effect at state n + m*", useful, for example, to concisely specify actions which are encapsulations of sequences of actions. For example if pressing a key on a keyboard is an action, then entering a password could be encoded as one action that encapsulates several other actions whose intermediate effects are not relevant. As we've mentioned, one way to extend the existing languages of updates in order to express such statements, is to allow the update statements not only to specify the set of logic program rules that belong to the KB produced by the "current" state transition, but to also specify a set of commands that belongs to the update that will govern the next state transition, i.e. we need commands to assert and retract, **assert** and **retract** commands, and we need to assert and retract these, in turn, i.e., we need nested (or embedded) commands. This can be achieved by allowing the explicit update of not only the object KB but also the set of statements that govern the future updates, i.e. the set PC_s. According to this framework, each knowledge state will contain the current object KB and a set of statements that, together with any external updates, specify its future evolution. We will be referring to this set of statements that specifies the future evolutions as the set of *Self Updates* (SU) in the sense that they do not require any external updates to change the knowledge state. This set of self updates replaces the previous set of persistent commands (PC).

It is worth stressing that, unlike in *KUL* (and *LUPS*), in this new update framework the knowledge states can in fact evolve without any external updates. In *KUL* (and *LUPS*), each "state transition" occurs only when a new external update is issued. In this new framework we assign a more operational view whereby an external cycle will drive the evolution of the knowledge base, be there an external update or otherwise.

Commands: In order to specify those updates mentioned before with the ability to encode state transitions that span several states, we need to enrich the set of available update commands and statements. In our new language, we need to include commands (and statements) that update the set of Self Updates. This will be achieved with very little cost by simply using the same set of commands, but allowing them to specify assertions and retractions of statements instead of just rules. In other words, we need to define update commands for statements: commands that assert or retract statements in SU_{s+1}. If S is a statement, we need commands of the form [**always_**]**assert**(S) and [**always_**]**retract**(S). As we will see below, at each state transition we shall have to somehow combine the self and external updates to determine the state transition. For this, it will be useful to allow the inhibition of statements, i.e. we need to be able to externally specify that, for this particular state transition, some self updates should be ignored, and vice versa, that some external updates should be inhibited, this being specified by statements belonging to the self updates. We should be able to state this "temporary" inhibition without retracting the inhibited statement. For this, we will introduce such inhibiting commands that will be indicated by prefixing each of the existing basic commands with the keyword "*not*". With commands that are able to retract statements from the set of Self Updates and the ability to specify the inhibition of commands, the *KUL* (and *LUPS*) commands for cancellation of persistent statements are no longer needed since their behaviour can be approximated as a combination of a retraction and an inhibition command. As we will see below, such encoding of the *KUL* (and *LUPS*) commands for cancellation has a slightly different behaviour. Briefly, in *KUL* (and *LUPS*), a cancellation commands such as

$$\textbf{cancel assert } L \leftarrow L_1, \ldots, L_k \textbf{ when } L_{k+1}, \ldots, L_m$$

will cancel every persistent command of the form

$$\textbf{always assert}[\textbf{ event}]\ L \leftarrow L_1, \ldots, L_k \textbf{ when } \mathit{Conditions}$$

if $L_{k+1}, \ldots, L_m$ holds. In the framework we are introducing now, cancellations are performed on selected persistent commands instead of on every persistent command whose specified rule is the same as the one specified by the cancellation command. Suppose for example, that we have the two, previously issued, persistent commands:

$$\textbf{always assert } L \leftarrow L_1, \ldots, L_k \textbf{ when } L_{k+1}$$
$$\textbf{always assert event } L \leftarrow L_1, \ldots, L_k \textbf{ when } L_{k+1}, L_{k+2}$$

With *KUL* (and *LUPS*) commands for cancellation, if one of these persistent commands is cancelled, the so is the other. Within the framework we are now introducing, cancellations are selectively performed i.e., each persistent commands is selectively, individually, cancelled.

We will also introduce a new type of command, which will be referred to as semi-persistent commands. Such semi-persistent commands also specify assertions and retractions, just as the persistent and non-persistent ones, but only persist until they are executed for the first time. Their purpose is to allow the specification of updates that are to be performed only once, at the first opportunity, i.e. at the first (current or future) state transition such that the set of conditions of the statement holds. Such statements should persist until they perform the update, after which they are removed. They will be identified by prefixing the keyword **once** before the keywords **assert** and **retract**, i.e. we have the commands **once_assert** [**_event**] (ρ) and **once_retract** [**_event**] (ρ).

Conditions: The update commands, together with their preconditions form update statements. In *KUL* (and *LUPS*), commands are executed if a set of conditions hold in the current knowledge state. These take the form of conjunctions of literals belonging to the object language. With the goal in mind of using this framework to specify an agent's behaviours, it is important to allow these conditions to refer to objects not necessarily part of the agent's knowledge base. One such case is an agent that is capable of sensing the environment (which can include anything from its physical position to incoming messages from other agents). We would like to specify updates that are conditional on some observations, without having to assert such observations into the knowledge base, either because they are not trustworthy, they are irrelevant, or any other reason for that matter. In the *KUL* (and *LUPS*) framework, one can only reason about (evaluate) conditions with respect to the knowledge base. An update that is conditional on an environment observation would require the previous assertion of the observation, with an extra state transition and, only then, the condition would hold and the command be executed. Add to this the fact that the observation is now in the knowledge base, something that may not be desirable. In EPI, such a notion of external observation exists. Although the language was designed to specify update policies to a knowledge base, its main objective is to have some degree of control over the updates that are actually performed, in face of a set of external events. Also, allowing such external events permits the specification of generic update policies for possible future observations that are as yet unknown [75]. To allow for updates conditional on environment observations, possibly unknown yet and without having to assert them in the knowledge base and wait for an extra cycle, we will introduce a similar notion of events which, to avoid any confusion with the **event** keyword of non-inertial commands, will be referred to as *environment observations*.

One other aspect of EPI that will be imported, though with a slightly different semantics, is the possibility of allowing commands to depend on the simultaneous execution of other commands. It is not difficult to imagine situations where we wish to perform an update only if another update is executed too. For example, we might want to retract some rule, but only if some other rule is asserted at the same time.

Finally, we will allow updates to be conditional on the "memorial" presence (resp. absence) of specified rules in the knowledge base, i.e. an update would only be executed if the specified rule has been asserted before and not retracted since the last assertion (resp. has never been asserted or has been retracted since). Note here the difference between this "memorial" presence or absence of rules and the notion of rejected rules in the semantics of DLP. A rule may have been asserted (and not retracted since), in which case this rule is memorially present, but may be rejected according to the underlying DLP semantics. For one particular knowledge state, the memorial presence (or absence) of rules, unlike their rejection, does not depend on whichever stable model we are considering. This concept was directly available already in the transformation of the previous section, in the form of the auxiliary predicate $N(R)$. At a given state, those rules for which $N(R)$ belongs to all stable models are precisely those that are memorially present at that state. In this extended framework, we shall allow statements to contain conditions on the memorial presence or absence of rules.

While *KUL* allows the specification of how an update mechanism should behave, the new language herein set forth also allows for the update of such behaviours i.e. it allows to update both knowledge and behaviours. Therefore, we call such language *KABUL* which stands for *Knowledge And Behaviour Update Language*.

5.2 *KABUL* - Framework

Forthwith, we describe the overall framework suitable for representing an agent's knowledge base with self, external, and observation based updating.

As mentioned before, at each state s, the knowledge base consists of a pair $\langle \mathcal{P}_s, SU_s \rangle$ where $\mathcal{P}_s = P_0 \oplus ... \oplus P_s$ is a dynamic logic program (also referred to as the object level KB) and SU_s is the self update at state s. The self update consists of a set of update statements, in the language that will be defined below, which will partially specify the future evolution of the knowledge base. At this point it is worth to mention why, if both are updatable, the object knowledge base is represented by a sequence (of logic programs) and the self update is not also a sequence (in this case of update programs): it is so because at each state transition some update actions are performed, making a commitment as to the change in the knowledge state. Once such a commitment is made, there is no way of going back i.e., unlike in DLP where the principle of inertia allows for a rule to be rejected and subsequently reused again, when we consider the self-update and the update actions it specifies, once executed (resp. not-executed) the command cannot be unexecuted (resp. executed) or, in other words, the principle of inertia does not make sense in the context of the more imperative part of this framework represented by the update commands.

An object level rule in a logic program within a DLP corresponds to a (possibly partial) definition, for some literal, that is true (the definition) at that state. Then, since we believe that such definitions tend not to change with time, we apply the principle of inertia. Unlike object level rules, update statements represent specifications for specific state transitions. We can specify one-time statements such as those representing the basic assertion or retraction, or we can specifically state that those commands are also to be part of future state transition specifications, i.e. the life span of one such statements is specifically encoded in its specification. One can thus see update statements, and in particular the set of self updates, as a set of facts, whose meaning will affect the object level knowledge base, but whose definition and updates are treated as purely extensional updates, in the sense that only its present state, and not its historical evolution, is needed to determine its present model and future definitions.

State transitions will be governed not only by the self update, but also by another set of incoming statements, the external update, and a set of environment observations. The external update can be seen as the means to provide the possibility of the knowledge base being changed (updated) by a user or another agent with such capabilities. The environment observations allow the agent to reason about input from possible existing sensors, incoming messages, etc. As will become apparent below, when the semantics is defined, the external updates are statements that can, by themselves, directly change the knowledge state, whereas the environment observations only serve to "activate" existing statements, be they self or external in origin, by allowing its preconditions to be verified.

With the purpose of having an operational view of this framework, whereby no explicit external update is needed in order for the knowledge base to evolve, we assume a synchronous clock that drives the entire process. At each tick of the clock, the following cycle is performed:

---

cycle $(s, \langle \mathcal{P}_s, SU_s \rangle)$
  record any external observations (EO_{s+1})
  record any external updates (EU_{s+1})
  determine the reduced statements of SU_s and EU_{s+1} wrt. $\mathcal{P}_s$ and EO_{s+1}
  combine the reduced statements to determine a set of executable commands
  determine the knowledge base at the next state $\langle \mathcal{P}_{s+1}, SU_{s+1} \rangle$
  cycle $(s+1, \langle \mathcal{P}_{s+1}, SU_{s+1} \rangle)$

According to this cycle, given a knowledge state $\langle \mathcal{P}_s, SU_s \rangle$ where $\mathcal{P}_s = P_0 \oplus ... \oplus P_s$ is a dynamic logic program and SU_s is the self update at state s, the state transition is produced according to an input consisting of a pair $\langle EU_{s+1}, E_{s+1} \rangle$ where EU_{s+1} is the external update program (set of statements) and EO_{s+1} is an environment observation, consisting of a sub-set of all possible environment observations.

In what concerns the environment observations, since we are dealing with rule updates of logic programs in the object language, it is only natural that such external observations be about such rules. But we also want to differentiate between distinct forms of rule observation: for example, in the context of Legal Reasoning, where object level rules represent laws, we want to be able to express that some law has been voted by parliament, and distinguish such an observation from the one about the same law but where it has now been approved by the president. To this purpose, following the usual tradition, we define a propositional language (of observations), $\mathcal{E}$, consisting of the ground terms of a first order language whose set of terms include the object level rules. We dub elements of $\mathcal{E}$ (environment) observations. Going back to the Legal Reasoning context, if r is an object level rule representing some law, then *voted*(r) and *approved*(r) would be examples of propositions in such a language of observations.

The next state of the knowledge base is $\langle \mathcal{P}_{s+1}, SU_{s+1} \rangle$, where $\mathcal{P}_{s+1} = P_0 \oplus ... \oplus P_s \oplus P_{s+1}$, i.e. each state transition produces a new generalized logic program P_{s+1} to be added to the already existing sequence, and a new set of statements corresponding to the self update at state $s+1$. Both P_{s+1} and SU_{s+1}, will depend on EO_{s+1}, $\mathcal{P}_s$, and a combination of both the self update (SU_s) and the external update (EU_{s+1}). Schematically we have:

$$\langle \mathcal{P}_s, SU_s \rangle \overset{\langle EU_{s+1}, EO_{s+1} \rangle}{\longrightarrow} \langle \mathcal{P}_{s+1}, SU_{s+1} \rangle$$

The initial state, $s = 0$, without loss of generality, is empty.

Definition 73 (Initial Knowledge State) *The* initial knowledge state *is the knowledge state at state* 0, $\langle \mathcal{P}_0, SU_0 \rangle$ *where:*

$$\mathcal{P}_0 = P_0$$
$$P_0 = \{\}$$
$$SU_0 = \{\}$$

Each knowledge state can be seen as the result of applying a sequence of state transitions specified by pairs of the form $\langle EU_{s+1}, EO_{s+1} \rangle$ to the initial (empty) knowledge state. We often use the notation $\langle \mathcal{P}_0, SU_0 \rangle \otimes \langle EU_1, EO_1 \rangle \otimes \langle EU_2, EO_2 \rangle \otimes ... \otimes \langle EU_s, EO_s \rangle$ to denote the knowledge state produced by such a sequence, i.e. the knowledge state $\langle \mathcal{P}_s, SU_s \rangle$.

There remains to be defined what such update programs (self and external) look like, how they combine and how they produce the state transitions. The following sections will be occupied with the syntax of such update programs and the semantics for those state transitions.

5.3 *KABUL* - Syntax

In this Section, we introduce the syntax of *KABUL*.

What kind of update commands do we need to specify the state transitions mentioned before? We certainly need the basic (non-persistent) commands of *KUL*, corresponding to the four basic update operations on the object knowledge base:

assert(R)	**retract**(R)
assert_event(R)	**retract_event**(R)

As in *KUL*, we also need the persistent version of these commands, obtained by prefixing any of the previous commands with the keyword "**always_**" such as for example **always_assert**(R), **always_retract_event**(R), etc.

Each of these commands will only be executed if some conditions hold. These conditions can refer to literals that must hold in the object level KB at the current state, presence or absence of concomitant environment observations, denoted by $in\,(E)$ or $out\,(E)$ where E is an external observation, the concurrent execution of another basic update operation, and the memorial presence or absence of rules in the object knowledge base, denoted by $in\,(R)$ or $out\,(R)$ where R is a rule. Each command together with its pre-conditions forms a statement, with the generic form

$$\mathbf{command}(\rho) \Leftarrow Conditions$$

As mentioned before, we also introduce a new type of commands that are persistent until executed for the first time, denoted by:

$$\textbf{once\_assert}(R) \qquad \textbf{once\_retract}(R)$$

together with their non-inertial versions denoted by:

$$\textbf{once\_assert\_event}(R) \qquad \textbf{once\_retract\_event}(R)$$

Its purpose is to allow the specification of updates that are to be performed just once, at the first opportunity, i.e. at the first (current or future) state transition such that *Conditions* hold. They should persist until they perform the update, after which they are removed.

So far we've only mentioned commands for rule manipulation. We also need commands to specify the self-update at the next state. In other words, we need to define update commands for statements: commands that assert or retract statements in SU_{s+1}. If S is a statement, we need the following basic (non-persistent) commands

$$\textbf{assert}(S) \qquad \textbf{retract}(S)$$

And their persistent versions:

$$\textbf{always\_assert}(S) \qquad \textbf{always\_retract}(S)$$
$$\textbf{once\_assert}(S) \qquad \textbf{once\_retract}(S)$$

Since each statement, unless specified by the **always** or **once** keyword, does not persist by inertia, there is no need for non-inertial commands for statements. In fact what could be the reading of one such non-inertial command for statements? That some statement should be asserted and retracted at the subsequent state? Such behaviour is already specifiable by asserting a (non-persistent) assert command. As we've mentioned before, inertia is a principle that we apply, by default, when combining the logic programs that constitute the object level DLP. Therefore, it is only fit that we allow the specification of object level rules to which we should not apply inertia. We have also explained that the life span of an update statement is encoded in its specification with the keywords **always** and **once**, besides the basic commands with none of such keywords. Since we do not apply inertia to update statements, besides the persistence already defined by those keywords, there is no need no define commands to override it.

It will be useful to allow for commands specifying the inhibition of a certain update. For this purpose, we introduce four inhibition commands, corresponding to the inhibition of the four basic updates (**assert**(ρ), **retract**(ρ), **assert_event**(ρ), **retract_event**(ρ)[1]). Such inhibition commands are obtained from the basic commands by prefixing them with the keyword "*not*". The intuitive meaning of such inhibition commands is to prevent the corresponding update specified by another command. Accordingly, the inhibition command *not* **assert**(ρ) will prevent the assertion of ρ, be it specified by a command **assert**(ρ), **always_assert**(ρ) or **once_assert**(ρ), according to the semantics below. Recall that, although the commands **assert**(ρ), **always_assert**(ρ) or **once_assert**(ρ) encode different behaviours in what their persistence is concerned, they all correspond to the same update operation. Similarly, the inhibition command *not* **retract_event**(ρ) will prevent the retraction of ρ, be it specified by a command **retract_event**(ρ), **always_retract_event**(ρ) or **once_retract_event**(ρ).

[1]Where ρ stands for a rule or a statement.

The **cancel** command of LUPS, whose purpose was to inhibit and remove a persistent statement, is similar to a combination of an inhibition command and a retraction (of the statement) command. For our purposes, we will restrict the initial object propositional language $\mathcal{L}$, as defined previously, not to contain any propositions of the forms: $N(\_)$, $Ev(\_,\_)$. If they do occur, they must be renamed. We now formalize the syntax of the language for updates.

Definition 74 (*KABUL* - Syntax) *Let $\mathcal{L}$ be a propositional language. Let $\mathcal{R}$ be the set of rules generated by $\mathcal{L}$. Let $\mathcal{E}$ be a language of observations.* A statement *is a propositional expression of the form*

$$\begin{aligned} C_0(\rho_0) \Leftarrow {} & C_1(\rho_1), ..., C_n(\rho_n), L_1, \ldots, L_k, \\ & \mathbf{R} : \mathbf{in}(R_1), ..., \mathbf{in}(R_m), \mathbf{out}(R_{m+1}), ..., \mathbf{out}(R_n), \\ & \mathbf{E} : \mathbf{in}\left(E_1\right), ..., \mathbf{in}\left(E_p\right), \mathbf{out}\left(E_{p+1}\right), ..., \mathbf{out}\left(E_q\right) \end{aligned}$$

where:

- *$C_0(\rho_0)$ is either a persistent command, a non-persistent command, or an inhibition command;*
- *each $C_1(\rho_1), ..., C_n(\rho_n)$ $(n \geq 0)$ is either a non-persistent command or an inhibition command. We restrict the conditions to the concurrent execution (or not) of a basic update operation, i.e., we do not differentiate if such a basic update operation originated in a persistent command or in a basic command.*
- *each $L_1, ..., L_k$ $(k \geq 0)$ is a literal from $\mathcal{L}$;*
- *each $R_1, ..., R_n$ $(n \geq 0)$ is a rule from $\mathcal{R}$;*
- *each $E_1, ..., E_q$ $(m \geq 0)$ is an observation from $\mathcal{E}$;*

Let $\mathcal{S}$ denote the set of all statements.
A command *is a propositional expression of any of the forms*[2]*:*

$$[\mathbf{always\_} \mid \mathbf{once\_}]\, \mathbf{assert}\, [\mathbf{\_event}]\, (R) \tag{5.1}$$
$$[\mathbf{always\_} \mid \mathbf{once\_}]\, \mathbf{retract}\, [\mathbf{\_event}]\, (R) \tag{5.2}$$
$$[\mathbf{always\_} \mid \mathbf{once\_}]\, \mathbf{assert}\, (S) \tag{5.3}$$
$$[\mathbf{always\_} \mid \mathbf{once\_}]\, \mathbf{retract}\, (S) \tag{5.4}$$

where R is a rule and S is a statement. A persistent command *is a command containing one of the keywords* **always** *or* **once**. *A* non-persistent command *is a command that is not persistent.*

An inhibition command *is a propositional expression of any of the forms:*

$$not\, \mathbf{assert}\, [\mathbf{\_event}]\, (R) \tag{5.5}$$
$$not\, \mathbf{retract}\, [\mathbf{\_event}]\, (R) \tag{5.6}$$
$$not\, \mathbf{assert}\, (S) \tag{5.7}$$
$$not\, \mathbf{retract}\, (S) \tag{5.8}$$

[2]Where [**a** | **b**] will be used for notational convenience denoting the presence of either **a**, or **b**, or neither.

where R is a rule and S is a statement.

We dub commands of forms (5.1) and (5.2) rule commands, *and those of forms (5.3) and (5.4)* statement commands.

Given a command or inhibition command $c = [not]\, C(\rho)$, by argument of c, *denoted by $Arg\,(c)$, we mean ρ.*

If S is a statement as above, then:

$$\begin{aligned}
&\mathbf{H}\,(S) = C_0(\rho_0)\\
&\mathbf{C}\,(S) = C_1(\rho_1), ..., C_n(\rho_n)\\
&\mathbf{L}\,(S) = L_1, \ldots, L_k\\
&\mathbf{R}\,(S) = \mathbf{in}(R_1), ..., \mathbf{in}(R_m), \mathbf{out}(R_{m+1}), ..., \mathbf{out}(R_n)\\
&\mathbf{E}\,(S) = \mathbf{in}\,(E_1)\,, ..., \mathbf{in}\,(E_p)\,, \mathbf{out}\,(E_{p+1})\,, ..., \mathbf{out}\,(E_q)
\end{aligned}$$

Each statement can specify from very simple state transitions, such as the ones that served as examples for LUPS, to rather more complex updates. Throughout, as usual, statements with variables stand for the set of all the ground instances, where variables starting with capital R (e.g. R_1,...,R_n) stand for rules in $\mathcal{R}$. Whenever unambiguous, when using environment observations in commands of the form $\mathbf{in}\,(E)$, we drop the $\mathbf{in}\,()$ and simply write E.

There follow some examples of statements:

Example 38 *In the context of legal reasoning, before a law is to be enforced, it must first be voted by parliament, then it must be approved (not vetoed) by the president, and finally it must be published. If these three steps were to be regarded as environment observations, this behaviour could be encoded by the following statement:*

$$\mathbf{always\_assert}\left(\begin{array}{r}\mathbf{once\_assert}\,(\mathbf{once\_assert}\,(R) \Leftarrow \mathbf{E} : \mathbf{in}\,(publ(R))) \Leftarrow\\ \mathbf{E} : \mathbf{in}\,(app(R))\end{array}\right) \Leftarrow \\ \mathbf{E} : \mathbf{in}\,(voted(R))$$

or using the simplification for observations:

$$\mathbf{always\_assert}\,(\mathbf{once\_assert}\,(\mathbf{once\_assert}\,(R) \Leftarrow \mathbf{E} : publ(R)) \Leftarrow \mathbf{E} : app(R)) \Leftarrow \\ \mathbf{E} : voted(R)$$

Below, a more elaborate example based on such legal knowledge bases will be presented.

Example 39 *Consider three actions: set, clear and go, where set enables go, clear disables go, and go causes some non-inertial effect (effect). The actions can be specified by the two statements:*

$$\begin{aligned}
&\mathbf{always_assert}\,(\mathbf{always_assert_event}\,(\mathit{effect}) \Leftarrow \mathbf{E} : go) \Leftarrow \mathbf{E} : set\\
&\mathbf{always_retract}\,(\mathbf{always_assert_event}\,(\mathit{effect}) \Leftarrow \mathbf{E} : go) \Leftarrow \mathbf{E} : reset
\end{aligned}$$

Example 40 *A behaviour specifying that the knowledge base must always be updated with any observed rule is specified by the statement:*

$$\mathbf{always\_assert}\,(R) \Leftarrow \mathbf{E} : rule(R)$$

If we only wish to assert the rule if it is not present in the knowledge base we would write:

$$\mathbf{always\_assert}\,(R) \Leftarrow \mathbf{R} : \mathbf{out}(R), \mathbf{E} : rule(R)$$

Example 41 *Specifying that a rule should never be asserted if a warning is observed can be specified by the following set of statements:*

$$\textbf{always\_assert}\,(\textit{not}\,\textbf{assert}\,(R) \Leftarrow \textbf{E}:\textit{warning}) \Leftarrow$$
$$\textit{not}\,\textbf{assert}\,(R) \Leftarrow \textbf{E}:\textit{warning}$$

As will become clearer when we set forth the semantics, since statements with inhibition commands are non-persistent, the specification of persistent inhibitions requires two statements: one to specify the inhibition at the initial state transition and the other to persistently assert such inhibition statement for future state transitions. As will be detailed below, $\textit{not}\,\textbf{assert}\,(r)$ *inhibits all assertions of* r*, be them specified by an* $\textbf{assert}\,(r)$, $\textbf{always\_assert}\,(r)$ *or* $\textbf{once\_assert}\,(r)$.

Example 42 *Specifying that a rule* r *should be asserted if another rule* r' *is, at the same time, non-initially retracted would be encoded by the statement:*

$$\textbf{assert}\,(r) \Leftarrow \textbf{retract\_event}\,(r')$$

In this example, rule r *would be asserted if any of the following commands was also executed:*

$$\textbf{retract\_event}\,(r') \qquad \textbf{always\_retract\_event}\,(r') \qquad \textbf{once\_retract\_event}\,(r')$$

i.e. as long as the rule r' *was retracted by any non-inertial command.*

Example 43 *Specifying that a rule* r *should not be retracted if another rule* r' *is, at the same time, also not retracted would be encoded by the following statement:*

$$\textit{not}\,\textbf{retract}\,(r) \Leftarrow \textit{not}\,\textbf{retract}\,(r')$$

In this example, rule r *would not be retracted unless any of the following commands was also executed:*

$$\textbf{retract}\,(r') \qquad \textbf{always\_retract}\,(r') \qquad \textbf{once\_retract}\,(r')$$

i.e. as long as the rule r' *was retracted by any non-inertial command.*

Example 44 *Specifying that any rule should not be asserted if it is not observed can be specified by the following statement:*

$$\textit{not}\,\textbf{assert}\,(R) \Leftarrow \textbf{E}:\textbf{out}(R)$$

The table below summarizes the syntax of *KABUL* in BNF [26].

⟨*statement*⟩	::=	⟨*command*⟩ [⇐ ⟨*conditions*⟩] ;
⟨*base_comm*⟩	::=	**assert** [**_event**] (⟨*rule*⟩) | **retract** [**_event**] (⟨*rule*⟩) |
		| **assert** (⟨*statement*⟩) | **retract** (⟨*statement*⟩) ;
⟨*per_comm*⟩	::=	**always_** ⟨*base_comm*⟩ | **once_** ⟨*base_comm*⟩ ;
⟨*inhib_comm*⟩	::=	*not* ⟨*base_comm*⟩ ;
⟨*command*⟩	::=	⟨*base_comm*⟩ | ⟨*per_comm*⟩ | ⟨*inhib_comm*⟩ ;
⟨*conditions*⟩	::=	[⟨*comm_conds*⟩ ,] [⟨*lit_conds*⟩ ,]
		[**R** : ⟨*rule_conds*⟩ ,] [**E** : ⟨*env_conds*⟩] ;
⟨*comm_conds*⟩	::=	⟨*base_comm*⟩ [, ⟨*comm_conds*⟩] |
		| ⟨*inhib_comm*⟩ [, ⟨*comm_conds*⟩] ;
⟨*lit_conds*⟩	::=	⟨*literal*⟩ [, ⟨*lit_conds*⟩] ;
⟨*rule_conds*⟩	::=	**in** (⟨*rule*⟩) [, ⟨*rule_conds*⟩] | **out** (⟨*rule*⟩) [, ⟨*rule_conds*⟩] ;
⟨*env_conds*⟩	::=	**in** (⟨*observ*⟩) [, ⟨*env_conds*⟩] | **out** (⟨*observ*⟩) [, ⟨*env_conds*⟩] ;

Let Ψ be the statement $C(\rho) \Leftarrow Cond$. The following list summarizes the intuition behind each command $C(\rho)$:

assert $(R \mid S)$: if the condition *Cond* holds at the current state, a given rule R is added to the successor state logic program (or statement S to the successor state self update).

retract $(R \mid S)$: if the condition *Cond* holds at the current state, the given rule R is deleted at the successor state logic program (or statement S is prevented from being added to the successor state self update).

always_assert $(R \mid S)$: same as **assert** $(R \mid S)$ and, also, statement Ψ will be added to the successor state self update program, independently of the condition *Cond* holding or not, unless a command of the form [**always_** | **once_**] **retract** (Ψ) is also executed.

always_retract $(R \mid S)$: same as **retract** $(R \mid S)$ and, also, statement Ψ will be added to the successor state self update, independently of the condition *Cond* holding or not, unless a command of the form [**always_** | **once_**] **retract** (Ψ) is also executed.

once_assert $(R \mid S)$: same as **assert** $(R \mid S)$ and, also, if the condition *Cond* does not hold at the current state, statement Ψ will be added to the successor state self update, unless a command of the form [**always_** | **once_**] **retract** (Ψ) is also executed.

once_retract $(R \mid S)$: same as **retract** $(R \mid S)$ and, also, if the condition *Cond* does not hold at the current state, statement Ψ will be added to the successor state self update, unless a command of the form [**always_** | **once_**] **retract** (Ψ) is also executed.

assert_event (R) : if the condition *Cond* holds at the current state, a given rule R is added to the successor state logic program, and its inertial effect is blocked at subsequent states.

retract_event (R) : if the condition *Cond* holds at the current state, the given rule R's inertial effect is temporarily blocked at the successor state logic program, this blockage being removed at subsequent states.

always_assert_event (R) : same as **assert_event** (R) and, also, statement Ψ will be added to the successor state self update, independently of the condition *Cond* holding or not, unless a command of the form [**always_** | **once_**] **retract** (Ψ) is also executed.

always_retract_event (R) : same as **retract_event** (R) and, also, statement Ψ will be added to the successor state self update, independently of the condition *Cond* holding or not, unless a command of the form [**always_** | **once_**] **retract** (Ψ) is also executed.

once_assert_event (R) : same as **assert_event** (R) and, also, if the condition *Cond* does not hold at the current state, statement Ψ will be added to the successor state self update, unless a command of the form [**always_** | **once_**] **retract** (Ψ) is also executed.

once_retract_event (R) : same as **retract_event** (R) and, also, if the condition *Cond* does not hold at the current state, statement Ψ will be added to the successor state self update, unless a command of the form [**always_** | **once_**] **retract** (Ψ) is also executed.

Definition 75 (Update Program) *An* update program *in* KABUL *is a set of statements.*

We will extend the notion of query to include the memorial presence or absence of rules.

Definition 76 (Query) *A query to the knowledge base is a propositional expression of the form:*

$$\mathbf{holds}(L_1, ..., L_k, in(R_1), ..., in(R_m), out(R_{m+1}), ..., out(R_n)) \text{ } \mathbf{at} \text{ } q \text{ ?}$$

*where $L_1, ..., L_k$ are literals and $R_1, ..., R_n$ are rules, and q is a state such that $q \leq s$ where s is the current state. If $q = s$ we often omit the "***at*** q" from the query.*

5.4 *KABUL* - Semantics

In this section we provide a semantics for the language of updates *KABUL*. Given a KB state $\langle \mathcal{P}_s, SU_s \rangle$, where $\mathcal{P}_s = P_0 \oplus ... \oplus P_s$, an external update program EU_{s+1} and a set of external observations, EO_{s+1}, we want to characterize the successor KB state $\langle \mathcal{P}_{s+1}, SU_{s+1} \rangle$, where $\mathcal{P}_{s+1} = P_0 \oplus ... \oplus P_s \oplus P_{s+1}$, i.e. we want to characterize P_{s+1} and SU_{s+1}, which will depend on a suitable combination of both update programs (self and external), as well as EO_{s+1} and $\mathcal{P}_s$. This will be achieved in three steps:

1. partially evaluate the statements in SU_s and EU_{s+1} with respect to the external set of observations and current object level KB to determine two update program reducts;

2. determine, based on the previously obtained reducts, a set of commands to be executed;

3. determine the next state knowledge base.

Before we continue, we introduce the notion of *transition frame*. A transition frame is a tuple $\langle \mathcal{P}_s, \models, SU_s, EU_{s+1}, EO_{s+1}, <, Sel(.) \rangle$ where $\mathcal{P}_s, SU_s, EU_{s+1}$ and EO_{s+1} are as defined above. The $\models$ is a consequence operator corresponding to the semantics assigned to the object knowledge base $\mathcal{P}_s$, which will be elaborated upon in the next subsection. As will become clear, the combination of SU_s and EU_{s+1} to determine the update to be performed may allow for more than one possible set of commands to be executed. We therefore assume a selection function, $Sel(.)$, that returns one of such sets of commands. When combining the statements and inhibition statements of both the self and external updates, different precedence relations can be assigned to them. To this purpose we need to establish how such a combination is to be accomplished, namely in what concerns the interaction between both the updates and the inhibition commands in the statements of both updates. For example, we can have assertion commands of the self update override the corresponding retraction command originated in the external update, or vice-versa. We can have inhibition commands of either update inhibit the corresponding command of either update, or any other similar policy. Since, for each update program, SU_s and EU_{s+1}, statements with commands in their heads and those with inhibition commands in their heads can be assigned a different role, with possibly different priorities when combining both sets to determine a set of executable commands, we need to split each update program into two sets, according to the heads of the statements.

Definition 77 *Let U be a set of statements. We define:*

$$U^+ = \{C_0(\rho) \Leftarrow \mathbf{Cond} \in U\}$$
$$U^- = \{not\, C_0(\rho) \Leftarrow \mathbf{Cond} \in U\}$$

We dub U^+ the positive update and U^- the inhibition update.

Example 45 *Let U be the update program containing the statements:*

$$\mathbf{always\_assert}\,(\mathbf{always\_assert\_event}\,(b \leftarrow d) \Leftarrow \mathbf{E} : \mathbf{in}(obs\,(d))) \Leftarrow \mathbf{E} : \mathbf{in}(obs\,(b))$$
$$\mathbf{always\_assert}\,(R) \Leftarrow \mathbf{R} : \mathbf{out}(R), \mathbf{E} : \mathbf{in}(rule(R))$$
$$\mathbf{always\_assert\_event}\,(b \leftarrow d) \Leftarrow not\,\mathbf{assert}\,(a)\,, a, not\, b$$
$$not\,\mathbf{assert}\,(c \leftarrow d) \Leftarrow not\, b, \mathbf{E} : \mathbf{in}(obs\,(b))$$
$$\mathbf{assert\_event}\,(a \leftarrow h) \Leftarrow not\,\mathbf{assert}\,(a)\,, not\, a, b$$

Then, U^+ contains the statements:

$$\mathbf{always\_assert}\,(\mathbf{always\_assert\_event}\,(b \leftarrow d) \Leftarrow \mathbf{E} : \mathbf{in}(obs\,(d))) \Leftarrow \mathbf{E} : \mathbf{in}(obs\,(b))$$
$$\mathbf{always\_assert}\,(R) \Leftarrow \mathbf{R} : \mathbf{out}(R), \mathbf{E} : \mathbf{in}(rule(R))$$
$$\mathbf{always\_assert\_event}\,(b \leftarrow d) \Leftarrow not\,\mathbf{assert}\,(a)\,, a, not\, b$$
$$\mathbf{assert\_event}\,(a \leftarrow h) \Leftarrow not\,\mathbf{assert}\,(a)\,, not\, a, b$$

and U^- the statement:

$$not\,\mathbf{assert}\,(c \leftarrow d) \Leftarrow not\, b, \mathbf{E} : \mathbf{in}(obs\,(b))$$

With the two updates, SU_s and EU_{s+1}, we obtain the following four sets of statements corresponding to the positive and inhibition updates of both the self and external updates:

$$SU_s^+ = \{C_0(\rho) \Leftarrow \mathbf{Cond} \in SU_s\}$$
$$SU_s^- = \{not\, C_0(\rho) \Leftarrow \mathbf{Cond} \in SU_s\}$$
$$EU_{s+1}^+ = \{C_0(\rho) \Leftarrow \mathbf{Cond} \in EU_{s+1}\}$$
$$EU_{s+1}^- = \{not\, C_0(\rho) \Leftarrow \mathbf{Cond} \in EU_{s+1}\}$$

It is over these four sets of statements that the order relation $<$, in the transition frame, is defined. Such order relation should be interpreted as follows: if $A < B$ then the statements in B should prevail over those in A.

In the following subsections we explain how each of the three steps needed to determine the next state of the knowledge base is accomplished.

5.4.1 Update Program Reduct

First we partially evaluate the statements in SU_s and EU_{s+1} (or SU_s^+, SU_s^-, EU_{s+1}^+ and EU_{s+1}^-) with respect to the external set of observations EO_{s+1} and current object level KB $\mathcal{P}_s$. In LUPS [15], as well as in KUL, the semantics assigned to the DLP $\mathcal{P}_s$ was based on the intersection of all stable models at state s, corresponding to the consequence operator $\models_{sm}$. According to this skeptical approach, an update would only be performed if it depends on literals that are true in all stable models. Suppose, for example, that we have a DLP at state 1, consisting of the logic program with the following rules:

$$a \leftarrow not\, b \qquad b \leftarrow not\, a \qquad c \leftarrow a \qquad c \leftarrow b \qquad not\, g \leftarrow d \qquad g \leftarrow e$$

Consider further an update with the three statements:

$$\textbf{assert}\,(d) \Leftarrow a \qquad \textbf{assert}\,(e) \Leftarrow b \qquad \textbf{assert}\,(f) \Leftarrow c$$

What is the expected result of performing such an update on such a program? The initial logic program has the following two stable models: $M_1 = \{a, c\}$ and $M_2 = \{b, c\}$. Therefore we have three possible ways of evaluating the conditions of the update statements. We can evaluate them in the intersection of all stable models, as before, corresponding to a skeptical approach; we can use the union of all stable models, corresponding to a credulous approach; or we can evaluate them for each particular stable model, corresponding to what will be referred to as a casuistic approach. Let us look at each of the three possibilities in turn for this example:

Skeptical Approach According to this approach, the intersection of all stable models is used when determining the executability of each statement, i.e. we would use the set of literals $\{c\}$ to evaluate the conditions. Consequently, only the conditions of the statement $\textbf{assert}\,(f) \Leftarrow c$ would be positively evaluated and f would be asserted in the knowledge base. The criticism levelled at this approach would be grounded on a line of argumentation based on that since the truth of c hinged on the truth of either a or b, then, if one asserts f on the basis of c, one should also expect to either assert d on the basis of a or assert e on the basis of b. In favour of this approach would be the argument according to which, since each of the stable models is a two-valued model then, in each of the possible worlds they represent, either a or b is true and, therefore, c is true in every world. Since we are only sure of the truth of c, we should only perform updates based on c, and not on a or b. According to this approach, saying that f indirectly depends on the presence of either d or e is an incorrect statement.

Credulous Approach According to this approach, the union of all stable models is used when determining the executability of each statement., i.e. we would use the set of literals $\{a, b, c\}$ to evaluate the conditions. Accordingly, the conditions of all three statements would be positively evaluated and all of d, e and f would be asserted in the knowledge base. This approach does not seem appropriate for updates. Note that in the above example, this would cause a contradiction at the next state because of the last two rules in the original program, i.e. both g and $not\, g$ would be "derivable". Since a and b cannot both be true, it seems strange that both d and e are asserted. And, on top of this, we get a contradiction that we never asked for. One advantage of this approach, also shared by the previous skeptical approach, is that the semantics assigns a single model. This does not happen with the next approach.

Casuistic Approach According to this approach, each stable model is individually considered, each of them giving rise to a (possibly) different set of commands to be executed. It solves the problems encountered in the previous approaches at the expense that each update would not produce a single knowledge base at the next state, but rather a family of them. According to this approach, if we consider the stable model $\{a, c\}$ we assert d and f. If we consider the stable model $\{b, c\}$ we assert e and f.

From the descriptions of the three possible approaches, it seems obvious that the credulous one is not appropriate for the kind of updates we want to perform and will not be further considered. Both of the remaining approaches could be used in our setting.

Throughout the remainder of this work we keep with the skeptical approach, for the following reasons:

- First and most important is that if we were to use the casuistic approach the number of knowledge bases to be considered would grow exponentially. For each knowledge base at some state s we would have to determine a set of executable commands for each of its models, producing, at the subsequent state $s+1$, one knowledge base for each model of each knowledge base at state s. Even though this could be a wise choice were our main concern to reason about updates, where it may have been advantageous to keep all possible states of the world and reason about them all, our stance is somewhat more on a pragmatic side: since one of our main goals is to use this framework to actually specify knowledge bases to be used, among others, in the context of agent systems, we consider it advantageous to define one single knowledge base after each state transition instead of requiring each agent (or knowledge base system) to keep track of an exponentially growing number of them;

- The definition of the semantics for the skeptical approach can be easily extended to the case where instead of a model we have a set of models, and instead of a set of executable commands we have a set of sets of executable commands, one for each truth valuation, i.e. we add some simplicity while keeping all the doors open for the casuistic approach.

- Historically, this was the initial option of the authors of LUPS. We say historically because in [16] Alferes et al. present an extended version of their early paper [15]. There, for reasons never fully explained, they abandon their original skeptical approach to adopt the credulous one which, as we have seen, is not appropriate to deal with this kind of updates.

The partial evaluation of the statements in SU_s and EU_{s+1} with respect to the external set of observations EO_{s+1} and current object level KB $\mathcal{P}_s$ allows us to obtain two sets of reduced statements whose conditions range only over the concurrent execution of other commands. The semantics for such partial evaluation depends on the type of conditions and is as follows:

Literals The evaluation of literals is performed as before, i.e. a conjunction of such literals $\mathbf{L}(S) = L_1, \ldots, L_k$ is evaluated to true iff $\bigoplus \mathcal{P}_s \models_{sm} L_1, \ldots, L_k$, or $\bigoplus \mathcal{P}_s \models_{sm} \mathbf{L}(S)$ for short.

Rules The evaluation of the conditions on the memorial presence or absence of rules in the object knowledge base, $\mathbf{R}(S)$, of a statement S, will be done by evaluating the corresponding auxiliary predicates $N(\_)$ in the object knowledge base. The predicate $N(r)$ is a unique identifier for rule r[3]. Intuitively, each $in(R)$ evaluates to true if the rule R has been inertially asserted in the knowledge base and not retracted since such latest assertion, or it has been non-inertially asserted during the previous state transition. Conversely, each $out(R)$ evaluates to true if the rule R has never been inertially asserted or has been inertially retracted since its latest inertial assertion, and it was not non-inertially asserted during the previous state transition, or it has been non-inertially retracted during the previous state transition. Accordingly, a condition of the form $\mathbf{R}(S) = \mathbf{in}(R_1), ..., \mathbf{in}(R_m), \mathbf{out}(R_{m+1}), ..., \mathbf{out}(R_n)$ evaluates to true, denoted by $\bigoplus \mathcal{P}_s \models_{rule} \mathbf{R}(S)$ iff $\bigoplus \mathcal{P}_s \models_{sm} N(R_1), ..., N(R_m), not\, N(R_{m+1}), ..., not\, N(R_n)$. Note that the evaluation of these conditions on rules does not depend on whether we choose the casuistic, skeptical, or credulous approaches because it is easily proved that if $\bigoplus \mathcal{P}_s \models_{sm} N(R)$ then $N(R)$ belongs to every stable model of $\mathcal{P}_s$ at state s. Similarly for $not\, N(R_n)$.

Observations The evaluation of conditions on external observations, $\mathbf{E}(S)$, of a statement S, will be done by simply checking for their presence or absence in the set EO_{s+1}. Accordingly, $\mathbf{E}(S) = \mathbf{in}(E_1), ..., \mathbf{in}(E_p), \mathbf{out}(E_{p+1}), ..., \mathbf{out}(E_q)$ evaluates to true, denoted by $EO_{s+1} \models_{obs} \mathbf{E}(S)$, iff $\{E_1, ..., E_p\} \subseteq EO_{s+1}$ and $\{E_{p+1}, ..., E_q\} \cap EO_{s+1} = \{\}$.

For a statement of the form:

$$\begin{aligned} C_0(\rho_0) \Leftarrow\ & C_1(\rho_1), ..., C_n(\rho_n), L_1, \ldots, L_k, \\ & \mathbf{R} : \mathbf{in}(R_1), ..., \mathbf{in}(R_m), \mathbf{out}(R_{m+1}), ..., \mathbf{out}(R_n), \\ & \mathbf{E} : \mathbf{in}(E_1), ..., \mathbf{in}(E_p), \mathbf{out}(E_{p+1}), ..., \mathbf{out}(E_q) \end{aligned}$$

a partial evaluated statement has the form:

$$C_0(\rho_0) \Leftarrow C_1(\rho_1), ..., C_n(\rho_n)$$

Each update program is reduced as per the following definition:

Definition 78 (Update Program Reduct) *The reduct of an update program U, with respect to a set of external observations EO and a dynamic logic program $\mathcal{P}_s$ at state s, is the set of (reduced) statements U^r, defined as follows:*

$$\begin{aligned} U^r = \{\mathbf{H}(S) \Leftarrow \mathbf{C}(S) : (\mathbf{H}(S) \Leftarrow \mathbf{C}(S), \mathbf{L}(S), \mathbf{R} : \mathbf{R}(S), \mathbf{E} : \mathbf{E}(S)) \in U \wedge \\ \bigoplus \mathcal{P}_s \models_{sm} \mathbf{L}(S) \wedge \bigoplus \mathcal{P}_s \models_{rule} \mathbf{R}(S) \wedge EO \models_{obs} \mathbf{E}(S)\Big\} \end{aligned}$$

Example 46 *Let $\mathcal{P}_s$ be a dynamic logic program at state s such that its only stable model is:*

$$M_s = \{a, not\, b, c, N(b \leftarrow a), not\, N(not\, b \leftarrow a), not\, N(a \leftarrow), ...\}$$

[3]To determine the unique identifier of a rule, we consider its head and the set of literals in its body. Accordingly, in line with the tradition of "pure" logic programming, the rules $a \leftarrow b, c$ and $a \leftarrow c, b$ are considered the same rule and would have the same identifier.

Let EO_{s+1} be the following set of external observations:

$$EO_{s+1} = \{obs\,(d)\,, obs\,(b)\,, rule(not\,b \leftarrow a), rule(b \leftarrow a)\}$$

Let U be the update program of example 45, i.e. containing the statements:

$$\begin{array}{l}
\textbf{always_assert}\,(\textbf{always_assert_event}\,(b \leftarrow d) \Leftarrow \mathbf{E} : \mathbf{in}(obs\,(d))) \Leftarrow \mathbf{E} : \mathbf{in}(obs\,(b)) \\
\textbf{always_assert}\,(R) \Leftarrow \mathbf{R} : \mathbf{out}(R), \mathbf{E} : \mathbf{in}(rule(R)) \\
\textbf{always_assert_event}\,(b \leftarrow d) \Leftarrow not\,\textbf{assert}\,(a)\,, a, not\,b \\
not\,\textbf{assert}\,(c \leftarrow d) \Leftarrow not\,b, \mathbf{E} : \mathbf{in}(obs\,(b)) \\
\textbf{assert_event}\,(a \leftarrow h) \Leftarrow not\,\textbf{assert}\,(a)\,, not\,a, b
\end{array}$$

The reduct of U, with respect to EO_{s+1} and $\bigoplus \mathcal{P}_s$, is U^r, containing the reduced statements:

$$\begin{array}{l}
\textbf{always_assert}\,(\textbf{always_assert_event}\,(b \leftarrow d) \Leftarrow \mathbf{E} : \mathbf{in}(obs\,(d))) \Leftarrow \\
\textbf{always_assert}\,(not\,b \leftarrow a) \Leftarrow \\
\textbf{always_assert_event}\,(b \leftarrow d) \Leftarrow not\,\textbf{assert}\,(a) \\
not\,\textbf{assert}\,(c \leftarrow d) \Leftarrow
\end{array}$$

which can be split into the positive (reduced) update U^{r+} containing the reduced statements

$$\begin{array}{l}
\textbf{always_assert}\,(\textbf{always_assert_event}\,(b \leftarrow d) \Leftarrow \mathbf{E} : \mathbf{in}(obs\,(d))) \Leftarrow \\
\textbf{always_assert}\,(not\,b \leftarrow a) \Leftarrow \\
\textbf{always_assert_event}\,(b \leftarrow d) \Leftarrow not\,\textbf{assert}\,(a)
\end{array}$$

and the inhibition (reduced) update U^{r-} containing the reduced statement:

$$not\,\textbf{assert}\,(c \leftarrow d) \Leftarrow$$

With a transition frame $\langle \mathcal{P}_s, \models_{sm}, SU_s, EU_{s+1}, EO_{s+1}, <, Sel(.)\rangle$, we can univocally determine SU_s^r and EU_{s+1}^r. If, instead, we had used each individual stable model of $\mathcal{P}_s$, we would obtain a pair of SU_s^r and EU_{s+1}^r for each such stable model.

5.4.2 Executable Commands

In this section we show how to combine the two sets of reduced statements, SU_s^r and EU_{s+1}^r, to determine a set of commands to be executed. To this purpose we need to establish how such a combination is to be accomplished, namely in what concerns the interaction between both updates and the inhibition commands in the statements of both updates, in line with the specified order relation.

Before we continue, we will set forth some definitions needed in the sequel, both throughout this Chapter as well as in a subsequent one. In such definitions, U^r stands for a set of reduced statements. In the following two definitions, we will included the optional construct $@X$, which has not been introduced yet. Its purpose is to allow these definitions to be reused, later on, when such construct is introduced.

Definition 79 (Rule Arguments with respect to U^r) *By the* set of rule arguments *of U^r, denoted by $Args_R(U^r)$, we mean the set of all rules appearing as arguments in the commands (and inhibition commands) of U^r, i.e.:*

$$\begin{array}{rl}
Args_R\,(U^r) = & \{Arg\,(H\,(S)) \mid Arg\,(H\,(S)) = \rho\,[@X]\,, \rho \in \mathcal{R}, S \in U^r\} \cup \\
& \cup \{Arg\,(C) \mid Arg\,(C) = \rho\,[@X]\,, \rho \in \mathcal{R}, C \in \mathbf{C}\,(S)\,, S \in U^r\}
\end{array}$$

Definition 80 (Statement Arguments with respect to U^r) *By the* set of statement arguments of U^r, *denoted by* $Args_S(U^r)$, *we mean the set of all statements appearing as arguments in the commands (and inhibition commands) of* U^r, *i.e.:*

$$Args_S(U^r) = \{Arg(H(S)) \mid Arg(H(S)) = \rho[@X], \rho \in \mathcal{S}, S \in U^r\} \cup \\ \cup \{Arg(C) \mid Arg(C) = \rho[@X], \rho \in \mathcal{S}, C \in \mathbf{C}(S), S \in U^r\}$$

Example 47 *With the set of reduced statements of Example 46, we have:*

$$Args_R(U^r) = \left\{ \begin{array}{c} not\, b \leftarrow a \\ b \leftarrow d \\ c \leftarrow d \\ a \end{array} \right\}$$

$$Args_S(U^r) = \{\textbf{always\_assert\_event}\,(b \leftarrow d) \Leftarrow \mathbf{E} : \textbf{in}(obs\,(d))\}$$

Definition 81 (Basic Rule Commands with respect to U^r) *By the set of basic rule commands, given* U^r, *we mean the set* $BasicComm_R(U^r)$ *defined as follows:*

$$BasicComm_R(U^r) = \left\{ \begin{array}{c} \textbf{assert}\,(\rho), \textbf{assert\_event}\,(\rho), \textbf{retract}\,(\rho), \\ \textbf{retract\_event}\,(\rho) : \rho \in Args_R(U^r) \end{array} \right\}$$

Definition 82 (Basic Statement Commands with respect to U^r) *By the set of basic statement commands, given* U^r, *we mean the set* $BasicComm_S(U^r)$ *defined as follows:*

$$BasicComm_S(U^r) = \{\textbf{assert}\,(\rho), \textbf{retract}\,(\rho) : \rho \in Args_S(U^r)\}$$

Definition 83 (Basic Commands with respect to U^r) *By the set of basic commands, given* U^r, *we mean the set* $BasicComm(U^r)$ *defined as follows:*

$$BasicComm(U^r) = BasicComm_R(U^r) \cup BasicComm_S(U^r)$$

Definition 84 (Persistent Commands with respect to U^r) *By the set of persistent commands, given* U^r, *we mean the set* $PerComm(U^r)$ *defined as follows:*

$$PerComm(U^r) = \left\{ \begin{array}{c} \textbf{always\_}\langle base\_comm\rangle, \textbf{once\_}\langle base\_comm\rangle : \\ : \langle base\_comm\rangle \in BasicComm(U^r) \end{array} \right\}$$

Definition 85 (Commands with respect to U^r) *By the set of commands, given* U^r, *we mean the set* $\mathcal{C}(U^r)$ *defined as follows:*

$$\mathcal{C}(U^r) = BasicComm(U^r) \cup PerComm(U^r)$$

Definition 86 (Command Language with respect to U^r) *By the command language, given* U^r, *we mean* $\mathcal{L}_{\mathcal{C}(U^r)}$, *defined as follows:*

$$\mathcal{L}(U^r) = \mathcal{C}(U^r) \cup \{not\, C(\rho) : C(\rho) \in \mathcal{C}(U^r)\}$$

Definition 87 (Assert and Retract Commands with respect to U^r) *By the set of assert (resp. retract) commands, given* U^r, *we mean the set* $AssertComm(U^r)$ *(resp.* $RetractComm(U^r)$*) defined as follows:*

$$AssertComm(U^r) = \left\{ \begin{array}{c} C(\rho) : C(\rho) = [\textbf{always\_} \mid \textbf{once\_}]\,\textbf{assert}\,[\textbf{\_event}]\,(\rho), \\ C(\rho) \in \mathcal{C}(U^r) \end{array} \right\}$$

$$RetractComm(U^r) = \left\{ \begin{array}{c} C(\rho) : C(\rho) = [\textbf{always\_} \mid \textbf{once\_}]\,\textbf{retract}\,[\textbf{\_event}]\,(\rho), \\ C(\rho) \in \mathcal{C}(U^r) \end{array} \right\}$$

Definition 88 (Corresponding Basic Command) *Let* $C(\rho) = [X\_]Y(\rho)$ *be a command such that* $Y(\rho)$ *is a basic command. Then, the basic command of* $C(\rho)$*, denoted by* $Basic(C(\rho))$*, is* $Y(\rho)$*.*

Since such combination of the reduced statements will be achieved in a manner similar to logic program updates, we start with a preliminary definition for converting sets of reduced statements into logic programs.

Definition 89 (Corresponding Logic Program) *Let* U^r *be a set of reduced statements. The logic program corresponding to* U^r *is* U^**, written in the language* $\mathcal{L}(U^r)$ *defined as follows:*

$$U^* = \{\mathbf{H}(S) \leftarrow \mathbf{C}(S) \mid S \in U^r\}$$

Example 48 *Consider the two sets of reduced statements,* U^{r+} *and* U^{r-}*, of Example 46. The corresponding logic programs are:*

$$U^{*+} = \left\{ \begin{array}{l} \textbf{always\_assert}\,(\textbf{always\_assert\_event}\,(b \leftarrow d) \Leftarrow \mathbf{E} : \mathbf{in}(obs\,(d))) \leftarrow \\ \textbf{always\_assert}\,(not\,b \leftarrow a) \leftarrow \\ \textbf{always\_assert\_event}\,(b \leftarrow d) \leftarrow not\,\textbf{assert}\,(a) \end{array} \right\}$$

$$U^{*-} = \{not\,\textbf{assert}\,(c \leftarrow d) \leftarrow\}$$

With a transition frame $\langle \mathcal{P}_s, \models_{sm}, SU_s, EU_{s+1}, EO_{s+1}, <, Sel(.)\rangle$, we can univocally determine SU_s^{*+}, SU_s^{*-}, EU_{s+1}^{*+} and EU_{s+1}^{*-}. We use W_{s+1} to denote the set of such four programs, i.e. $W_{s+1} = \{SU_s^{*+}, SU_s^{*-}, EU_{s+1}^{*+}, EU_{s+1}^{*-}\}$. Again, if instead, we had used each individual stable model of $\mathcal{P}_s$, we would obtain a W_{s+1} for each such stable model. We also assume that the order $<$ will carry over to the programs in W_{s+1}. Also, since after translating the sets of reduced statements into logic programs we will no longer deal with the former, we will often use U^* as argument, when using Definitions 79-87, instead of U^r. Accordingly, for example, instead of $BasicComm(U^r)$ we will write $BasicComm(U^*)$.

Since we will be dealing with interpretations and models of such logic programs, for each transition frame, we define its language, as being $\mathcal{L}(SU_s^* \cup EU_{s+1}^*)$.

Over the language $\mathcal{L}(SU_s^* \cup EU_{s+1}^*)$, the notion of interpretation is defined as for logic programs, i.e. an interpretation in the language $\mathcal{L}(SU_s^* \cup EU_{s+1}^*)$ is any set I_Δ such that

$$I_\Delta = \Delta \cup \{not\,C(\rho) : C(\rho) \in \mathcal{C}(SU_s^* \cup EU_{s+1}^*) \wedge C(\rho) \notin \Delta\}$$

where Δ is a set of commands such that $\Delta \subseteq \mathcal{C}(SU_s^* \cup EU_{s+1}^*)$. We say that I_Δ is the command interpretation (uniquely) corresponding to Δ, given the underlying language $\mathcal{C}(SU_s^* \cup EU_{s+1}^*)$.

Definition 90 (Coherent Set of Commands) *A set of commands* Δ *is coherent iff for any* ρ*:*

$$\{[\textbf{always\_} \mid \textbf{once\_}]\,\textbf{assert}\,[\textbf{\_event}]\,(\rho), [\textbf{always\_} \mid \textbf{once\_}]\,\textbf{retract}\,[\textbf{\_event}]\,(\rho)\} \nsubseteq \Delta$$

An interpretation I_Δ *is coherent if and only if it corresponds to a coherent set of commands.*

With these preliminary definitions in hand, we can now tackle the main problem of combining the self and external updates to determine the set of commands to be executed. This will be attained in a manner similar to the one employed to determine the stable models of a dynamic logic program. As a result, some rules will be rejected by other rules in case there is a conflict. But now the notion of conflicting rules cannot be the same as for DLP, where two rules were conflicting if $H(R) = not\, H(R)$. This is so because we now have propositions in the heads of rules that should be treated as conflicting, but are not simply related as one being the default negation of the other. For example, if a set of inhibition statements is to have higher priority than a set of positive statements, then we want a statement in the former, whose head is *not* **assert** (ρ), to reject a statement in the latter, whose head is **always_assert** (ρ). Recall that the persistent statement denoted by the **always_assert** keyword corresponds to the basic assertion update operation, denoted by the keyword **assert**, and should therefore be rejected. Note, however, that this rejection is only at the execution of the command level. Being rejected at this level does not mean that the statement will not be part of the self update of the next state. This would only be the case if there was a retraction command for the statement. In what concerns the rejection of rules to determine the sets of executable commands, we define a notion of *conflicting commands*, denoted by the symbol $\dot{\bowtie}$. We write $C_1(\rho)\,\dot{\bowtie}\,C_2(\rho)$ to denote that commands $C_1(\rho)$ and $C_2(\rho)$ are conflicting. If $C_1(\rho)\,\dot{\bowtie}\,C_2(\rho)$ then $C_2(\rho)\,\dot{\bowtie}\,C_1(\rho)$. Any assertion and retraction commands with the same argument are mutually conflicting, i.e.:

$$[\textbf{always\_} \mid \textbf{once\_}]\,\textbf{assert}\,[\textbf{\_event}]\,(\rho) \quad \dot{\bowtie} \quad [\textbf{always\_} \mid \textbf{once\_}]\,\textbf{retract}\,[\textbf{\_event}]\,(\rho)$$

It is a condition for conflict between commands that they have the same argument. Also, any command conflicts with the inhibition command of its basic update operation. Since we have four basic update operations, they correspond to the following cases:

$$\begin{array}{lcl}
[\textbf{always_} \mid \textbf{once_}]\,\textbf{assert}\,(\rho) & \dot{\bowtie} & not\,\textbf{assert}\,(\rho) \\
[\textbf{always_} \mid \textbf{once_}]\,\textbf{assert_event}\,(\rho) & \dot{\bowtie} & not\,\textbf{assert_event}\,(\rho) \\
[\textbf{always_} \mid \textbf{once_}]\,\textbf{retract}\,(\rho) & \dot{\bowtie} & not\,\textbf{retract}\,(\rho) \\
[\textbf{always_} \mid \textbf{once_}]\,\textbf{retract_event}\,(\rho) & \dot{\bowtie} & not\,\textbf{retract_event}\,(\rho)
\end{array}$$

With this notion of conflicting commands, the notion of rejected rules follows, as expected:

Definition 91 (Rejected Rules) *Let W be a set of logic programs corresponding to a set of reduced statements. Let $<$ be a partial order on the elements of W, and let Δ a set of commands. The set of rejected rules given $W, <$ and Δ is:*

$$Rejected\,(W, <, \Delta) = \left\{ \begin{array}{c} r : r \in U, U \in W, \exists r' \in U', U' \in W, H(r)\,\dot{\bowtie}\,H(r'), \\ U < U', I_\Delta \models B(r'), r' \notin Rejected\,(W, <, \Delta) \end{array} \right\}$$

Proposition 64 *Let W be a set of logic programs corresponding to a set of reduced statements. Let $<$ be a partial order on the elements of W, and let Δ a set of commands. The set $Rejected\,(W, <, \Delta)$ always exists and is unique.*

Proof. *The algorithm:*

Input: $W, \Delta, <$
Output: $Rejected\,(W, <, \Delta)$
begin
$Rejected\,(W, <, \Delta) := \{\}$
repeat
  $P :=$ *select a maximal element of* W
  $W := W - \{P\}$
  for every $U \in W$ ***do***
    $Dif := \{r : r \in U, \exists r' \in P, U < P, H(r) \bowtie H(r'), I_\Delta \models B(r')\}$
    $U := U - Dif$
    $Rejected\,(W, <, \Delta) := Rejected\,(W, <, \Delta) \cup Dif$
until $W = \{\}$
return $Rejected\,(W, <, \Delta)$
end

---

can be used to compute the set $Rejected\,(W, <, \Delta)$. ■

With a transition frame $\langle \mathcal{P}_s, \models_{sm}, SU_s, EU_{s+1}, EO_{s+1}, <, Sel(.)\rangle$ we have that $W = W_{s+1} = \{SU_s^{*+}, SU_s^{*-}, EU_{s+1}^{*+}, EU_{s+1}^{*-}\}$.

The reader may have noticed that, unlike for DLP, we require that any rule, to reject another one, is not itself rejected. To show why this is a desirable behaviour, suppose we have the following logic programs: $SU_s^{*+} = \{\mathbf{assert}(a \leftarrow) \leftarrow\}$, $SU_s^{*-} = \{not\,\mathbf{retract}(a \leftarrow) \leftarrow\}$, and $EU_{s+1}^{*+} = \{\mathbf{retract}(a \leftarrow) \leftarrow\}$, together with an order such that $SU_s^{*+} < EU_{s+1}^{*+} < SU_s^{*-}$. Since the command $\mathbf{retract}(a \leftarrow) \leftarrow$ is inhibited by the command $not\,\mathbf{retract}(a \leftarrow) \leftarrow$, there is no reason not to execute the command $\mathbf{assert}(a \leftarrow)$ and effectively assert $a \leftarrow$ in the knowledge state. The reader may see some similarity between this and the case of DLP with strong negation, inasmuch as a retraction command is in conflict with an assertion command the same way as an atom a is conflict with a strongly negated $-a$, but the outcome is different. The reason for this is that in DLP there is a notion of state transition implicit between two different programs whereas in this situation we are "statically" determining a set of commands to be executed to determine the next state. If we have what could be seen as the "DLP with strong negation" equivalent to this scenario, i.e. $P_1 = \{a \leftarrow\}$, $P_2 = \{-a \leftarrow\}$ and $P_3 = \{not\ -a \leftarrow\}$, at state 3, atom a would not be true. This is so because the rule of P_3 rejects that of P_2. If $a =$ "*the_train_is_approaching*", then at state 1 we know that the train is approaching; at state 2, possibly after listening and looking both ways, we know that the train is not approaching; then, at state 3, we say that we no longer know that the train is not approaching: should we conclude that, at state 3, the train is approaching? Clearly not. We should simply conclude that it cannot be assumed that the train is approaching and it cannot be assumed that the train is not approaching. When we deal with commands, we need to recall that inhibition commands serve to inhibit other commands. These inhibited commands should not only be inhibited from executing but also from rejecting other commands. To sum up, the way the rejection of rules, and the entire process of determining executable commands, is *only similar*, and not equal to DLP. Here we need to require that a rule (statement) to be able to reject another one must itself not be rejected.

Whenever some update command depends on any of the four basic update operations, to be executed, i.e. whenever the command depends on any of **assert**(ρ), **assert_event**(ρ), **retract**(ρ) or **retract_event**(ρ), it should be executed if any of the commands [**always_** | **once_**] **assert**(ρ), [**always_** | **once_**] **assert_event**(ρ) , [**always_** | **once_**] **retract**(ρ) or [**always_** | **once_**] **retract_event**(ρ), respectively, is also executed (assuming, of course, that the remaining conditions in the command also hold) . The following set of rules, Ω, ensure this behaviour. We call them subsumption rules because they establish that any persistent command subsumes its corresponding basic command.

Definition 92 (Subsumption Rules) *Let U^* be a logic program corresponding to a set of reduced statements. The set of* subsumption rules, *given U^*, is:*

$$\Omega(U^*) = \{Base(C(\rho)) \leftarrow C(\rho) : C(\rho) \in PerComm(U^*)\}$$

To ensure coherence of the models, we define the coherence rules:

Definition 93 (Coherence Rules) *Let U^* be a logic program corresponding to a set of reduced statements. The set of* coherence rules, *given U^*, is:*

$$\begin{aligned} Coh(U^*) = & \left\{ \begin{array}{c} not\, C(\rho) \leftarrow C'(\rho) : C(\rho) \in AssertComm(U^*), \\ C'(\rho) \in RetractComm(U^*) \end{array} \right\} \cup \\ & \cup \left\{ \begin{array}{c} not\, C(\rho) \leftarrow C'(\rho) : C(\rho) \in RetractComm(U^*), \\ C'(\rho) \in AssertComm(U^*) \end{array} \right\} \end{aligned}$$

where $C(\rho), C'(\rho) \in BasicComm(U^*)$.

Finally we define, as for DLP, the set of defaults.

Definition 94 (Default Rules) *Let U^* be the logic program corresponding to a set of reduced statements. Let $\Delta \subseteq \mathcal{C}(U^*)$ be a set of commands. The set of* default rules, *given U^* and Δ, is:*

$$\begin{aligned} Default(U^*, \Delta) = & \left\{ \begin{array}{c} not\, C(\rho) \leftarrow: \nexists (C'(\rho) \leftarrow Cond) \in U^*, I_\Delta \models Cond, \\ C(\rho) \in \mathcal{C}(U^*), Basic(C'(\rho)) = C(\rho) \end{array} \right\} \cup \\ & \cup \left\{ \begin{array}{c} not\, C(\rho) \leftarrow: \nexists (C(\rho) \leftarrow Cond) \in U^*, I_\Delta \models Cond, \\ C(\rho) \in PerComm(U^*) \end{array} \right\} \end{aligned}$$

The default rules simply state that the default of a command $C(\rho)$ i.e. $not\, C(\rho)$, should be assumed if there is no rule, with a true body, for command $C(\rho)$ or any command that subsumes it.

Finally we present the notion of executable commands:

Definition 95 (Executable Commands) *Let W be a set of logic programs corresponding to a set of reduced statements. Let $<$ be a partial order on the elements of W. A coherent set of commands Δ is a set of* executable commands *given W and $<$ iff this condition holds:*

$$I_\Delta = least(\mathcal{W}^* - Rejected(W, <, \Delta) \cup Common(\mathcal{W}^*, \Delta))$$

where

$$\mathcal{W}^* = \bigcup_{U^* \in W} U^*$$

$$Common\,(\mathcal{W}^*, \Delta) = \Omega\,(\mathcal{W}^*) \cup Coh\,(\mathcal{W}^*) \cup Default\,(\mathcal{W}^*, \Delta)$$

If W contains the logic program corresponding to the self update at state s and the external update at state $s+1$, and $<$ is the order relating them, in some transition frame TF_s, we say that Δ is a set of executable commands of TF_s or, if TF_s is implicit, we simply say that Δ is a set of executable commands at state s.

There follows an example to show how different order relations affect the set of executable commands:

Example 49 *Let $TF_s = \langle \mathcal{P}_s, \models_{sm}, SU_s, EU_{s+1}, EO_{s+1}, <, Sel(.) \rangle$ be a transition frame at state s. Let $SU_s^* = SU_s^{*+} \cup SU_s^{*-}$ and $EU_{s+1}^* = EU_{s+1}^{*+} \cup EU_{s+1}^{*-}$ be the corresponding logic programs of the two sets of reduced statements such that:*

$$SU_s^{*+} = \left\{ \begin{array}{l} r_1 : \textbf{always\_assert}\,(\textbf{always\_assert\_event}\,(b \leftarrow d) \Leftarrow \textbf{E} : \textbf{in}(obs\,(d))) \leftarrow \\ r_2 : \textbf{always\_assert}\,(not\, b \leftarrow a) \leftarrow \\ r_3 : \textbf{always\_assert\_event}\,(b \leftarrow d) \leftarrow not\, \textbf{assert}\,(a) \end{array} \right\}$$

$$SU_s^{*-} = \left\{ \; r_4 : not\, \textbf{assert}\,(c \leftarrow d) \leftarrow \; \right\}$$

$$EU_{s+1}^{*+} = \left\{ \begin{array}{l} r_5 : \textbf{always\_retract}\,(not\, b \leftarrow a) \leftarrow not\, \textbf{assert}\,(c \leftarrow d) \\ r_6 : \textbf{always\_assert}\,(c \leftarrow d) \leftarrow \end{array} \right\}$$

$$EU_{s+1}^{*-} = \left\{ \begin{array}{l} r_7 : not\, \textbf{assert\_event}\,(b \leftarrow d) \leftarrow \\ r_8 : not\, \textbf{assert}\,(not\, b \leftarrow a) \leftarrow not\, \textbf{assert}\,(c \leftarrow d) \end{array} \right\}$$

We now determine the sets of executable commands according to some distinct order relations:

SU < EU : *According to this operation mode, all external updates prevail over the self updating ones. This corresponds to the order: $SU_s^{*+} < EU_{s+1}^{*+}$, $SU_s^{*-} < EU_{s+1}^{*-}$, $SU_s^{*+} < EU_{s+1}^{*-}$, $SU_s^{*-} < EU_{s+1}^{*+}$. The only set of executable commands is:*

$$\Delta_{s+1} = \left\{ \begin{array}{c} [\textbf{always\_}]\,\textbf{assert}\,(c \leftarrow d)\,; [\textbf{always\_}]\,\textbf{assert}\,(not\, b \leftarrow a)\,; \\ [\textbf{always\_}]\,\textbf{assert}\,(\textbf{always\_assert\_event}\,(b \leftarrow d) \Leftarrow \textbf{E} : \textbf{in}(obs\,(d))) \end{array} \right\}$$

The reader can check that the set $Rejected\,(W_{s+1}, <, \Delta_{s+1})$ contains the following rules:

$$Rejected\,(W_{s+1}, <, \Delta_{s+1}) = \left\{ \begin{array}{ll} r_3 : & \textbf{always\_assert\_event}\,(b \leftarrow d) \leftarrow not\, \textbf{assert}\,(a) \\ r_4 : & not\, \textbf{assert}\,(c \leftarrow d) \leftarrow \end{array} \right\}$$

and that, indeed,

$$I_{\Delta_{s+1}} = least\left(\mathcal{W}_{s+1}^* - Rejected\,(W_{s+1}, <, \Delta_{s+1}) \cup Common\left(\mathcal{W}_{s+1}^*, \Delta_{s+1}\right)\right)$$

EU < SU : *According to this operation mode, all self updates prevail over the external ones. This corresponds to the order: $SU_s^{*+} > EU_{s+1}^{*+}$, $SU_s^{*-} > EU_{s+1}^{*-}$, $SU_s^{*+} > EU_{s+1}^{*-}$, $SU_s^{*-} > EU_{s+1}^{*+}$. The only set of executable commands is:*

$$\Delta_{s+1} = \left\{ \begin{array}{c} [\textbf{always\_}]\,\textbf{assert}\,(not\, b \leftarrow a)\,; \textbf{always\_assert\_event}\,(b \leftarrow d) \\ [\textbf{always\_}]\,\textbf{assert}\,(\textbf{always\_assert\_event}\,(b \leftarrow d) \Leftarrow \textbf{E} : \textbf{in}(obs\,(d))) \end{array} \right\}$$

The reader can check that the set $Rejected\,(W_{s+1}, <, \Delta_{s+1})$ *contains the rules:*

$$\begin{aligned} r_5 &: \mathbf{always\_retract}\,(not\, b \leftarrow a) \leftarrow not\,\mathbf{assert}\,(c \leftarrow d) \\ r_6 &: \mathbf{always\_assert}\,(c \leftarrow d) \leftarrow \\ r_7 &: not\,\mathbf{assert\_event}\,(b \leftarrow d) \leftarrow \\ r_8 &: not\,\mathbf{assert}\,(not\, b \leftarrow a) \leftarrow not\,\mathbf{assert}\,(c \leftarrow d) \end{aligned}$$

and that, indeed,

$$I_{\Delta_{s+1}} = least\left(\mathcal{W}^*_{s+1} - Rejected\,(W_{s+1}, <, \Delta_{s+1}) \cup Common\left(\mathcal{W}^*_{s+1}, \Delta_{s+1}\right)\right)$$

$\mathbf{U}^- > \mathbf{U}^+$: *According to this operation mode, all inhibition commands prevail over any other commands. There is no distinction between self and external updates. This corresponds to the order:* $SU^{*-}_s > EU^{*+}_{s+1}$, $SU^{*-}_s > SU^{*+}_s$, $EU^{*-}_{s+1} > EU^{*+}_{s+1}$, $EU^{*-}_{s+1} > SU^{*+}_s$. *The only set of executable commands is:*

$$\Delta_{s+1} = \left\{ \begin{array}{c} [\mathbf{always\_}]\,\mathbf{assert}\,(\mathbf{always\_assert\_event}\,(b \leftarrow d) \Leftarrow \mathbf{E} : \mathbf{in}(obs\,(d))) \\ [\mathbf{always\_}]\,\mathbf{retract}\,(not\, b \leftarrow a) \end{array} \right\}$$

The reader can check that the set $Rejected\,(W_{s+1}, <, \Delta_{s+1})$ *contains the rules:*

$$\begin{aligned} r_2 &: \mathbf{always\_assert}\,(not\, b \leftarrow a) \leftarrow \\ r_3 &: \mathbf{always\_assert\_event}\,(b \leftarrow d) \leftarrow not\,\mathbf{assert}\,(a) \\ r_6 &: \mathbf{always\_assert}\,(c \leftarrow d) \leftarrow \end{aligned}$$

and that, indeed,

$$I_{\Delta_{s+1}} = least\left(\mathcal{W}^*_{s+1} - Rejected\,(W_{s+1}, <, \Delta_{s+1}) \cup Common\left(\mathcal{W}^*_{s+1}, \Delta_{s+1}\right)\right)$$

We will leave to the reader checking the outcome of other possible order relations.

Throughout the remainder of this work, in particular when illustrating with examples, and unless otherwise stated, we will be using the operation mode according to which all inhibition commands prevail over all other commands. This amounts to a more skeptical approach to combining self and external updates whereby we "prefer" not to perform an update operation if there is an inhibition command of any nature, i.e. originating in either the self or external updates. As to the order relation between the positive external and self update statements, it will be explicitly stated whenever necessary. This order relation between positive statements affects the set of executable commands when an assertion command is present in one update and a corresponding retraction command is present in the other update, since one can reject the other if there is an ordering between both.

In the previous example we did not show the operation mode corresponding to the order $U^- < U^+$, i.e. when the positive statements prevail over the inhibition ones. This mode is not particularly interesting because the executable commands are simply the same, as if no inhibition commands were present. Formally:

Proposition 65 *Let* $TF_s = \langle \mathcal{P}_s, \models, SU_s, EU_{s+1}, EO_{s+1}, <, Sel(.)\rangle$ *be an arbitrary transition frame at state s, such that the order relation contains* $SU^-_s < EU^+_{s+1}$, $SU^-_s < SU^+_s$, $EU^-_{s+1} < EU^+_{s+1}$ *and* $EU^-_{s+1} < SU^+_s$. *Then, a set of commands* Δ_{s+1} *is a set of* executable commands *at state s of* TF_s *iff* Δ_{s+1} *is a set of* executable commands *at state s of* $TF'_s = \langle \mathcal{P}_s, \models, SU_s^+, EU_{s+1}^+, EO_{s+1}, <, Sel(.) \rangle$.

Proof. *First note that although the languages of both frames are different, this does not constitute a problem. The set of commands* Δ_{s+1} *will correspond to different interpretations* $I_{\Delta_{s+1}}$ *and* $I'_{\Delta_{s+1}}$ *depending on which frame* TF_s *and* TF'_s*, respectively, we are considering. Furthermore we have that* $I_{\Delta_{s+1}} = I'_{\Delta_{s+1}} \cup \{not\, C(\rho) : C(\rho) \in \mathcal{C}(\mathcal{W}^*_{s+1}) - \mathcal{C}(\mathcal{W}'^*_{s+1})\}$. *To simplify, without loss of generality, let us assume that both languages are equal and coincide with the one generated by* $\mathcal{C}(\mathcal{W}^*_{s+1})$.

($\Longrightarrow$) *Let* Δ_{s+1} *be a set of executable commands of* TF_s*. Then,*

$$I_{\Delta_{s+1}} = least\left(\mathcal{W}^*_{s+1} - Rejected\left(W_{s+1}, <, \Delta_{s+1}\right) \cup Common\left(\mathcal{W}^*_{s+1}, \Delta_{s+1}\right)\right)$$

First note that $Common\left(\mathcal{W}^*_{s+1}, \Delta_{s+1}\right) = Common\left(\mathcal{W}'^*_{s+1}, \Delta_{s+1}\right)$ *because we are assuming the same language. Denote by* $Inhib\left(W_{s+1}, <, \Delta_{s+1}\right) \subseteq Rejected\left(W_{s+1}, <, \Delta_{s+1}\right)$ *the set of rules r such that* $h(r) = not\, C$*, i.e.* $Inhib\left(W_{s+1}, <, \Delta_{s+1}\right) = Rejected\left(W_{s+1}, <, \Delta_{s+1}\right) \cap \left(EU^{*-}_{s+1} \cup SU^{*-}_s\right)$. *Note that the other remaining rules that belong to the set* $Rejected\left(W_{s+1}, <, \Delta_{s+1}\right)$ *are precisely those rejected in frame* TF'_s*, i.e.* $Rejected\left(W_{s+1}, <, \Delta_{s+1}\right) = Rejected\left(W'_{s+1}, <, \Delta_{s+1}\right) \cup Inhib\left(W_{s+1}, <, \Delta_{s+1}\right)$. *Then, the previous equation can be rewritten as:*

$$I_{\Delta_{s+1}} = least\left(\begin{array}{c}\left(SU^{*+}_s \cup EU^{*+}_{s+1} - Rejected\left(W'_{s+1}, <, \Delta_{s+1}\right)\right) \cup \\ \left(SU^{*-}_s \cup EU^{*-}_{s+1} - Inhib\left(W_{s+1}, <, \Delta_{s+1}\right)\right) \cup Common\left(\mathcal{W}'^*_{s+1}, \Delta_{s+1}\right)\end{array}\right)$$

if we analyze the set of rules $SU^{*-}_s \cup EU^{*-}_{s+1} - Inhib\left(W_{s+1}, <, \Delta_{s+1}\right)$ *we can see that every rule* $r = not\, C(\rho) \leftarrow \mathbf{C}$ *in it, shares the property that* $\nexists r' \in \left(SU^{*+}_s \cup EU^{*+}_{s+1} - Rejected\left(W'_{s+1}, <, \Delta_{s+1}\right)\right)$ *such that* $H(r') = C(\rho)$ *and* $I_\Delta \models B(r')$*. But if this is the case, then there are rules in* $Common\left(\mathcal{W}'^*_{s+1}, \Delta_{s+1}\right)$ *that, for every such* $C(\rho)$*, will allow the derivation of* $not\, C(\rho)$ *when determining the least model in the equation above. We can thus remove those rules in the previous equation to obtain:*

$$I_{\Delta_{s+1}} = least\left(\mathcal{W}'^*_{s+1} - Rejected\left(W'_{s+1}, <, \Delta_{s+1}\right) \cup Common\left(\mathcal{W}'^*_{s+1}, \Delta_{s+1}\right)\right)$$

Which is the fixed point condition for Δ_{s+1} *being a set of executable commands of* TF'_s*. The proof in the opposite direction is analogous and is omitted.* ■

Note that the previous proposition is also valid if we add an order between the positive self and external updates.

In general we may have more than one Δ_{s+1}, or no Δ_{s+1} at all. As in [75] we assume a selection function $Sel(.)$ that returns one set of executable commands Δ_{s+1}. If there are no sets of executable commands, the selection function $Sel(.)$ returns the set $\{\mathbf{assert}(\bot_{s+1})\}$, where $\bot_{s+1}$ is a reserved proposition that will be asserted in the KB to signal that no executable set of commands was possible, and so be easily filtered out if necessary.

If there are no statements with command conditions in both the self and external updates, then determining the set of executable commands becomes quite simpler, given the set of reduced statements. In such cases, if a set of commands exists it is unique and can be determined by the following algorithm. If a set of executable commands does not exist, the algorithm returns $\{\mathbf{assert}(\bot_{s+1})\}$.

Input: $SU_s^{r+}, EU_{s+1}^{r+}, SU_s^{r-}, EU_{s+1}^{r-}, <$
Output: Δ_{s+1}
begin
$\Delta_{s+1} := \{\}$
$W := \{SU_s^{r+}, EU_{s+1}^{r+}, SU_s^{r-}, EU_{s+1}^{r-}\}$
repeat
  $P :=$ select a maximal element of W
  $W := W - \{P\}$
  for every $U \in W$ **do**
    $U := U - \{s \in U : \exists [not]\, C(\rho) \in P, U < P, [not]\, C(\rho) \dot{\bowtie} H(s)\}$
  $\Delta_{s+1} := \Delta_{s+1} \cup \{[not]\, C(\rho) : [not]\, C(\rho) \Leftarrow\in P\}$
  if Δ_{s+1} is not coherent **then return** $\{$**assert** $(\bot_{s+1})\}$
until $W = \{\}$
$\Delta_{s+1} := \Delta_{s+1} \cup \{Base(C)(\rho) : C(\rho) \in \Delta_{s+1}\}$
return Δ_{s+1}
end

Proposition 66 *Let* $TF_s = \langle \bigoplus \mathcal{P}_s, \models, SU_s, EU_{s+1}, EO_{s+1}, <, Sel(.)\rangle$ *be an arbitrary transition frame at state s, such that for every statement in* SU_s *and* EU_{s+1} *does not contain any command conditions. Then the previous algorithm returns the unique set of executable commands if it exists, and otherwise returns* $\{$**assert** $(\bot_{s+1})\}$.

Proof. (Sketch) *Since this is almost obvious, we will just appeal to the intuition of the reader. Of the common rules necessary to check whether a coherent set of commands is an executable set of commands,* $\Omega(\mathcal{W}^*)$ *guarantees that all subsumed commands belong to* Δ_{s+1} *and that any command that depends on a command that is subsumed by another command that is also executed, is also executed. This last part is irrelevant because we don't have command conditions. The first part is ensured by the last step of the algorithm, before returning. As for the coherence rules,* $Coh(\mathcal{W}^*)$*, they ensure coherence, which is also explicitly checked by the algorithm, at every step. The default rules* $Default(\mathcal{W}^*, \Delta)$*, only serve the purpose of allowing the verification of the conditions in other rules which, in our case, are not needed. We are left with the facts in* $SU_s^{r+}, EU_{s+1}^{r+}, SU_s^{r-}$ *and* EU_{s+1}^{r-}*. It is quite trivial to see that adding non-rejected facts, from the maximal set down, according to the order relation, is equivalent to obtaining the least* $(\mathcal{W}^* - Rejected(W_{s+1}, <, \Delta_{s+1}))$*. Just note that in the definition of* $Rejected(W_{s+1}, <, \Delta_{s+1})$

$$Rejected(W_{s+1}, <, \Delta_{s+1}) = \left\{ \begin{array}{c} r : r \in U \in W_{s+1}, \exists r' \in U' \in W_{s+1}, H(r) \dot{\bowtie} H(r'), \\ U < U', I_{\Delta_{s+1}} \models B(r'), r' \notin Rejected(W_{s+1}, <, \Delta_{s+1}) \end{array} \right\}$$

the condition $r' \notin Rejected(W_{s+1}, <, \Delta_{s+1})$ *is achieved by always choosing a maximal element to perform the rejections. The condition* $I_{\Delta_{s+1}} \models B(r')$ *is trivially verified. The other conditions amount to the ones checked by the algorithm.* ■

As when determining the stable models of a Dynamic Logic Program, the sets of executable commands can also be determined by calculating the stable models of a GLP obtained by a suitable syntactical transformation of SU_s^* and U_{s+1}^*, which we now present:

Definition 96 (Executable Commands Transformation) *Consider the transition frame at state s* $TF_s = \langle \mathcal{P}_s, \models_{sm}, SU_s, EU_{s+1}, EO_{s+1}, <, Sel(.)\rangle$. *The executable command program at state s is the logic program consisting of the following rules:*

(RS) Rewritten self update clauses

$$C(\rho)_{SU^+} \leftarrow C_1(\rho_1), ..., C_m(\rho_m), C_{m+1}(\rho_{m+1})^-, ..., C_n(\rho_n)^-$$
$$C(\rho)_{SU^-} \leftarrow C_1(\rho_1), ..., C_m(\rho_m), C_{m+1}(\rho_{m+1})^-, ..., C_n(\rho_n)^-$$

for any clause:

$$C(\rho) \leftarrow C_1(\rho_1), ..., C_m(\rho_m), not\, C_{m+1}(\rho_{m+1}), ..., not\, C_n(\rho_n)$$

respectively,

$$not\, C(\rho) \leftarrow C_1(\rho_1), ..., C_m(\rho_m), not\, C_{m+1}(\rho_{m+1}), ..., not\, C_n(\rho_n)$$

in the program SU_s^*. *The rewritten self update rules encode the specifications originated in the self update program.*

(RU) Rewritten external update clauses:

$$C(\rho)_{EU^+} \leftarrow C_1(\rho_1), ..., C_m(\rho_m), C_{m+1}(\rho_{m+1})^-, ..., C_n(\rho_n)^-$$
$$C(\rho)_{EU^-} \leftarrow C_1(\rho_1), ..., C_m(\rho_m), C_{m+1}(\rho_{m+1})^-, ..., C_n(\rho_n)^-$$

for any clause:

$$C(\rho) \leftarrow C_1(\rho_1), ..., C_m(\rho_m), not\, C_{m+1}(\rho_{m+1}), ..., not\, C_n(\rho_n)$$

respectively,

$$not\, C(\rho) \leftarrow C_1(\rho_1), ..., C_m(\rho_m), not\, C_{m+1}(\rho_{m+1}), ..., not\, C_n(\rho_n)$$

in the program EU_{s+1}^*. *The rewritten external update rules encode the specifications originated in the external update program.*

(DR) Defining rules:

$$C(\rho) \leftarrow C(\rho)_{EU^+},\ not\, reject(C(\rho)_{EU^+})$$
$$C(\rho) \leftarrow C(\rho)_{SU^+},\ not\, reject(C(\rho)_{SU^+})$$
$$C(\rho)^- \leftarrow C(\rho)_{EU^-},\ not\, reject(C(\rho)_{EU^-})$$
$$C(\rho)^- \leftarrow C(\rho)_{SU^-},\ not\, reject(C(\rho)_{SU^-})$$

for all commands $\mathcal{C}(\mathcal{W}_{s+1}^*)$. *The defining rules state that each command should contribute to the set of executable commands if it can be concluded by a rule in one of the programs and is not rejected by another command.*

(OR) Order Rules

$$less(a, b) \leftarrow$$
$$less(X, Y) \leftarrow less(X, Z), less(Z, Y)$$

for all $a, b \in W_s$ *and* $a < b$. *The order rules simply state the order relation and define its transitive closure.*

(RR) Rejection rules:

$$reject(C(\rho)_{X^+}) \leftarrow C(\rho)_{Y^-}, less(X^+, Y^-), not\, reject(C(\rho)_{Y^-})$$
$$reject(C(\rho)_{X^-}) \leftarrow C(\rho)_{Y^+}, less(X^-, Y^+), not\, reject(C(\rho)_{Y^+})$$
$$reject(C_{assert}(\rho)_{X^+}) \leftarrow C_{retract}(\rho)_{Y^+}, less(X^+, Y^+), not\, reject(C_{retract}(\rho)_{Y^+})$$
$$reject(C_{retract}(\rho)_{X^+}) \leftarrow C_{assert}(\rho)_{Y^+}, less(X^+, Y^+), not\, reject(C_{retract}(\rho)_{Y^+})$$

for all $X, Y \in \{SU, EU\}$ *and all commands* $C_{assert}(\rho) \in AssertComm(\mathcal{W}^*_{s+1})$, $C(\rho) \in \mathcal{C}(\mathcal{W}^*_{s+1})$ *and* $C_{retract}(\rho) \in RetractComm(\mathcal{W}^*_{s+1})$. *The rejection rules encode the conditions under which a command can reject another one. In particular, the first two rules say that any command (resp. inhibition command) can reject the corresponding inhibition command (resp. command) if it has not been rejected and originates in a program of higher priority order. The last two rules state that any retraction (resp. assertion) command can reject the corresponding assertion (resp. retraction) command if it has not been rejected and originates in a program of higher priority order.*

(SubR) Subsumption Rules:

$$Basic(C(\rho)) \leftarrow C(\rho)$$

for all $C(\rho) \in PerComm(\mathcal{W}^*_{s+1})$. *The subsumption rules correspond to the previously defined* $\Omega(\mathcal{W}^*_{s+1})$ *rules.*

(CohR) Coherence Rules

$$not\, C(\rho)^- \leftarrow C'(\rho)$$

for all $C(\rho) \in AssertComm(\mathcal{W}^*_{s+1}), C'(\rho) \in RetractComm(\mathcal{W}^*_{s+1})$, *and all* $C(\rho) \in RetractComm(\mathcal{W}^*_{s+1}), C'(\rho) \in AssertComm(\mathcal{W}^*_{s+1})$, *and such that* $C(\rho), C'(\rho) \in BasicComm(U^*)$. *The coherence rules correspond to the previously defined* $Coh(\mathcal{W}^*_{s+1})$ *rules and ensure the coherence of every stable model.*

(DR) Default rules:

$$C(\rho)^- \leftarrow not\, C'(\rho)_{SU^+}, not\, C''(\rho)_{EU^+}$$
$$C'''(\rho)^- \leftarrow not\, C'''(\rho)_{SU^+}, not\, C'''(\rho)_{EU^+}$$
$$not\, C(\rho) \leftarrow C(\rho)^-$$

for all $C(\rho), C'(\rho), C''(\rho) \in \mathcal{C}(\mathcal{W}^*_{s+1})$ *such that* $Base(C'(\rho)) = Base(C''(\rho)) = C(\rho)$ *and all* $C'''(\rho) \in PerComm(\mathcal{W}^*_{s+1})$. *The default rules correspond to the previously defined* $Default(\mathcal{W}^*, \_)$ *rules.*

Proposition 67 *Every stable model of the executable command program at state s is coherent.*

Proof. *The Coherence rules, together with the Subsumption and the final Default rule ensure coherency of any stable model.* ■

Theorem 68 *Let* $TF_s = \langle \mathcal{P}_s, \models_{sm}, SU_s, EU_{s+1}, EO_{s+1}, <, Sel(.) \rangle$ *be a transition frame at state s. A set of commands* Δ_{s+1} *is a set of* executable commands *iff* $I_{\Delta_{s+1}} \subset M$ *and M is a stable model of the executable command program at state s.*

Proof. *The proof is similar to that of theorem 40 and is omitted.* ■

5.4.3 Successor State

In the previous Subsections we have started with a transition frame, partially evaluated the statements in both the self and external updates with respect to the current state and the external observations. Subsequently, we have combined the reduced self and external statements, taking into account the specified order relation, to characterize the sets of executable updates, of which we select one according to some selection function. With a coherent set of commands, we are now ready to determine the successor state of the KB, according to the next definitions:

Definition 97 (Logic Program Corresponding to a Set of Rule Commands) *Let Δ be a set of rule commands and s $(s \geq 0)$ a state. Then, the Logic Program Corresponding to Δ at state $s+1$ is $\Gamma_R(\Delta, s+1)$ defined as follows:*

$$\begin{aligned}
&\Gamma_R(\Delta, s+1) = \{N(r) \leftarrow; H(r) \leftarrow B(r), N(r) : \textbf{assert}\,(r) \in \Delta\} \cup \\
&\cup \{not\, N(r) \leftarrow : \textbf{retract}\,(r) \in \Delta\} \cup \\
&\cup \{Ev(r, s+1) \leftarrow; H(r) \leftarrow B(r), Ev(r, s+1) : \textbf{assert_event}\,(r) \in \Delta\} \cup \\
&\cup \{not\, N(r) \leftarrow Ev(r, s+1); Ev(r, s+1) \leftarrow : \textbf{retract_event}\,(r) \in \Delta\} \cup \\
&\cup \{not\, Ev(R, s) \leftarrow\}
\end{aligned}$$

This operator will be used to construct the logic program of the object level KB at the successor state, given a set of rule commands. The construction of the next state of the object level knowledge base is quite simple and is based on the basic rule commands in the set of executable commands previously determined. The first set in the equation contains the rules that are to be asserted, augmented with its corresponding identifier, $N(r)$. Furthermore, the identifier of each asserted rule is also asserted as a fact. The second set in the equation corresponds to the retraction of rules, a behaviour that can be achieved simply by making its corresponding identifier false, i.e. by including the fact not $N(r)$ for all retracted rules. The third and fourth sets in the equation are similar but, since they correspond to non-inertial assertions and retractions, all involved rules must be augmented with the atom $Ev(r, s+1)$. Each asserted atom $Ev(r, s+1)$ will only be true for the duration of one state. This is ensured by the last set of the definition where not $Ev(R, s)$ is asserted.

Definition 98 (Self Update Corresponding to a Set of Commands) *Let Δ be a set of commands. Let $\Delta^S \subseteq \Delta$ be the set of all statement commands in Δ. Let Λ be a set of statements. Then, the Self Update Corresponding to Δ, given Λ, is $\Gamma_S(\Delta, \Lambda)$ defined as follows:*

$$\begin{aligned}
&\Gamma_S(\Delta, \Lambda) = \{\psi : \psi = (\textbf{always_}\langle base_comm\rangle \Leftarrow Cd), \psi \in \Lambda\} \cup \\
&\cup \{\psi : \psi = (\textbf{once_}\langle base_comm\rangle \Leftarrow Cd), \psi \in \Lambda, \textbf{once_}\langle base_comm\rangle \notin \Delta\} \cup \\
&\cup \{\psi : \textbf{assert}\,(\psi) \in \Delta^S\} - \\
&- \{\psi : \textbf{retract}\,(\psi) \in \Delta^S\}
\end{aligned}$$

This operator will be used to construct the self update of the KB at the successor state, given a set of commands and a set of statements (containing the self update at the previous state and the external update statements). The construction of the self update at the next state is based on the executable commands Δ, together with the set of statements Λ which will be equal to the union of both the self and external updates, i.e. $\Lambda = EU \cup SU$. Accordingly, first we add all persistent statements except for those with *the keyword* **once** *that have been executed. This is achieved by the first two sets in the equation. Then, we add all statements that should be asserted and delete all those that should be retracted, as specified in* Δ^S.

Definition 99 (Knowledge Base at the Successor State) *Let* $\langle \mathcal{P}_s, SU_s \rangle$ *be a KB at state* s*, where* $\mathcal{P}_s = P_0 \oplus ... \oplus P_s$ *and let* Δ_{s+1} *be a set of executable commands. Let* $\Delta^R_{s+1} \subseteq \Delta_{s+1}$ *be the set of all rule commands in* Δ_{s+1}*. Let* $\Lambda_{s+1} = EU_{s+1} \cup SU_s$*. Then, the KB at state* $s+1$ *is*

$$\langle \mathcal{P}_{s+1}, SU_{s+1} \rangle$$

where

$$\begin{aligned} \mathcal{P}_{s+1} &= P_0 \oplus ... \oplus P_s \oplus P_{s+1} \\ P_{s+1} &= \Gamma_R \left(\Delta^R_{s+1}, s+1 \right) \\ SU_{s+1} &= \Gamma_S \left(\Delta_{s+1}, \Lambda_{s+1} \right) \end{aligned}$$

Definition 100 (*KABUL* Semantics) *Let* $\langle \mathcal{P}_s, SU_s \rangle$ *be a KB at state* s*. A query (where* $q \leq s$*)*

$$\mathbf{holds}(L_1, ..., L_k, \mathbf{in}(R_1), ..., \mathbf{in}(R_m), \mathbf{out}(R_{m+1}), ..., \mathbf{out}(R_n)) \text{ } \mathbf{at} \text{ } q \text{ ?}$$

is true iff

$$\begin{aligned} &\bigoplus\nolimits_q \mathcal{P}_s \models_{sm} L_1, ..., L_k \wedge \\ &\bigoplus\nolimits_q \mathcal{P}_s \models_{rule} \mathbf{in}(R_1), ..., \mathbf{in}(R_m), \mathbf{out}(R_{m+1}), ..., \mathbf{out}(R_n) \end{aligned}$$

In the next Section we present illustrative examples.

5.5 Illustrative Examples

We first present an example to illustrate the complete process of determining the next state of a knowledge base, given an initial state, a set of external observations and an external update. Next we show examples of application of this framework.

Example 50 *Let* $\langle \mathcal{P}_1, SU_1 \rangle$ *be a KB at state* 1*, where* $\mathcal{P}_1 = P_0 \oplus P_1$ *such that* $P_0 = \{\}$ *and* P_1 *contains the rules*[4]*:*

$$\begin{aligned} P_1 : \quad & a \leftarrow b, n\,(a \leftarrow b) \\ & b \leftarrow not\, c, n\,(b \leftarrow not\, c) \\ & n\,(a \leftarrow b) \leftarrow \\ & n\,(b \leftarrow not\, c) \leftarrow \\ & not\, ev\,(R, 0) \leftarrow \end{aligned}$$

and the self update contains the statements:

$$\begin{aligned} SU_1 : \quad & \mathbf{once\_assert\_event}\,(not\, a \leftarrow b) \Leftarrow a, \mathbf{R} : \mathbf{in}(a \leftarrow b) \\ & \mathbf{always\_retract}\,(b \leftarrow not\, c) \Leftarrow not\, \mathbf{assert\_event}\,(not\, a \leftarrow b), \mathbf{E} : \mathbf{in}(obs\,(b)) \\ & \mathbf{always\_assert}\,(c \leftarrow) \Leftarrow not\, \mathbf{assert}\,(d \leftarrow), not\, c \end{aligned}$$

[4]This KB would have been obtained by starting from the initial (empty) state and updating it with the assertion of the rules and statements in both P_1 and SU_1.

At state 2 we receive an external update, EU_2, containing the statements:

$$\begin{array}{ll} EU_2: & \mathbf{assert}\,(\mathbf{always\_assert\_event}\,(d \leftarrow) \Leftarrow \mathbf{E}:\mathbf{in}(obs\,(d))) \Leftarrow b \\ & \mathbf{retract}\,(\mathbf{always\_assert}\,(c \leftarrow) \Leftarrow not\,\mathbf{assert}\,(d \leftarrow), not\,c) \Leftarrow \\ & not\,\mathbf{assert}\,(c \leftarrow) \Leftarrow \mathbf{assert\_event}\,(not\,a \leftarrow b) \\ & not\,\mathbf{assert}\,(not\,a \leftarrow b) \Leftarrow \mathbf{E}:\mathbf{out}(obs\,(b)) \\ & \mathbf{always\_assert}\,(c \leftarrow a, d) \Leftarrow not\,a, not\,d \end{array}$$

together with the set of external observations:

$$EO_2 = \{obs\,(a)\,, obs\,(b)\}$$

In this particular example we assume that $EU > SU$, i.e. all statements in the external update may override those in the self update. We will not prefer between positive and inhibition statements.

The only stable model at state 1, of $\mathcal{P}_1$ is

$$M_1 = \{a, b, not\,c, not\,d, n\,(a \leftarrow b)\,, n\,(b \leftarrow not\,c)\}$$

where we do not include those irrelevant elements of the form $ev\,(\_,\_)$. According to the set of external observations EO_2 and the stable model M_1, we determine the set of reduced self update statements, SU_1^r, which contains the reduced statements:

$$\begin{array}{ll} SU_1^r: & \mathbf{once\_assert\_event}\,(not\,a \leftarrow b) \Leftarrow \\ & \mathbf{always\_retract}\,(b \leftarrow not\,c) \Leftarrow not\,\mathbf{assert\_event}\,(not\,a \leftarrow b) \\ & \mathbf{always\_assert}\,(c \leftarrow) \Leftarrow not\,\mathbf{assert}\,(d \leftarrow) \end{array}$$

and the set of reduced external update statements, EU_2^r, which contains the reduced statements:

$$\begin{array}{ll} EU_2^r: & \mathbf{assert}\,(\mathbf{always\_assert\_event}\,(d \leftarrow) \Leftarrow \mathbf{E}:\mathbf{in}(obs\,(d))) \Leftarrow \\ & \mathbf{retract}\,(\mathbf{always\_assert}\,(c \leftarrow) \Leftarrow not\,\mathbf{assert}\,(d \leftarrow), not\,c) \Leftarrow \\ & not\,\mathbf{assert}\,(c \leftarrow) \Leftarrow \mathbf{assert\_event}\,(not\,a \leftarrow b) \end{array}$$

These correspond to the logic programs (where $SU_1^{*-} = \{\}$):

$$\begin{array}{ll} SU_1^{*+}: & \mathbf{once\_assert\_event}\,(not\,a \leftarrow b) \leftarrow \\ & \mathbf{always\_retract}\,(b \leftarrow not\,c) \leftarrow not\,\mathbf{assert\_event}\,(not\,a \leftarrow b) \\ & \mathbf{always\_assert}\,(c \leftarrow) \leftarrow not\,\mathbf{assert}\,(d \leftarrow) \end{array}$$

$$\begin{array}{ll} EU_2^{*+}: & \mathbf{assert}\,(\mathbf{always\_assert\_event}\,(d \leftarrow) \Leftarrow \mathbf{E}:\mathbf{in}(obs\,(d))) \leftarrow \\ & \mathbf{retract}\,(\mathbf{always\_assert}\,(c \leftarrow) \Leftarrow not\,\mathbf{assert}\,(d \leftarrow), not\,c) \leftarrow \end{array}$$

$$EU_2^{*-}: \quad not\,\mathbf{assert}\,(c \leftarrow) \leftarrow \mathbf{assert\_event}\,(not\,a \leftarrow b)$$

and the set of arguments that generates the command language is:

$$Args_R\,(SU_1^* \cup EU_2^*) = \left\{ \begin{array}{c} not\,a \leftarrow b \\ b \leftarrow not\,c \\ c \leftarrow \\ d \leftarrow \end{array} \right\}$$

$$Args_S\,(SU_1^* \cup EU_2^*) = \left\{ \begin{array}{c} \mathbf{always\_assert\_event}\,(d \leftarrow) \Leftarrow \mathbf{E}:\mathbf{in}(obs\,(d)) \\ \mathbf{always\_assert}\,(c \leftarrow) \Leftarrow not\,\mathbf{assert}\,(d \leftarrow), not\,c \end{array} \right\}$$

the command language, which we omit, is just the set of all commands and inhibition commands generated with these arguments.

Let Δ_2 be the coherent set of executable commands:

$$\Delta_2 = \left\{ \begin{array}{c} [\textbf{once\_}]\,\textbf{assert\_event}\,(not\,a \leftarrow b) \\ \textbf{assert}\,(\textbf{always\_assert\_event}\,(d \leftarrow) \Leftarrow \mathbf{E} : \textbf{in}(obs\,(d))) \\ \textbf{retract}\,(\textbf{always\_assert}\,(c \leftarrow) \Leftarrow not\,\textbf{assert}\,(d \leftarrow), not\,c) \end{array} \right\}$$

This corresponds to a set of executable commands. We leave to the reader the check that, indeed, this is a set of executable commands and, furthermore, the only such set. With this set of commands we are ready to determine the next state of our knowledge base. The successor state is $\langle \mathcal{P}_2, SU_2 \rangle$, where $\mathcal{P}_2 = P_0 \oplus P_1 \oplus P_2$ and P_2 contains the rules:

$$\begin{array}{rl} P_2 : & not\,a \leftarrow b, ev\,(not\,a \leftarrow b, 2) \\ & ev\,(not\,a \leftarrow b, 2) \leftarrow \\ & not\,ev\,(R, 1) \leftarrow \end{array}$$

and where SU_2 contains the statements:

$$\begin{array}{rl} SU_2 : & \textbf{always\_retract}\,(b \leftarrow not\,c) \Leftarrow not\,\textbf{assert\_event}\,(not\,a \leftarrow b), \mathbf{E} : \textbf{in}(obs\,(b)) \\ & \textbf{always\_assert\_event}\,(d \leftarrow) \Leftarrow \mathbf{E} : \textbf{in}(obs\,(d)) \\ & \textbf{always\_assert}\,(c \leftarrow a, d) \Leftarrow not\,a, not\,d \end{array}$$

Note that the statement **once_assert_event** $(not\,a \leftarrow b) \Leftarrow a, \mathbf{R} : \textbf{in}(a \leftarrow b)$ *in SU_1 does not belong to SU_2 since it was executed at this state transition. The object knowledge base at state 2 has the following single stable model, modulo irrelevant elements of the form $ev\,(\_,\_)$.:*

$$M_2 = \{not\,a, b, not\,c, not\,d, n\,(a \leftarrow b), n\,(b \leftarrow not\,c), ev\,(not\,a \leftarrow b, 2)\}$$

If, at the next state transition, both the external update and the set of external observations are empty, we would obtain the only set of executable commands

$$\Delta_3 = \{[\textbf{always\_}]\,\textbf{assert}\,(c \leftarrow a, d)\}$$

which would produce the successor state $\langle \mathcal{P}_3, SU_3 \rangle$, where $\mathcal{P}_3 = P_0 \oplus P_1 \oplus P_2 \oplus P_3$ and P_3 contains the rules:

$$\begin{array}{rl} P_3 : & c \leftarrow a, d, n\,(c \leftarrow a, d) \\ & n\,(c \leftarrow a, d) \leftarrow \\ & not\,ev\,(R, 2) \leftarrow \end{array}$$

and where SU_3 contains the statements:

$$\begin{array}{rl} SU_3 : & \textbf{always\_retract}\,(b \leftarrow not\,c) \Leftarrow not\,\textbf{assert\_event}\,(not\,a \leftarrow b), \mathbf{E} : \textbf{in}(obs\,(b)) \\ & \textbf{always\_assert\_event}\,(d \leftarrow) \Leftarrow \mathbf{E} : \textbf{in}(obs\,(d)) \\ & \textbf{always\_assert}\,(c \leftarrow a, d) \Leftarrow not\,a, not\,d \end{array}$$

Now, at state 3, the object knowledge base has the following single stable model, modulo irrelevant elements of the form $ev\,(\_,\_)$:

$$M_3 = \{a, b, not\,c, not\,d, n\,(a \leftarrow b), n\,(b \leftarrow not\,c), n\,(c \leftarrow a, d)\}$$

Note that even though the truth values of a, b, c and d are the same as at state 1, this new state is significantly different because the rule $c \leftarrow a, d$ is now in place in the knowledge base. Its assertion was made possible because of the presence of the non-inertial rule $not\,a \leftarrow b$ at state 2, which caused a to be false during one state (given that is the duration of a non-inertial rule) and allowed the execution of the command in the statement: **always_assert** $(c \leftarrow a, d) \Leftarrow not\,a, not\,d$.

The next example illustrates how to specify update policies to a knowledge base, where the updates depend on sequences of external observations. We have chosen a legal reasoning scenario because of the suitability of DLP to represent the evolution of laws in time, in particular in what concerns the temporal collision principle *Lex Posterior* (*Lex Posterior Derogat Legi Priori*) according to which the rule enacted at a later point in time overrides the earlier one.

Example 51 *Consider a knowledge base whose purpose is to represent the laws of a country, and their evolution in time. The object knowledge base will contain the rules and the self update will contain the statements that represent the specification of how the knowledge base should evolve according to the passing of laws by parliament, approval by the president, and any rulings by the court regarding the constitutionality of such laws. The knowledge base will evolve according to external observations. Such external observations represent, for any law encoded as a logic program rule* (R)*: its voting by parliament represented by the predicate* $voted(R)$*; its approval by the president represented by predicate* $approved(R)$*; its veto by the president represented by predicate* $vetoed(R)$*; and its ruling as unconstitutional by a higher court of law represented by predicate* $unconst(R)$*. Accordingly, if* $\mathcal{R}$ *is the set of all possible rules, a set of external observations at each state is a subset of* $\mathcal{E}$*, where*

$$\mathcal{E} = \{voted(R), approved(R), vetoed(R), unconst(R) : R \in \mathcal{R}\}$$

Consider the following scenario:

- *A law* (R)*, to be in force, has to first be voted by parliament, and then sent to the president for approval. To represent this we have chosen a persistent assertion statement* (s_1) *that, every time a new law is voted, asserts a statement into the self update of the next state that will await for the law to be approved to assert it into the object knowledge base, and then cease to persist in the self update.*

$$s_1 : \textbf{always\_assert}\,(\textbf{once\_assert}\,(R) \Leftarrow \mathbf{E} : approved(R)) \Leftarrow \mathbf{E} : voted(R)$$

- *If the law is vetoed by the president, the process is aborted. This behaviour can be represented by a statement with a persistent retraction command* (s_2) *that retracts the statement asserted by* (s_1) *if a* $vetoed(R)$ *is observed.*

$$s_2 : \textbf{always\_retract}\,(\textbf{once\_assert}\,(R) \Leftarrow \mathbf{E} : approved(R)) \Leftarrow \mathbf{E} : vetoed(R)$$

- *After being voted by parliament, a law can be found unconstitutional by a higher court. In these cases, the assertion of such a law in the knowledge base should be immediately inhibited . Such permanent inhibition commands are accomplished by always asserting them into the self update of the next state* (s_3)*(recall that statements with inhibition commands are non-persistent).*

$$s_3 : \textbf{always\_assert}\,(not\;\textbf{assert}\,(R) \Leftarrow \mathbf{E} : unconst(R)) \Leftarrow$$

- *If the law that was found unconstitutional had already been asserted in the knowledge base it should be removed from it. This is accomplished by a statement with a persistent retraction command* (s_4) *that tests for the presence of the law in the object level knowledge base.*

$$s_4 : \textbf{always\_retract}\,(R) \Leftarrow \textbf{in}\,(R)\,, \mathbf{E} : unconst(R)$$

- *If the law has not been approved by the president, the process should be aborted. This is accomplished by a statement (s_5) in all respects similar to statement (s_2).*

$$s_5 : \textbf{always\_retract}\,(\textbf{once\_assert}\,(R) \Leftarrow \mathbf{E} : approved(R)) \Leftarrow \mathbf{E} : unconst(R)$$

We now show the evolution of a knowledge base construed on such a scenario. The knowledge state at s is represented by the pair $\langle \mathcal{P}_s, SU_s \rangle$ where $\mathcal{P}_s = P_0 \oplus ... \oplus P_s$. At state 0 everything is empty, i.e. $P_0 = \{\}$ and $SU_s = \{\}$. Then we perform an external update to program *the knowledge base with the desired behaviour, i.e., we assert statements s_1 through s_5. We should also assert any previously existing laws. As an example, we assert the rule*

$$r_1 : not\, jail\_for\_abortion(X) \leftarrow abortion(X)$$

representing a law ruling that abortions are not punished with jail. The external update at this state is, thus:

$$EU_1 = \left\{ \begin{array}{lllll} \textbf{assert}\,(s_1) \Leftarrow & ; & \textbf{assert}\,(s_2) \Leftarrow & ; & \textbf{assert}\,(s_3) \Leftarrow \\ \textbf{assert}\,(s_4) \Leftarrow & ; & \textbf{assert}\,(s_5) \Leftarrow & ; & \textbf{assert}\,(r_1) \Leftarrow \end{array} \right\}$$

The set of external observations is empty, i.e. $E_1 = \{\}$. At this state the (unique) set of executable commands is:

$$\Delta_1 = \{\textbf{assert}\,(s_1), \textbf{assert}\,(s_2), \textbf{assert}\,(s_3), \textbf{assert}\,(s_4), \textbf{assert}\,(s_5), \textbf{assert}\,(r_1)\}$$

and we obtain:

$$P_1 = \left\{ \begin{array}{l} not\, jail\_for\_abortion(X) \leftarrow abortion(X), n\,(r_1\,(X)) \\ n\,(r_1\,(X)) \leftarrow \\ not\, ev(R, 0) \leftarrow \end{array} \right\}$$

$$SU_1 = \{s_1, s_2, s_3, s_4, s_5\}$$

At this state, anyone who performs an abortion would not go to jail. For example if, together with the previous external update, the fact abortion(mary) was also asserted, representing that Mary had an abortion, we would have that $\bigoplus \mathcal{P}_1 \models_{sm} not\, jail\_for\_abortion(mary)$, i.e. Mary would not go to jail for it.

At the subsequent state, parliament enacts three laws to the effect that: (r_2) abortions become a crime punishable with jail unless there is danger for the pregnant woman; (r_3) a suspect is automatically guilty; (r_4) the Kyoto protocol is to be adopted. These laws are represented by the rules:

$$\begin{array}{l} r_2 : jail\_for\_abortion(X) \leftarrow abortion(X), not\, danger(X) \\ r_3 : guilty(X) \leftarrow suspect(X) \\ r_4 : kyoto\_protocol \leftarrow \end{array}$$

This is represented by the set of external observations:

$$EO_2 = \{voted(r_2), voted(r_3), voted(r_4)\}$$

There was no external update at this state. So the (unique) set of executable commands is:

$$\Delta_2 = \left\{ \begin{array}{l} [\textbf{always\_}]\,\textbf{assert}\,(\textbf{once\_assert}\,(r_2) \Leftarrow \mathbf{E} : approved(r_2)) \\ [\textbf{always\_}]\,\textbf{assert}\,(\textbf{once\_assert}\,(r_3) \Leftarrow \mathbf{E} : approved(r_3)) \\ [\textbf{always\_}]\,\textbf{assert}\,(\textbf{once\_assert}\,(r_4) \Leftarrow \mathbf{E} : approved(r_4)) \\ [\textbf{always\_}]\,\textbf{assert}\,(not\,\textbf{assert}\,(R) \Leftarrow \mathbf{E} : unconst(R)) \end{array} \right\}$$

and we obtain:

$$P_2 = \{not\, ev(R,1) \leftarrow\}$$

$$SU_2 = \{s_1, s_2, s_3, s_4, s_5, s_6, s_7, s_8, s_9\}$$

Where:

$$s_6 : not\, \textbf{assert}\,(R) \Leftarrow \textbf{E} : unconst(R)$$
$$s_7 : \textbf{once\_assert}\,(r_2) \Leftarrow \textbf{E} : approved(r_2)$$
$$s_8 : \textbf{once\_assert}\,(r_3) \Leftarrow \textbf{E} : approved(r_3)$$
$$s_9 : \textbf{once\_assert}\,(r_4) \Leftarrow \textbf{E} : approved(r_4)$$

At the immediately subsequent state, the president approves laws r_2 and r_3, and the court finds r_3 unconstitutional. Furthermore, parliament votes a law stating that a suspected terrorist could be tortured, represented by the rule:

$$r_5 : torture(X) \leftarrow suspected\_terrorist(X)$$

This is represented by the set of external observations:

$$EO_3 = \{approved(r_2), approved(r_3), unconst(r_3), voted(r_5)\}$$

There was no external update at this state. So the (unique) set of executable commands is:

$$\Delta_3 = \left\{ \begin{array}{l} [\textbf{once\_}]\,\textbf{assert}\,(r_2) \\ [\textbf{always\_}]\,\textbf{retract}\,(\textbf{once\_assert}\,(r_3) \Leftarrow \textbf{E} : approved(r_3)) \\ [\textbf{always\_}]\,\textbf{assert}\,(not\,\textbf{assert}\,(R) \Leftarrow \textbf{E} : unconst(R)) \\ [\textbf{always\_}]\,\textbf{assert}\,(\textbf{once\_assert}\,(r_5) \Leftarrow \textbf{E} : approved(r_5)) \end{array} \right\}$$

and we obtain:

$$P_3 = \left\{ \begin{array}{l} jail\_for\_abortion(X) \leftarrow abortion(X), not\, danger(X), n\,(r_2\,(X)) \\ n\,(r_2\,(X)) \leftarrow \\ not\, ev(R,2) \leftarrow \end{array} \right\}$$

$$SU_3 = \{s_1, s_2, s_3, s_4, s_5, s_9, s_{10}, s_{11}\}$$

Where:

$$s_{10} : not\,\textbf{assert}\,(R) \Leftarrow \textbf{E} : unconst(R)$$
$$s_{11} : \textbf{once\_assert}\,(r_5) \Leftarrow \textbf{E} : approved(r_5)$$

At this state, anyone who performs an abortion and is not in danger would go to jail. For example if, together with the previous external update, the facts abortion(mary), abortion(jane) and danger(jane) were also asserted, representing that Mary and Jane had an abortion and that Jane was in danger, we would have that $\bigoplus \mathcal{P}_3 \models_{sm}$ $not\, jail\_for\_abortion(jane)$, and $\bigoplus \mathcal{P}_3 \models_{sm} jail\_for\_abortion(mary)$ i.e. Jane would not go to jail while Mary would. Note that, at this state, any person who is a suspect would not be found guilty even though such a law was approved by the president. This is so because the observation that the law was unconstitutional "enabled" the inhibition command not **assert** (r_3) *preventing its assertion in the knowledge base.*

At the subsequent state, the president approves law r_5 and vetoes law r_4. This is represented by the next set of external observations:

$$EO_4 = \{vetoed(r_4), approved(r_5)\}$$

There was no external update at this state. So the (unique) set of executable commands is:

$$\Delta_4 = \left\{ \begin{array}{l} [\mathbf{always\_}]\, \mathbf{retract}\, (\mathbf{once\_assert}\, (r_4) \Leftarrow \mathbf{E} : approved(r_4)) \\ [\mathbf{always\_}]\, \mathbf{assert}\, (not\, \mathbf{assert}\, (R) \Leftarrow \mathbf{E} : unconst(R)) \\ [\mathbf{once\_}]\, \mathbf{assert}\, (r_5) \end{array} \right\}$$

and we obtain:

$$P_4 = \left\{ \begin{array}{l} not\, ev(R,3) \leftarrow \\ torture(X) \leftarrow suspected\_terrorist(X), n\,(r_5\,(X)) \\ n\,(r_5\,(X)) \leftarrow \end{array} \right\}$$

$$SU_4 = \{s_1, s_2, s_3, s_4, s_5, s_{12}\}$$

Where:

$$s_{12} : not\, \mathbf{assert}\, (R) \Leftarrow \mathbf{E} : unconst(R)$$

At this state, anyone who is a suspected terrorist could be tortured. For example if, together with the previous external update, the fact suspected_terrorist(john), was also asserted, representing that John is a suspected terrorist, we would have that $\bigoplus \mathcal{P}_4 \models_{sm} torture(john)$*, i.e. John could be tortured.*

At the subsequent state, the torture law (r_5) is found unconstitutional. This is represented by the set of external observations:

$$EO_5 = \{unconst(r_5)\}$$

There was no external update at this state. So the (unique) set of executable commands is:

$$\Delta_5 = \left\{ \begin{array}{l} [\mathbf{always\_}]\, \mathbf{retract}\, (r_5) \\ [\mathbf{always\_}]\, \mathbf{retract}\, (\mathbf{once\_assert}\, (r_5) \Leftarrow \mathbf{E} : approved(r_5)) \\ [\mathbf{always\_}]\, \mathbf{assert}\, (not\, \mathbf{assert}\, (R) \Leftarrow \mathbf{E} : unconst(R)) \end{array} \right\}$$

and we obtain:

$$P_5 = \left\{ \begin{array}{l} not\, ev(R,4) \leftarrow \\ not\, n\,(r_5\,(X)) \leftarrow \end{array} \right\}$$

$$SU_4 = \{s_1, s_2, s_3, s_4, s_5, s_{13}\}$$

Where:

$$s_{13} : not\, \mathbf{assert}\, (R) \Leftarrow \mathbf{E} : unconst(R)$$

At this state, the suspected terrorist John, asserted at the previous state, could no longer be tortured, i.e. $\bigoplus \mathcal{P}_5 \models_{sm} not\, torture(john)$.

Next, we illustrate the representation of "delayed" effects of actions, i.e. actions whose effects take a number of state transitions before becoming observable.

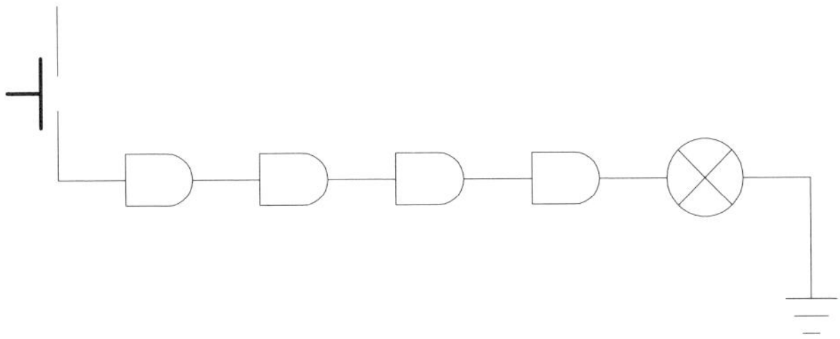

Figure 5.1: Circuit with four delays

Example 52 *Suppose we have a circuit such that an action (external observation)* push *lights up a lamp, for the duration of one state, but only after a delay of four states, as depicted in Figure 5.1. The specification of the effects of the action* push *can be expressed by the statement:*

$$\textbf{always\_assert}\,(\textbf{assert}\,(\textbf{assert}\,(\textbf{assert\_event}\,(light\_on) \Leftarrow) \Leftarrow) \Leftarrow) \Leftarrow \mathbf{E} : push \tag{5.9}$$

If at state 3 *we have the set of events* $EO_3 = \{push\}$, *then at states* $s = 4, 5, 6$ *we have* $\bigoplus \mathcal{P}_s \models_{sm} not\, light\_on$, *at state* $s = 7$ *we have* $\bigoplus \mathcal{P}_7 \models_{sm} light\_on$, *and at states* $s \geq 8$ *we have* $\bigoplus \mathcal{P}_s \models_{sm} not\, light\_on$, *again. Note that, in (5.9), the* **always** *specifies that the action push is always available, and the* **event** *specifies that light_on should only be asserted during one state.*

The next example illustrates the representation of actions whose effect is to enable or disable other actions.

Example 53 *Consider three actions:* set, clear *and* go, *where* set *enables* go, clear *disables* go, *and* go *causes some non-inertial effect (effect). The actions can be specified by the two statements:*

$$\textbf{always\_assert}\,(\textbf{always\_assert\_event}\,(effect) \Leftarrow \mathbf{E} :go) \Leftarrow \mathbf{E} :set$$
$$\textbf{always\_retract}\,(\textbf{always\_assert\_event}\,(effect) \Leftarrow \mathbf{E} :go) \Leftarrow \mathbf{E} :reset$$

Note that a simultaneous set *and* reset *would be signaled by an assertion of* $\bot_s$ *into the KB.*

Example 54 *The Yale Shooting scenario of Example 37 would be encoded by the statements:*

$$\textbf{always\_assert}\,(loaded) \Leftarrow \mathbf{E} :load$$
$$\textbf{always\_assert}\,(not\, loaded) \Leftarrow loaded, \mathbf{E} :shoot$$
$$\textbf{always\_assert}\,(not\, alive) \Leftarrow loaded, \mathbf{E} :shoot$$

The initial situation is asserted by the statements:

$$\textbf{assert}\,(alive)$$
$$\textbf{assert}\,(not\, loaded)$$

The sequence of four actions would be represented by the sets of external observations:

$$EO_2 = \{load\} \qquad EO_3 = \{wait\} \qquad EO_4 = \{shoot\} \qquad EO_5 = \{wait\}$$

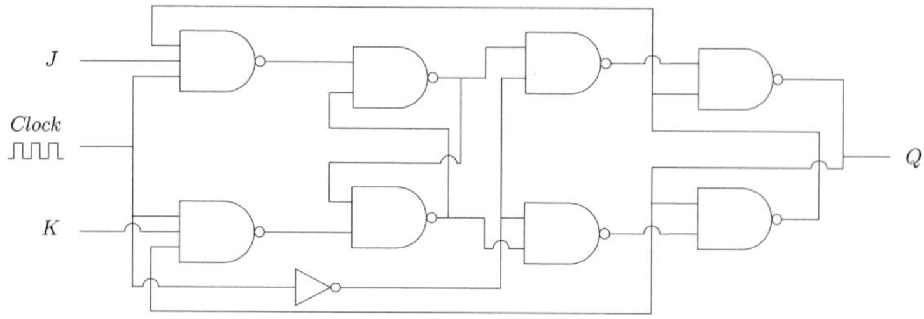

Figure 5.2: Falling Edge JK Flip-Flop

Finally we show how sequential logic circuits can be encoded.

Example 55 *In this example we show how to represent the behaviour of a JK flip-flop circuit. First we consider the falling edge version of such circuit, depicted in Figure 5.2, according to which the changes in the outputs of the circuit (Q) depend on the inputs (J and K) and occur when the clock changes from 1 (true) to 0 (false), as per the truth table:*

J	K	*Clock*	Q
0	0	$^1\searrow_0$	*no change*
0	1	$^1\searrow_0$	0
1	0	$^1\searrow_0$	1
1	1	$^1\searrow_0$	*toggle*

If all three inputs (J, K and Clock) are external observations, we can encode the behaviour with the set of statements:

$$\begin{array}{l}
\textbf{always_assert}\,(\textbf{always_assert}\,(q) \Leftarrow not\, q, \mathbf{E}:j, k, not\; clock) \Leftarrow \mathbf{E}:clock \\
\textbf{always_assert}\,(\textbf{always_assert}\,(not\, q) \Leftarrow q, \mathbf{E}:j, k, not\; clock) \Leftarrow \mathbf{E}:clock \\
\textbf{always_assert}\,(\textbf{always_assert}\,(q) \Leftarrow \mathbf{E}:j, not\, k, not\; clock) \Leftarrow \mathbf{E}:clock \\
\textbf{always_assert}\,(\textbf{always_assert}\,(not\, q) \Leftarrow \mathbf{E}:not\, j, k, not\; clock) \Leftarrow \mathbf{E}:clock \\
\textbf{always_retract}\,(\textbf{always_assert}\,(q) \Leftarrow not\, q, \mathbf{E}:j, k, not\; clock) \Leftarrow \mathbf{E}:not\; clock \\
\textbf{always_retract}\,(\textbf{always_assert}\,(not\, q) \Leftarrow q, \mathbf{E}:j, k, not\; clock) \Leftarrow \mathbf{E}:not\; clock \\
\textbf{always_retract}\,(\textbf{always_assert}\,(q) \Leftarrow \mathbf{E}:j, not\, k, not\; clock) \Leftarrow \mathbf{E}:not\; clock \\
\textbf{always_retract}\,(\textbf{always_assert}\,(not\, q) \Leftarrow \mathbf{E}:not\, j, k, not\; clock) \Leftarrow \mathbf{E}:not\; clock
\end{array}$$

Alternatively, we can use the language to program a non-stop pulsing clock, with the set of statements:

$$\begin{array}{c}
\textbf{always_assert}\,(clock) \Leftarrow not\; clock \\
\textbf{always_assert}\,(not\; clock) \Leftarrow clock
\end{array}$$

With this clock, the falling edge JK flip flop would be specified by the statements:

$$\begin{array}{l}
\textbf{always_assert}\,(q) \Leftarrow \textbf{assert}\,(not\; clock), clock, not\, q, \mathbf{E}:j, k \\
\textbf{always_assert}\,(not\, q) \Leftarrow \textbf{assert}\,(not\; clock), clock, q, \mathbf{E}:j, k \\
\textbf{always_assert}\,(q) \Leftarrow \textbf{assert}\,(not\; clock), clock, \mathbf{E}:j, not\, k \\
\textbf{always_assert}\,(not\, q) \Leftarrow \textbf{assert}\,(not\; clock), clock, \mathbf{E}:not\, j, k
\end{array}$$

A rising edge JK flip-flop, depicted in Figure 5.3, is in all respects similar to the

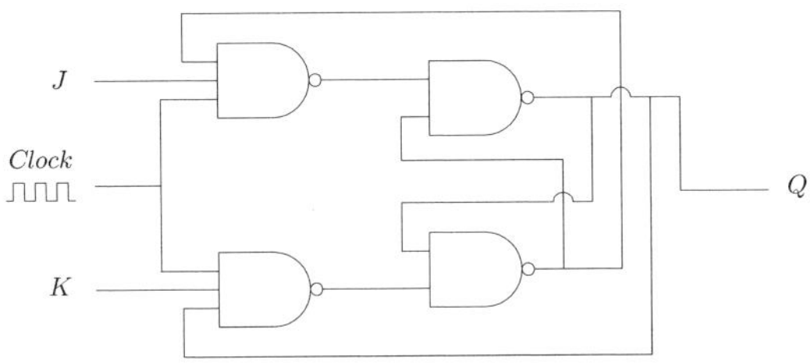

Figure 5.3: Rising Edge JK Flip-Flop

previous one but the changes in the outputs occur when the clock changes from 0 (false) to 1 (true), as per the truth table:

J	K	$Clock$	Q
0	0	$_0\nearrow^1$	*no change*
0	1	$_0\nearrow^1$	0
1	0	$_0\nearrow^1$	1
1	1	$_0\nearrow^1$	*toggle*

Without the internal clock the behaviour would be encoded by the set of statements:

$$\begin{array}{l}
\textbf{always_assert}\,(\textbf{always_assert}\,(q) \Leftarrow not\, q, \mathbf{E}:j, k, clock) \Leftarrow \mathbf{E}:not\, clock \\
\textbf{always_assert}\,(\textbf{always_assert}\,(not\, q) \Leftarrow q, \mathbf{E}:j, k, clock) \Leftarrow \mathbf{E}:not\, clock \\
\textbf{always_assert}\,(\textbf{always_assert}\,(q) \Leftarrow \mathbf{E}:j, not\, k, clock) \Leftarrow \mathbf{E}:not\, clock \\
\textbf{always_assert}\,(\textbf{always_assert}\,(not\, q) \Leftarrow \mathbf{E}:not\, j, k, clock) \Leftarrow \mathbf{E}:not\, clock \\
\textbf{always_retract}\,(\textbf{always_assert}\,(q) \Leftarrow not\, q, \mathbf{E}:j, k, clock) \Leftarrow \mathbf{E}:clock \\
\textbf{always_retract}\,(\textbf{always_assert}\,(not\, q) \Leftarrow q, \mathbf{E}:j, k, clock) \Leftarrow \mathbf{E}:clock \\
\textbf{always_retract}\,(\textbf{always_assert}\,(q) \Leftarrow \mathbf{E}:j, not\, k, clock) \Leftarrow \mathbf{E}:clock \\
\textbf{always_retract}\,(\textbf{always_assert}\,(not\, q) \Leftarrow \mathbf{E}:not\, j, k, clock) \Leftarrow \mathbf{E}:clock
\end{array}$$

To the internal clock previously specified, we would add this set of statements to obtain the rising edge JK Flip Flop:

$$\begin{array}{l}
\textbf{always_assert}\,(q) \Leftarrow \textbf{assert}\,(clock), not\, clock, not\, q, \mathbf{E}:j, k \\
\textbf{always_assert}\,(not\, q) \Leftarrow \textbf{assert}\,(clock), not\, clock, q, \mathbf{E}:j, k \\
\textbf{always_assert}\,(q) \Leftarrow \textbf{assert}\,(clock), not\, clock, \mathbf{E}:j, not\, k \\
\textbf{always_assert}\,(not\, q) \Leftarrow \textbf{assert}\,(clock), not\, clock, \mathbf{E}:not\, j, k
\end{array}$$

5.6 Properties

In this Section we explore some basic properties of KABUL.

One important issue when dealing with updates of knowledge bases, such as those specified by KABUL, concerns possible simplifications to the object level knowledge base. Since size matters in what concerns the computational complexity of determining the stable models of the object level DLP necessary to perform each state transition, and even for state transitions where the set of executable commands is empty a new non-empty program is added to the object level DLP (with the rule $not\, Ev(R, s) \leftarrow$), it is important to define simplifications to the DLP that are not computationally expensive, but preserve some notion of equivalence between the original knowledge state and the simplified one. Throughout, we assume that the selection function $Sel(.)$ does not take into account the syntactic structure of the knowledge state, but rather its semantics only. This is important for otherwise no simplifications would be possible, because they would necessarily affect the syntax of knowledge states. We start by defining a notion of equivalence between knowledge states:

Definition 101 (K-Update Equivalence) *Let $\langle \mathcal{P}_s, SU_s \rangle$ be a knowledge state. A knowledge state $\langle \mathcal{P}'_s, SU'_s \rangle$ is k-update equivalent to $\langle \mathcal{P}_s, SU_s \rangle$, denoted by $\langle \mathcal{P}_s, SU_s \rangle \overset{k}{\equiv} \langle \mathcal{P}'_s, SU'_s \rangle$, iff for every external input $\langle EU_{s+1}, EO_{s+1} \rangle, ..., \langle EU_{s+n}, EO_{s+n} \rangle$ and every query Q:*

$$Q = \mathbf{holds}(L_1, ..., L_k, in(R_1), ..., in(R_m), out(R_{m+1}), ..., out(R_n)) \text{ } \mathbf{at} \text{ } q \text{ ?}$$

where $s \leq q \leq s+n$, Q is true in $\langle \mathcal{P}_s, SU_s \rangle \otimes \langle EU_{s+1}, EO_{s+1} \rangle \otimes ... \otimes \langle EU_{s+n}, EO_{s+n} \rangle$ iff Q is true in $\langle \mathcal{P}'_s, SU'_s \rangle \otimes \langle EU_{s+1}, EO_{s+1} \rangle \otimes ... \otimes \langle EU_{s+n}, EO_{s+n} \rangle$.

Recall that we use the notation $\langle \mathcal{P}_0, SU_0 \rangle \otimes \langle EU_1, EO_1 \rangle \otimes \langle EU_2, EO_2 \rangle \otimes ... \otimes \langle EU_s, EO_s \rangle$ to denote the knowledge state produced by such sequence, i.e. the knowledge state $\langle \mathcal{P}_s, SU_s \rangle$.

Since it is not possible to simplify the set of self updates, unless for some trivial simplifications such as removing a statement whose body can never be true (e.g. contains a pair of complementary literals), we will concentrate on simplifications of the object level DLP $\mathcal{P}_s$, i.e. given a knowledge state $\langle \mathcal{P}_s, SU_s \rangle$ we will try to find knowledge states of the form $\langle \mathcal{P}'_s, SU_s \rangle$ such that $\langle \mathcal{P}_s, SU_s \rangle \overset{k}{\equiv} \langle \mathcal{P}'_s, SU_s \rangle$. In Chapter 3, we set forth several properties specifying simplifications to a DLP that preserve update equivalence. Trivially we have:

Proposition 69 *Let $\langle \mathcal{P}_s, SU_s \rangle$ and $\langle \mathcal{P}'_s, SU_s \rangle$ be two knowledge states. Then, if $\mathcal{P}_s \overset{\oplus}{\equiv} \mathcal{P}'_s$ then $\langle \mathcal{P}_s, SU_s \rangle \overset{k}{\equiv} \langle \mathcal{P}'_s, SU_s \rangle$.*

Even though it is clear that if $\mathcal{P}_s \overset{\oplus}{\equiv} \mathcal{P}'_s$ holds then so does $\langle \mathcal{P}_s, SU_s \rangle \overset{k}{\equiv} \langle \mathcal{P}'_s, SU_s \rangle$, the simplifications previously defined do not produce very good results when applied to knowledge states produced in KABUL. This is so because all object level rules that have been asserted by the KABUL commands are augmented with their corresponding naming predicate and, more important, can be retracted. For example, if the rule $a \leftarrow b$ has been asserted at some state i, and subsequently, the rule $a \leftarrow$ is asserted at state $i+j$, then, Proposition 38 would suggest that rule $a \leftarrow b$ could be removed. But since, in KABUL, any rule can be retracted, we cannot remove such a rule without losing equivalence. In fact, Proposition 38 does not actually apply because these two rules would be augmented with their names $(N(r))$ and $B(a \leftarrow b, N(a \leftarrow b)) \not\supseteq B(a \leftarrow N(a \leftarrow))$. Nevertheless, some of those propositions can effectively be applied to yield some simplifications. Some can be applied directly while others require us to take into account the particular construction of the object level DLP of KABUL. To clarify their application within the KABUL framework, we now present the relevant instances:

The first simplification concerns the possibility to delete rules that have been inertially retracted:

Proposition 70 *Let $\langle \mathcal{P}_s, SU_s \rangle$ be a knowledge state, let $P_i \in \mathcal{P}_s$ and let $H(r) \leftarrow B(r), N(r) \in P_i$ be a rule such that $\mathcal{P}_s \models_{sm} not\, N(r), not\, Ev(r,s)$. Let $\mathcal{P}'_s$ be obtained from $\mathcal{P}_s$ by replacing P_i with $P'_i = P_i \backslash \{H(r) \leftarrow B(r), N(r)\}$. Then, $\langle \mathcal{P}_s, SU_s \rangle \overset{k}{\equiv} \langle \mathcal{P}'_s, SU_s \rangle$.*

Proof. *From the way the object level DLP is constructed, if r belongs to P_i and we have that at state s both $not\, N(r)$ and $not\, Ev(r,s)$ are both true, then $N(r)$ will only become true again in a command of the form* **assert** (r) *is executed at a subsequent state transition. If $Ev(r,s)$ were true (due to a non-inertial retraction), then $N(r)$ could become true at the subsequent state thus invalidating this reasoning. But since when* **assert** (r) *is executed at some state $s+n$ the rule $H(r) \leftarrow B(r), N(r)$ will also belong to P_{s+n}, the rule r in P_i will have a false body until state $s+n$, and after such state, we can remove it due to Proposition 37.* ■

Under the same conditions one can also remove facts of the form $N(r)$.

Proposition 71 *Let $\langle \mathcal{P}_s, SU_s \rangle$ be a knowledge state, let $P_i \in \mathcal{P}_s$ and let $N(r) \leftarrow \in P_i$ be a rule such that $\mathcal{P}_s \models_{sm} not\, N(r), not\, Ev(r,s)$. Let $\mathcal{P}'_s$ be obtained from $\mathcal{P}_s$ by replacing P_i with $P'_i = P_i \setminus \{N(r) \leftarrow\}$. Then, $\langle \mathcal{P}_s, SU_s \rangle \overset{k}{\equiv} \langle \mathcal{P}'_s, SU_s \rangle$.*

Proof. *If $N(r) \leftarrow \in P_i$ and $\mathcal{P}_s \models_{sm} not\, N(r), not\, Ev(r,s)$, then there is a $not\, N(r) \leftarrow \in P_j$, $j > i$. Then, by Proposition 39, this proposition follows.* ■

As the reader may have noticed, in this proposition we did not have to consider the semantics of $\mathcal{P}_s$. We could have just syntactically checked for instances of $N(r) \leftarrow$ belonging to states prior to the latest instance of $not\, N(r) \leftarrow$. But since any state transition already requires the semantics determination, we opted for this version of the proposition. Otherwise it would be the direct application of Proposition 39.

The next proposition allows us to remove any non-inertially asserted rule after the state at which it was valid. This is in fact an expected result because of the very motivation for non-inertial commands:

Proposition 72 *Let $\langle \mathcal{P}_s, SU_s \rangle$ be a knowledge state, let $P_i \in \mathcal{P}_s$, $i < s$, and let $r \in P_i$ be a rule such that $Ev(r,i) \in B(r)$. Let $\mathcal{P}'_s$ be obtained from $\mathcal{P}_s$ by replacing P_i with $P'_i = P_i \setminus \{r\}$. Then, $\langle \mathcal{P}_s, SU_s \rangle \overset{k}{\equiv} \langle \mathcal{P}'_s, SU_s \rangle$.*

Proof. *Since every $P_i \in \mathcal{P}_s$ contains the rule $not\, Ev(r, i-1) \leftarrow$, and there will be no subsequent occurrences of $Ev(r, i-1)$, $B(r)$ will always be false and the rule can be safely removed.* ■

Proposition 73 *Let $\langle \mathcal{P}_s, SU_s \rangle$ be a knowledge state, let $P_i \in \mathcal{P}_s$, $i < s$. Let $\mathcal{P}'_s$ be obtained from $\mathcal{P}_s$ by replacing P_i with $P'_i = P_i \setminus \{Ev(r,i) \leftarrow\}$. Then, $\langle \mathcal{P}_s, SU_s \rangle \overset{k}{\equiv} \langle \mathcal{P}'_s, SU_s \rangle$.*

Proof. *Since P_{i+1} contains $not\, Ev(r,i) \leftarrow$, it amounts to the direct application of Proposition 39.* ■

Next we establish the relationship between KABUL and other frameworks, starting with the expected Theorem according to which it embeds DLP:

Theorem 74 (Embedding of DLP) *Let $\mathcal{P} = P_1 \oplus ... \oplus P_s$ be a Dynamic Logic Program. Let $\langle EU_1, \{\} \rangle, ..., \langle EU_s, \{\} \rangle$ be such that*

$$EU_i = \{\mathbf{assert}\,(r) \Leftarrow: r \in P_i\}$$

for every $1 \leq i \leq s$. *Let* ϕ *be a conjunction of literals of the underlying object language of* $\mathcal{P}$. *Then,* $\bigoplus_i \mathcal{P} \models_{sm} \phi$ *iff* **holds** ϕ **at** i? *is true in* $\langle \mathcal{P}_i, SU_i \rangle = \langle \mathcal{P}_0, SU_0 \rangle \otimes \langle EU_1, \{\} \rangle \otimes \ldots \otimes \langle EU_i, \{\} \rangle$. *Furthermore,* $SM(\mathcal{P}_i) = SM(P_1 \oplus \ldots \oplus P_i)$ *when restricted to the underlying object language of* $\mathcal{P}$.

Proof. *Let* $\mathcal{P}$ *and* $\langle EU_1, \{\} \rangle, \ldots, \langle EU_s, \{\} \rangle$ *be as defined above. Then,* $\langle \mathcal{P}_0, SU_0 \rangle \otimes \langle EU_1, \{\} \rangle \otimes \ldots \otimes \langle EU_i, \{\} \rangle = \langle \mathcal{P}_i, \{\} \rangle$ *where* $\mathcal{P}_i = P'_0 \oplus P'_1 \oplus \cdots \oplus P'_i$ *is such that* $(1 \leq n \leq i)$:

$$P'_0 = \{\}$$
$$P'_n = \{N(r) \leftarrow; H(r) \leftarrow B(r), N(r) : r \in P_n\} \cup \{not\, Ev(R, t-1) \leftarrow; Ev(R, t) \leftarrow\}$$

since the literals not $Ev(R, t-1)$ *and* $Ev(R, t)$ *cannot belong to* ϕ, *nor those of the form* $N(R)$, *and there are no rules for not* $N(R)$, *and since* P'_0 *can be simply eliminated for being empty,* $SM(\mathcal{P}_i) = SM(P''_1 \oplus \cdots \oplus P''_i)$ *where*

$$P''_n = \{H(r) \leftarrow B(r) : r \in P_n\}$$

Note that $P''_n = P_n$. *It follows that* $\bigoplus_i \mathcal{P} \models_{sm} \phi$ *iff* $\bigoplus \mathcal{P}_i \models_{sm} \phi$ *iff* $P''_1 \oplus \cdots \oplus P''_i \models_{sm} \phi$. ■

Immediately we obtain that KABUL embeds both Interpretation Updates and Logic Programs under the stable model semantics.

Corollary 75 *KABUL embeds interpretation updates [157].*

Corollary 76 *KABUL embeds logic programs under the stable model semantics.*

We now draw some brief remarks about the complexity of KABUL. We first consider the complexity of reasoning about a knowledge state $\langle \mathcal{P}_s, SU_s \rangle$.

Theorem 77 (Complexity of Query Evaluation) *Consider the KABUL knowledge state* $\langle \mathcal{P}_s, SU_s \rangle$ *and the query:*

$$Q = \textbf{holds}(L_1, \ldots, L_k, in(R_1), \ldots, in(R_m), out(R_{m+1}), \ldots, out(R_n)) \textbf{ at } s\ ?$$

Deciding whether Q *is true is* $coNP-complete$.

Proof. *Since to determine if the query is true we have to decide if*

$$L_1, \ldots, L_k, N(R_1), \ldots, N(R_m), not\, N(R_{m+1}), \ldots, not\, N(R_n)$$

is true in every stable model of $\mathcal{P}_s$, *the complexity result is the same as for DLP (Theorem 41).* ■

For each state, we can also perform brave reasoning i.e., determine if some atom belongs to some stable model of $\mathcal{P}_s$, as well as determine whether some interpretation is a stable model of $\mathcal{P}_s$. The complexity of these tasks is as for DLP, presented in Theorem 41 i.e.:

1. deciding whether $\mathcal{P}_s$ has a stable model is $NP-complete$;
2. deciding whether a given interpretation is a stable model of $\mathcal{P}_s$ is P;

3. deciding whether a given atom is true in at least one stable model of $\mathcal{P}_s$ is $NP-complete$;

We now turn to the complexity of determining the next state $\langle \mathcal{P}_{s+1}, SU_{s+1} \rangle$, given some state $\langle \mathcal{P}_s, SU_s \rangle$ and an input $\langle EU_{s+1}, EO_{s+1} \rangle$. To determine the next state, one first has to partially evaluate the statements to obtain the reduced statements. This step requires the determination of the stable models semantics of the object level DLP together with the partial evaluation of observations which is obtained by a simple check on the presence or absence of elements in a set. Therefore, this step is in the $coNP-complete$ class. Given the set of reduced statements, determining if a coherent set of commands is a set of executable commands is, as for DLP, in P. If the selection function can be polynomial-time computable with an NP oracle, then deciding which set of coherent commands is to be executed is in $NP-complete$. Given a set of executable commands, determining the next state is obtained in linear time.

Of course these are worst case complexity results. Under certain common conditions better results can be achieved. For example, if the statements involved do not contain command conditions, then determining the set of executable commands can be achieved polynomially, as per the algorithm presented before. Note that the selection function is redundant here. For the case where only factual updates exist, i.e. the case where all command arguments are either statements or facts, then the stable model semantics is total and can be determined in polynomial time.

5.7 Comparisons

Even though we have extensively referred LUPS which, together with KUL and EPI, served as the seed for KABUL, we have not presented a formal relationship between them. Although a straightforward embedding of LUPS by KABUL is not possible because of the way the semantics of LUPS deals with non-inertial commands, as shown in the previous Chapter, it would be reasonable to expect such embedding of KUL by KABUL. But such an embedding does not exist for the general case. This is so essentially because when evolving from KUL to KABUL we have abandoned the cancellation commands and introduced inhibition commands. In KUL, the effect of a cancellation statement[5] such as **cancel assert** *rule* **when** *conds*, if *conds* holds, is to remove from the set of persistent statements every statement of the form **always assert** *rule* **when** X, where X stands for any conjunction of literals. We believe that this cancellation command is too strong in its effects because it does not allow for selective cancellation of persistent statements. In KUL (as well as in LUPS), if the following two persistent statements are present:

always assert *rule* **when** a
always assert *rule* **when** b

it is not possible to cancel one of them without cancelling the other. In KABUL, there is no cancellation command, but rather a retraction command that allows the user to retract any particular statement, and an inhibition command that prevents some update operation from being carried out. If one knows which persistent commands have been previously issued for some particular rule, then one can obtain the same effect as

[5] To avoid confusion, we keep the KABUL designation and call a command with its preconditions a statement.

the KUL cancellation command by issuing a combination of retraction commands and inhibition commands. For example, if in KABUL we have the following two statements in the self update of some state:

$$\textbf{always\_assert}\,(rule) \Leftarrow a$$
$$\textbf{always\_assert}\,(rule) \Leftarrow b$$

and we want to perform a cancellation (*à la KUL*), subject to conditions *conds*, we can issue the following three statements (assuming that external updates prevail over self updates):

$$\textbf{retract}\,(\textbf{always\_assert}\,(rule) \Leftarrow a) \Leftarrow conds$$
$$\textbf{retract}\,(\textbf{always\_assert}\,(rule) \Leftarrow b) \Leftarrow conds$$
$$not\ \textbf{assert}\,(rule) \Leftarrow conds$$

Note however that an extension to KABUL to cater for such cancellation commands would be straightforward, either by explicitly introducing such commands and extending the semantics accordingly, or by allowing for the use of variables ranging in the domain of all possible statement conditions, i.e. by allowing statements of the form:

$$\textbf{retract}\,(\textbf{always\_assert}\,(rule) \Leftarrow X) \Leftarrow conds$$

One other issue that distinguishes KUL (and LUPS) from KABUL is the way incoherent updates are dealt with. Suppose we perform an update consisting of the following two statements:

$$\textbf{assert}\,(rule) \Leftarrow$$
$$\textbf{retract}\,(rule) \Leftarrow$$

In KUL (and LUPS), these statements would produce a contradictory object level DLP because both the facts *not* $N(R)$ and $N(R)$ would belong to the next state object level logic program. Accordingly, at such a state there are no stable models. On the contrary, and to avoid the situation where such an update causes the knowledge base to become such that it has no stable models, in KABUL such a pair of update statements would produce a set of executable commands only containing the command $\textbf{assert}\,(\bot_{s+1})$ to signal the fact. With this semantics, in KABUL, we can determine, if needed, whether such incoherent updates were attempted without causing such a knowledge state without stable models.

Given these intrinsic differences between KABUL and KUL, we can still embed the fragment of KUL consisting of the language without the cancellation command and no incoherent updates, in KABUL, as per the following Theorem:

Theorem 78 *Let* $\mathcal{U} = U_1 \otimes ... \otimes U_n$ *be a* KUL *program and* $\langle \mathcal{P}_n, SU_n \rangle = \langle \mathcal{P}_0, SU_0 \rangle \otimes \langle U_1', \{\} \rangle \otimes ... \otimes \langle U_n', \{\} \rangle$ *where each* U_i' *is obtained from* U_i *by simply replacing the keyword* **when** *with the arrow* $\Leftarrow$*, be such that for every* $s : 1 \leq s \leq n$ $\Delta_s \neq \{\textbf{assert}\,(\bot_s)\}$*. A query* $Q =$ **holds** $L_1, \ldots, L_k$ **at** $t?$*,* $1 \leq t \leq n$*, is true in* $\mathcal{U}$ *iff* Q *is true in* $\langle \mathcal{P}_n, SU_n \rangle$ *(with* $EU^+ = SU^+$*).*

Proof. *The KABUL next state constructive definitions (Definitions 97 and 98) can be easily reduced to their KUL inductive counterparts (Definition 68), coinciding if no cancellation commands are present and an executable set of commands different from* $\{\textbf{assert}\,(\bot_s)\}$ *exists at every state transition.* ■

We have stated that a straightforward embedding of LUPS is not possible because of the way LUPS handles non-inertial commands, it is possible to simulate such behaviour in KABUL. Recall that a non-inertial assertion would cause, when its effect ceases to persist, the retraction of all syntactically equal, previously asserted, rules. The effect of one such LUPS statement, of the form

$$\textbf{assert event } Rule \textbf{ when } Condition$$

could be achieved with the following KABUL statements:

$$\begin{aligned} \textbf{assert\_event}\,(Rule) &\Leftarrow Condition \\ \textbf{assert}\,(\textbf{retract}\,(Rule) \Leftarrow) &\Leftarrow Condition \end{aligned}$$

In what concerns EPI, we have mentioned before that the way persistent assertion commands are treated is somewhat unnatural inasmuch the rule specified by them will be asserted at every state after the first state at which their preconditions are met. Accordingly, if the statement

$$\textbf{always } Rule \textbf{ when } Condition$$

is present in the update policy and, for example at state 2 the pre-conditions *Condition* hold then, the rule *Rule* will be asserted at each program of every subsequent state transition. Even though we cannot understand the usefulness of such behaviour, it can be encoded in KABUL by the statements:

$$\begin{aligned} \textbf{always\_assert}\,(\textbf{always\_assert}\,(Rule) \Leftarrow) &\Leftarrow Condition \\ \textbf{assert}\,(Rule) &\Leftarrow Condition \end{aligned}$$

The second statement is needed for the first state transition, so that *Rule* is immediately asserted if *Condition* holds at the first state.

We now turn our attention to other existing frameworks which somehow share a relationship with KABUL, and draw remarks on their similarities and differences.

Providing relational database systems with production rules to activate their otherwise static nature has been extensively investigated, giving rise to what is commonly known as active databases [227]. The AI originated production rule paradigm [42] has been modified, to suit the relational database context, so that rules correspond to database operations, occurrences of database states, etc, and explicit specification of events is facilitated. Such active rules take the generic form:

on *event*
if *condition*
then *action*

The way a set of these rules is processed depends on the system, but usually follows a variation of the recognize-act cycle:

---

initial match (test rule conditions)
repeat until no rules match
  perform conflict resolution (pick a triggered rule)
  act (execute the rule's action)
  match (test rule conditions)
end.

One can easily identify resemblances between such active rules and KABUL statements. In fact, they are both triggered by events (external observations in the case of KABUL), and they both depend on conditions that have to be met. Actions in such active rules could be seen as update commands in KABUL, i.e. operations on the knowledge base. Here is where the similarities end and differences begin:

- first, the data part of active databases consists of relations whereas, in KABUL the object level knowledge base is a dynamic logic program. In some sense a DLP is closer to the traditional paradigm of deductive databases rather than the relational ones;
- second, in active databases only one rule is picked and executed at each cycle, while in KABUL all rules are evaluated and a set of update operations is determined for being executed. The process of picking a particular rule is somehow less declarative, in some sense resembling some of the main differences between PROLOG and "pure" Logic Programming in what concerns rule selection. In KABUL, conditions on rules can refer to the concurrent execution of other update actions, something not possible in active databases because of their "one rule at a time" policy;
- third, statements in KABUL allow the update operations to modify the set of statements that specify future updates, i.e. they allow the update of the behaviour specification. In active databases, this would be like having one such active rule to specify the introduction or removal of another such rule, something not possible in any active database system we are aware of.

In deductive databases (cf [200] for a survey), data is divided into two categories: extensional data (containing the facts) and intensional data (containing the rules). As we have mentioned before, update operations on these databases are only allowed on its extensional part. *DLP* overcomes this for logic programs (which can be seen as a deductive database). Accordingly, *KABUL* can be seen as an extension to such deductive databases allowing for the declarative specification of updates to both data and rules in a uniform manner, as well as introducing the concept of behaviour specification by means of the self update statements. In some sense, the concept of *Evolving Knowledge Bases* supported by *KABUL* has the knowledge representation capabilities of deductive databases (with SM semantics), together with the update semantics of *DLP*, plus a notion of declarative active rules (statements) encoding both external and internal updates, which can not only update the object level knowledge but also specify changes to such statements. All this together with access to external observations such as in active databases. At a higher abstraction level, we can see *Evolving Knowledge Bases* as a combination of the knowledge representation of *Deductive Databases*, the active rules of *Active Databases*, and full blown updates to either the object knowledge and the active rules:

$$EKB = DDB + ADB + \textit{Full Updates}$$

We have mentioned before the relationship between update languages (*LUPS*, *EPI* and *KUL*) and action languages such as $\mathcal{A}$ and $\mathcal{C}$, noting that they differ in their motivation and underlying assumptions, the former to specify updates and the latter to reason about actions and causality more suitable for planning purposes rather than to exhibit a reactive behaviour both to events and knowledge states consisting of rules - note that the notion of event is not present in action languages and states are just sets of facts (fluents). Such action languages have been applied to active databases [29] and later served as the inspiration for the *Policy Description Language* (*PDL*)[151]. Informally, *PDL* is a language in which one can declaratively specify policies (mappings of events into actions). In the authors' own words, "*PDL* can be described as a real time specialized production rule system to define policies" or, in other words, as an extension of action languages to incorporate events. In *PDL*, policies are specified by rules of the form:

$$event\ \textbf{causes}\ action\ \textbf{if}\ condition$$
$$event\ \textbf{triggers}\ policy\ defined\ event\ \textbf{if}\ condition$$

and event histories produce policies in the form of sequences of actions. Again, some similarities between *PDL* and update languages exist if assertions and retractions are to be seen as actions. Since *PDL* allows for *event* to refer to rather elaborate combinations of events, some of the expressions allowed by nesting in *KABUL* statements can be achieved, as for example actions that depend on sequences of events. But in *PDL*, policies are fixed, i.e. policies cannot change policies. For example, an action cannot specify the retraction of another policy.

However, *PDL* as well as other languages that deal with events such as the *Composite Temporal Event Language* of Motakis and Zaniolo [171] suggest the need for further investigation in what concerns the incorporation of ways to deal with complex composition of events in *KABUL*, possibly leading to more flexibility and syntactical simplifications in *KABUL*.

Synchronous Declarative Languages have been designed (e.g. [32, 45]) with the purpose of modelling reactive systems, providing idealized primitives allowing users to think of their programs as reacting instantaneously to external events, and variables are functions of multiform time each having an associated clock defining the sequence of instants where the variable takes its values. *KABUL* shares with these the declarativity and the ability to deal with changing environments. Being based on DLP, its approach allows for modelling environments where the governing laws change over time, and where it is possible to reason with incomplete information (via non-monotonic default negation). Both these aspects are beyond the scope of the synchronous declarative languages. On the other hand, the ability of these languages to deal with various clocks, and the synchronization primitives, cannot be handled by *KABUL* as it stands. The usefulness of these features for the problems we want to model, and the possibility of incorporating them in *KABUL*, should be considered.

Transaction Logic (*TL*) [34] is also a LP language for knowledge base updates. *TL* is concerned with finding, given a goal, the appropriate transactions (or updates) to an underlying knowledge base in order to satisfy the goal. In *TL*, unlike in *KABUL*, the rules that specify changes are not updatable. Also, the whole process in *TL* is query driven, and thus depends on goals. On the contrary, in *KABUL* there is no need for goals to start an update process: an *Evolving Knowledge Base* specified in *KABUL* evolves by itself. Also, in *KABUL* there is no notion of finding updates to satisfy a goal: the updates are given, and *KABUL* is concerned with determining the meaning of the EKB after such updates. Determining such updates would amount to some form of abduction over *KABUL* programs. Similar arguments apply when comparing *KABUL* to PROLOG asserts, though in this case there is the additional argument of there not being a clear semantics (with attending problems when asserts are subject to backtracking over them).

5.8 Concluding Remarks and Open Issues

In this Chapter we have modified and extended the LUPS based KUL language by introducing the language KABUL. Within this new framework we are able to express all the desirable update statements mentioned at the beginning of this Chapter, namely:

- to directly specify updates that depend on a sequence of conditions as we have seen in Example 51;
- to directly specify delayed effects of actions as we have seen in Example 52, as well as other action specifications not expressible in KUL as we've seen in Example 53.
- to express the specification of future updates with a good degree of flexibility, this being provided by the self-update and the possibility to write nested statements, and illustrated in Examples 50, 51 and 53;
- to directly specify an update that should be executed only once, at the first state transition on which its conditions are verified, and then cease to persist, this being accomplished by the newly introduced semi-persistent commands, and illustrated in Examples 50 and 51;
- to specify an update that depends on the concurrent execution of other commands. The solution being inspired by *EPI*, with its semantics corrected, and illustrated in Examples 50 and 55;
- to specify an update that depends on the "*memorial*" presence (or absence) of a specific rule in the object knowledge base, this being accomplished with the introduction of rule conditions, and illustrated in Examples 50 and 51;
- there is no longer the need, when reasoning about actions, for an intermediate state transition for the atom representing the action to be asserted, before its effects are verified, this being accomplished with the introduction of the access to external observations, and illustrated in Examples 50, 51, 52, 53, 54 and 55;
- to directly specify the inhibition of a command, this being attained with the introduction of inhibition commands and illustrated in Examples 50 and 51.

But most importantly, KABUL supports the concept of *Evolving Knowledge Bases* i.e., a knowledge base which can not only be externally updated, but is capable of self evolution by means of its internally specified behaviour.

Although we believe that KABUL achieves its proposed purpose, much remains to be done. We now elaborate on several issues which should be further investigated, some of them being the subject of our current research:

Well Founded Based Semantics: one of the most important features of the well founded semantics for logic programs is its amenability to implementation, namely in what concerns its complexity and possibility to have solely top down computation (relevancy). One way to reduce the computational complexity of KABUL is to use a well founded semantics for DLP, thus reducing the complexity of the partial evaluation step, followed by a well founded version of the semantics of executable commands. Also, when such unique well founded set of executable commands is specified, we no longer need the selection function. Achieving a polynomial implementable semantics of KABUL is certainly one of the most important subjects of further research.

Syntactical Simplifications: in order to have an expressive language in which rather complex update statements are representable in a uniform way, we often lose simplicity when writing some rather simple updates. This is true for example of updates that just specify the assertion of some rule when a certain sequence of conditions hold, where a statement with deep nesting is required for that. One promising way to solve this issue is to adapt existing frameworks, specialized in the representation of such temporal composition of events, to KABUL. We have already mentioned one such language, the Composite Temporal Event Language of Motakis and Zaniolo [171].

Minimalist Approach: in the introductory section of this Chapter, we have mentioned two alternatives to develop a language such as KABUL. The one we have opted for consists in incorporating in the language and its semantics the syntactical constructs that allow for an intuitive representation of the kind of statements we identify as required. The alternative consists in identifying a rather more minimalist language, with the same representation power, and build libraries of macros to allow for the use of other intuitive constructs. By opting for the former, we do by no means discard the latter. In fact, what we have learned from developing KABUL as we have, has provided us with a great insight into this problem, supplying us with the necessary knowledge to embark on the other task. This is the subject of our current research, of which the first results can be found in [2].

Chapter 6

Multi-dimensional Dynamic Logic Programming

According to Dynamic Logic Programming (DLP), *knowledge may be given by a sequence of theories (encoded as logic programs) representing different states of knowledge. These may represent time (e.g. in updates), specificity (e.g. in taxonomies), strength of updating instance (e.g. in the legislative domain), hierarchical position of knowledge source (e.g. in organizations), etc. The mutual relationships extant among states are used to determine the semantics of the combined theory composed of all the individual theories. Although suitable to encode a single dimension (e.g. time, hierarchies...),* DLP *cannot deal with more than one simultaneously because it is defined only for a linear sequence of states. To overcome this limitation, in this Chapter we introduce the notion of* Multi-dimensional Dynamic Logic Programming ($\mathcal{MDLP}$), *which generalizes* DLP *to collections of states organized in arbitrary acyclic digraphs representing precedence. In this setting, $\mathcal{MDLP}$ assigns semantics to sets and subsets of such logic programs. By dint of this natural generalization, $\mathcal{MDLP}$ affords extra expressiveness, in effect enlarging the latitude of logic programming applications unifiable under a single framework. The generality and flexibility provided by the acyclic digraphs ensure a wide scope and variety of application possibilities. Parts of this Chapter appeared in [132–134, 136, 137].*

6.1 Introduction and Motivation

Even though the main motivation behind the introduction of *DLP* was to represent the evolution of knowledge in time, the relationship between the different states can encode other aspects of a system. In fact, since its introduction, *DLP* (and *LUPS*) has been employed to represent a stock of features of a system, namely as a means to represent and reason about the evolution of knowledge in time; combine rules learnt by a diversity of agents [127]; reason about updates of agents' beliefs [57]; model agent interaction [198, 199]; model and reason about actions [9] and even resolve inconsistencies in metaphorical reasoning.

The common property among these applications of *DLP* is that the states associated with the given set of theories encode only one of several possible representational dimensions (e.g. time, hierarchies, domains,...). This is so inasmuch *DLP* is defined for linear sequences of states alone.

For example, *DLP* can be used to model the relationship of a hierarchical related group of agents, and *DLP* can be used to model the evolution of a single agent over time. But *DLP*, as it stands, cannot deal with both settings at once, and model the evolution of one such group of agents over time. An instance of such a multi-dimensional scenario can be found in legal reasoning, where the legislative agency is divided conforming to a hierarchy of power, governed by the principle *Lex Superior (Lex Superior Derogat Legi Inferiori)* according to which the rule issued by a higher hierarchical authority overrides the one issued by a lower one, and the evolution of law in time is governed by the principle *Lex Posterior (Lex Posterior Derogat Legi Priori)* according to which the rule enacted at a later point in time overrides the earlier one. *DLP* can be used to model each of these principles separately, by using the sequence of states to represent either the hierarchy or time, but is unable to cope with both at once when they interact.

In effect, knowledge updating is not to be simply envisaged as taking place in the time dimension alone. Several updating dimensions may combine simultaneously, with or without the temporal one, such as specificity (as in taxonomies), strength of the updating instance (as in the legislative domain), hierarchical position of knowledge source (as in organizations), credibility of the source (as in uncertain, mined, or learnt knowledge), or opinion precedence (as in a society of agents). Some of these examples will be further elaborated upon in a subsequent section. For this to be possible, *DLP* needs to be extended to allow for a more general structure of states.

In this Chapter we introduce the notion of *Multi-dimensional Dynamic Logic Programming* ($\mathcal{MDLP}$), which generalizes *DLP* to allow for collections of states represented by arbitrary acyclic digraphs. In this setting, $\mathcal{MDLP}$ assigns semantics to sets and subsets of logic programs, depending on how they stand in relation to one another, these relations being defined by the acyclic digraph (*DAG*) that represents the states. By dint of such natural generalization, $\mathcal{MDLP}$ affords extra expressiveness, thereby enlarging the latitude of logic programming applications unifiable under a single framework. The generality and flexibility provided by the *DAG*s ensure a wide scope and variety of possibilities, of which some will be expounded in the sequel.

It is our opinion that, by virtue of these newly added characteristics of multiplicity and composition, $\mathcal{MDLP}$ provides a "societal" viewpoint in *Logic Programming*, important in these web and agent days, for combining knowledge in general.

The remainder of this Chapter is structured as follows: first we provide the necessary definitions related to graph theory that will be used throughout. Next, we introduce the notion of *Multi-dimensional Dynamic Logic Programming* ($\mathcal{MDLP}$) and characterize its stable models. Then, we present an alternative semantical characterization based on a purely syntactical transformation. Finally we draw some properties of $\mathcal{MDLP}$ and present several illustrative examples.

6.2 Graphs

A *directed graph*, or *digraph*, $D = (V, E, \delta)$ is a composite notion of two finite or infinite sets $V = V_D$ of *vertices* and $E = E_D$ of (*directed*) *edges* and a mapping $\delta : E \rightarrow V \times V$. If $\delta(e) = (v, w)$ then v is called the *initial vertex* and w the *final vertex* of the edge e. A *directed edge sequence from v_0 to v_n* in a digraph is a sequence of edges $e_1, e_2, ..., e_n$

such that $\delta(e_i) = (v_{i-1}, v_i)$ for $i = 1, ..., n$. A *directed path* is a directed edge sequence in which all the edges are distinct. A *directed acyclic graph*, or *acyclic digraph (DAG)*, is a digraph D such that there are no directed edge sequences from v to v, for all vertices v of D. A *source* is a vertex with in-valency 0 (number of edges for which it is a final vertex) and a *sink* is a vertex with out-valency 0 (number of edges for which it is an initial vertex). We say that $v <_D w$ if there is a directed path from v to w and that $v \leq_D w$ if $v <_D w$ or $v = w$.

For simplicity, we will omit the explicit representation of the mapping δ of a graph, and represent its edges $e \in E$ by their corresponding pairs of vertices (v, w) such that $(v, w) = \delta(e)$. Therefore, a graph D will be represented by the pair (V, E) where V is a set of vertices and E is a set of pairs of vertices. The *transitive closure* of a graph D is a graph $D^+ = (V, E^+)$ such that for all $v, w \in V$ there is an edge (v, w) in E^+ if and only if $v <_D w$.

Follows the notion of relevancy DAG, D_v, of a DAG D, with respect to a vertex v of D.

Definition 102 (Relevancy DAG with respect to a vertex) *Let $D = (V, E)$ be an acyclic digraph. Let v be a vertex of D, i.e. $v \in V$. The relevancy DAG of D with respect to v is $D_v = (V_v, E_v)$ where:*

$$V_v = \{v_i : v_i \in V \text{ and } v_i \leq_D v\} \tag{6.1}$$

$$E_v = \{(v_i, v_j) : (v_i, v_j) \in E \text{ and } v_i, v_j \in V_v\} \tag{6.2}$$

Intuitively the relevancy DAG of D with respect to v is the subgraph of D consisting of all vertices and edges contained in all directed paths to v. We will also need the notion of Relevancy DAG with respect to a set of vertices:

Definition 103 (Relevancy DAG with respect to a set of vertices) *Let $D = (V, E)$ be an acyclic digraph. Let S be a set of vertices of D, i.e. $S \subseteq V$, and for every $v \in S$ let $D_v = (V_v, E_v)$ be the relevancy DAG of D with respect to v. The relevancy DAG of D with respect to S is $D_S = (V_S, E_S)$ where:*

$$V_S = \bigcup_{v \in S} V_v \tag{6.3}$$

$$E_S = \bigcup_{v \in S} E_v \tag{6.4}$$

Intuitively the relevancy *DAG* of D with respect to S is the subgraph of D consisting of the union of the relevancy *DAG*s with respect to all vertices in S.

6.3 Multi-dimensional Dynamic Logic Programming

As noted in the introduction of this Chapter, allowing the individual theories of a dynamic program update to relate via a linear sequence of states only, delimits the use of *DLP* to represent and reason about a single evolving aspect of a system (e.g. time, hierarchy,...). In this section we generalize *DLP* to allow for states to be represented by the vertices of an acyclic digraph (*DAG*) and their precedence relations by the corresponding graph edges, thus enabling to concurrently represent, depending on the choice

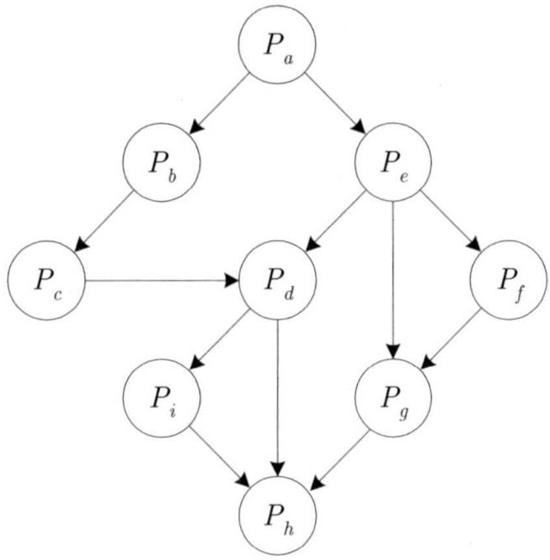

Figure 6.1: A Directed Acyclic Digraph

of a particular *DAG*, several interrelated dimensions of a representational updatable system. In particular, the *DAG* can stand not only for a system with n independent dimensions, but also encompass inter-dimensional dependencies. In this setting, $\mathcal{MDLP}$ assigns semantics to sets and to subsets of logic programs, depending on how they stand in relation to one another.

We start by defining the framework consisting of the generalized logic programs indexed by a *DAG*. Throughout this Chapter, we will restrict ourselves to *DAG*'s such that for every vertex v of the *DAG*, any path to v is finite.

Definition 104 (Multi-dimensional Dynamic Logic Program) *Let $\mathcal{L}_\mathcal{K}$ be a propositional language as described before. A* Multi-dimensional Dynamic Logic Program (MDLP), $\mathcal{P}$, *is a pair $(\mathcal{P}_D, D)$ where $D = (V, E)$ is an acyclic digraph and $\mathcal{P}_D = \{P_v : v \in V\}$ is a finite or infinite set of generalized logic programs in the language $\mathcal{L}_\mathcal{K}$, indexed by the vertices $v \in V$ of D. We call* states *such vertices of D. For simplicity, we will often leave the language $\mathcal{L}_\mathcal{K}$ implicit.*

6.3.1 Declarative Semantics

We want to characterize the models of $\mathcal{P}$ at any given state. To this purpose, we will keep to the basic intuition of logic program updates, whereby an interpretation is a stable model of the update of a program P by a program U iff it is a stable model of a program consisting of the rules of U together with the subset of rules of P comprised by those that are not rejected, i.e.do not carry over by inertia due to their being overridden by update program U. With the introduction of a *DAG* to index the programs, it is no longer the case that a given program has a single ancestor or a single descendent. This has to be dealt with, the desired intuition being that a program $P_v \in \mathcal{P}_D$ can be used to reject rules of program $P_u \in \mathcal{P}_D$, at v or some descendant of v, if there is a directed path from u to v. In the example depicted in Fig.6.1, rules of P_i can be used to reject rules from P_c but not to reject rules from P_f.

Formally, the models of the *Multi-dimensional Dynamic Logic Program* are characterized according to this definition:

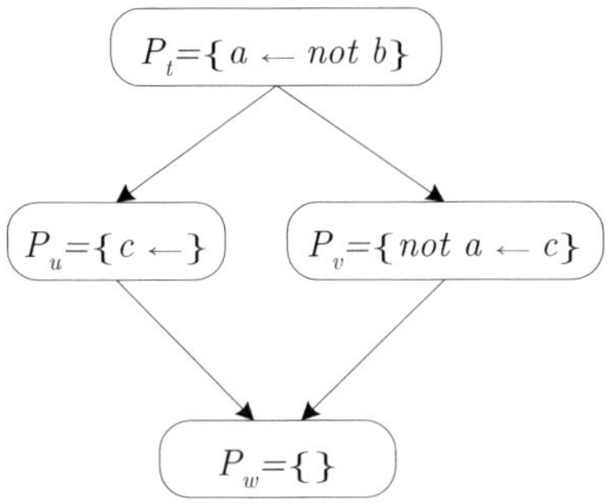

Figure 6.2: *MDLP* of Example 56

Definition 105 (Stable Models at state s) *Let* $\mathcal{P} = (\mathcal{P}_D, D)$ *be a* Multi-dimensional Dynamic Logic Program, *where* $\mathcal{P}_D = \{P_v : v \in V\}$ *and* $D = (V, E)$. *An interpretation* M_s *is a* stable model of $\mathcal{P}$ at state $s \in V$, *iff:*

$$M_s = least\left([\rho(\mathcal{P})_s - Reject(\mathcal{P}, s, M_s)] \cup Default\left(\rho(\mathcal{P})_s, M_s\right)\right) \tag{6.5}$$

where

$$\rho(\mathcal{P})_s = \bigcup_{i \leq_D s} P_i \tag{6.6}$$

$$Reject(\mathcal{P}, s, M_s) = \{r \in P_i \mid \exists r' \in P_j, i <_D j \leq_D s, r \bowtie r' \wedge M_s \vDash B(r')\} \tag{6.7}$$

$$Default\left(\rho(\mathcal{P})_s, M_s\right) = \{not\, A \mid \nexists r \in \rho(\mathcal{P})_s : (H(r) = A) \wedge M_s \vDash B(r)\} \tag{6.8}$$

By $SM\left(\bigoplus_s \mathcal{P}\right)$ *we mean the set of all stable models of* $\mathcal{P}$ *at state* s. *If some literal or conjunction of literals* ϕ *holds in all stable models of* $\mathcal{P}$ *at state* s, *we write* $\bigoplus_s \mathcal{P} \models_{sm} \phi$.

Intuitively, the set $Reject(\mathcal{P}, s, M_s)$ contains those rules belonging to a program indexed by a state i that are overridden by the head of another rule with true body in state j along any path to state s. $\rho(\mathcal{P})_s$ contains all rules of all programs that are indexed by a state along all paths leading to state s, i.e. all rules that are potentially relevant to determine the semantics at state s. The set $Default\left(\rho(\mathcal{P})_s, M_s\right)$ contains default negations $not\, A$ of all unsupported atoms A, i.e., those atoms A for which there is no rule in $\rho(\mathcal{P})_s$ whose body is true in M_s.

Example 56 *Consider the MDLP* $\mathcal{P} = (\mathcal{P}_D, D)$ *such that* $\mathcal{P}_D = \{P_t, P_u, P_v, P_w\}$ *where:*

$$\begin{array}{ll} P_t = \{a \leftarrow not\, b\} & P_u = \{c \leftarrow\} \\ P_v = \{not\, a \leftarrow c\} & P_w = \{\} \end{array} \tag{6.9}$$

and $D = (V, E)$ *where*

$$V = \{t, u, v, w\} \tag{6.10}$$

$$E = \{(t, u), (t, v), (u, w), (v, w)\} \tag{6.11}$$

as depicted in Fig.6.2. The only stable model at state w *is* $M_w = \{not\, a, not\, b, c\}$. *To confirm, we have that:*

$$Reject(\mathcal{P}, w, M_w) = \{a \leftarrow not\, b\} \qquad Default\left(\rho(\mathcal{P})_w, M_w\right) = \{not\, b\} \tag{6.12}$$

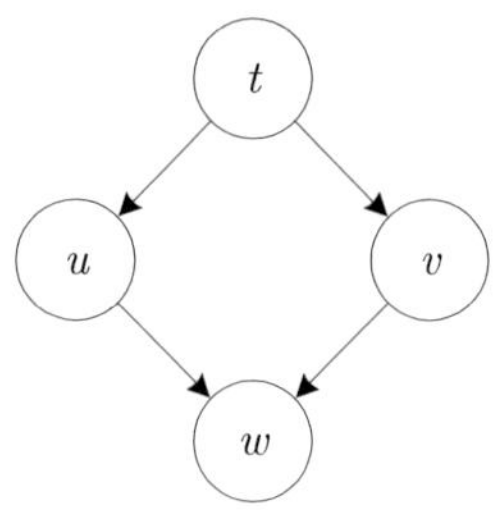

Figure 6.3: *MDLP* of Example 57

and, finally,

$$[\rho(\mathcal{P})_w - Reject(\mathcal{P}, w, M_w)] \cup Default(\rho(\mathcal{P})_w, M_w) = \{not\, a \leftarrow c; c \leftarrow; not\, b\} \quad (6.13)$$

whose least model is M_w. *Note that at state* v *the only stable model is* $M_v = \{a, not\, b, not\, c\}$ *because the rule* $not\, a \leftarrow c$ *only rejects the rule* $a \leftarrow not\, b$ *at state* w*, that is, when both the rules* $not\, a \leftarrow c$ *and* $c \leftarrow$ *are present.*

Example 57 *Consider the* MDLP $\mathcal{P} = (\mathcal{P}_D, D)$ *such that* $\mathcal{P}_D = \{P_t, P_u, P_v, P_w\}$ *where*

$$\begin{array}{llll} P_t = & \{d \leftarrow\} & P_w = & \{not\, a \leftarrow b \\ P_u = & \{a \leftarrow not\, e\} & & b \leftarrow not\, c \\ P_v = & \{not\, a \leftarrow d\} & & c \leftarrow not\, b\} \end{array} \quad (6.14)$$

and $D = (V, E)$ *where*

$$V = \{t, u, v, w\} \quad (6.15)$$
$$E = \{(t, u), (t, v), (u, w), (v, w)\} \quad (6.16)$$

as depicted in Fig. 6.3. The only stable model at state w *is*

$$M_w = \{not\, a, b, not\, c, d, not\, e\}$$

To confirm, we have that

$$Reject(\mathcal{P}, w, M_w) = \{a \leftarrow not\, e\} \qquad Default(\rho(\mathcal{P})_w, M_w) = \{not\, c, not\, e\} \quad (6.17)$$

and, finally,

$$\begin{array}{l} [\rho(\mathcal{P})_w - Reject(\mathcal{P}, w, M_w)] \cup Default(\rho(\mathcal{P})_w, M_w) = \\ = \{d \leftarrow; not\, a \leftarrow d; not\, a \leftarrow b; b \leftarrow not\, c; c \leftarrow not\, b\} \cup \{not\, c, not\, e\} \end{array} \quad (6.18)$$

whose least model is M_w. *The reader can check that* M_w *is* the only *stable model at state* w.

The next proposition establishes that when determining the models of a $MDLP$ at state s, we need only consider the part of the $MDLP$ corresponding to the relevancy graph with respect to state s.

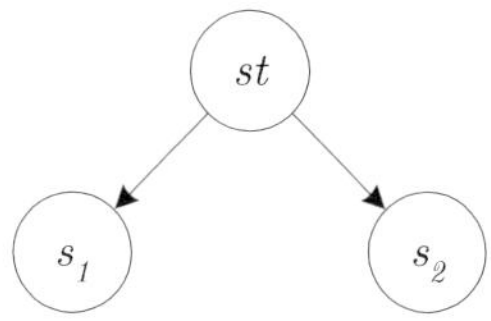

Figure 6.4: A DAG with one student and two supervisors

Proposition 79 *Let* $\mathcal{P} = (\mathcal{P}_D, D)$ *be a* Multi-dimensional Dynamic Logic Program, *where* $\mathcal{P}_D = \{P_v : v \in V\}$ *and* $D = (V, E)$. *Let* s *be a state in* V. *Let* $\mathcal{P}' = (\mathcal{P}_{D_s}, D_s)$ *be a Multi-dimensional Dynamic Logic Program where* $D_s = (V_s, E_s)$ *is the relevancy DAG of* D *with respect to* s. *and* $\mathcal{P}_{D_s} = \{P_v : v \in V_s\}$. M *is a* stable model of $\mathcal{P}$ at state s *iff* M *is a* stable model of $\mathcal{P}'$ at state s.

Proof. Simply recall that in Def. 105 the sets of rules $\rho(\mathcal{P})_s$, $Reject(\mathcal{P}, s, M)$, and $Default(\rho(\mathcal{P})_s, M)$, that completely characterize the stable models at state s, only depend on the rules of the programs indexed by the relevancy DAG with respect to s and on the relevancy DAG itself. Since they all coincide for $\mathcal{P}$ and $\mathcal{P}'$, the proposition follows. ∎

6.3.2 Multiple State Semantics

In the previous section we presented the semantics of a *Multi-dimensional Dynamic Logic Program* at a given state, by characterizing its stable models. But we might have a situation where we desire to determine the semantics jointly at more than one state. If all these states belong to the relevancy graph of one of them, we may simply determine the models at that state (Prop. 79). But this might not be the case. For example, imagine a student (st) with two supervisors (s_1 and s_2) whose opinion on something prevails over that of the student, as depicted in Fig.6.4. If we determine the models at state s_1 we do not consider the rules from s_2, and vice-versa. The student however might be interested in determining the semantics taking into account both supervisors, i.e. determining the models at a set of states.

For this purpose, we need to characterize the models at a set of states. Formally, the semantics of a $MDLP$ at an arbitrary set of its states is determined according to the following definition:

Definition 106 (Stable Models at a set of states S) *Let* $\mathcal{P} = (\mathcal{P}_D, D)$ *be a* Multi-dimensional Dynamic Logic Program, *where* $\mathcal{P}_D = \{P_v : v \in V\}$ *and* $D = (V, E)$. *Let* S *be a set of states such that* $S \subseteq V$. *An interpretation* M_S *is a* stable model of $\mathcal{P}$ at the set of states S *iff*

$$M_S = least\left(\left[\rho(\mathcal{P})_S - Reject(\mathcal{P}, S, M_S)\right] \cup Default\left(\rho(\mathcal{P})_S, M_S\right)\right) \tag{6.19}$$

where

$$\rho(\mathcal{P})_S = \bigcup_{s \in S}\left(\bigcup_{i \leq_D s} P_i\right) \tag{6.20}$$

$$Reject(\mathcal{P}, S, M_S) = \{r \in P_i \mid \exists s \in S, \exists r' \in P_j, i <_D j \leq_D s, r \bowtie r' \wedge M_S \vDash B(r')\} \tag{6.21}$$

$$Default\left(\rho(\mathcal{P})_S, M_S\right) = \{not\ A \mid \nexists r \in \rho(\mathcal{P})_S : (H(r) = A) \wedge M_S \vDash B(r)\} \tag{6.22}$$

By $SM(\bigoplus_S \mathcal{P})$ *we mean the set of all stable models of* $\mathcal{P}$ *at the set of states* S. *If some literal or conjunction of literals* ϕ *holds in all stable models of* $\mathcal{P}$ *at the set of states* S, *we write* $\bigoplus_S \mathcal{P} \models_{sm} \phi$. *If* $S = V$ *we simply omit the reference and write* $\bigoplus \mathcal{P} \models_{sm} \phi$. *Similarly, if* $S = V$, *instead of* $SM(\bigoplus_S \mathcal{P})$ *we write* $SM(\bigoplus \mathcal{P})$, *or simply* $SM(\mathcal{P})$, *and instead of* $\rho(\mathcal{P})_S$ *we simply write* $\rho(\mathcal{P})$.

If S contains only one state, then Def. 106 is equivalent to Def. 105:

Proposition 80 *Let* $\mathcal{P} = (\mathcal{P}_D, D)$ *be a* Multi-dimensional Dynamic Logic Program, *where* $\mathcal{P}_D = \{P_v : v \in V\}$ *and* $D = (V, E)$. *Let* $s \in V$ *be a state and* $S = \{s\}$. *The* stable models of $\mathcal{P}$ at the set of states S *coincide with the* stable models of $\mathcal{P}$ at state s.

Proof. Just note that (6.19), (6.20), (6.21) and (6.22) reduce to (6.5), (6.6), (6.7) and (6.8) respectively, when S contains only one state s. ∎

Intuitively, Def. 106 considers the relevancy graphs with respect to all states belonging to the set whose models are being determined.

In fact, this is equivalent to the addition of a new vertex α to the DAG, and connecting to α, by addition of edges, all states we wish to consider. Furthermore, the program indexed by α is empty. We then determine the stable models of this new *MDLP* at state α, as condoned by the following theorem:

Theorem 81 *Let* $\mathcal{P} = (\mathcal{P}_D, D)$ *be a* Multi-dimensional Dynamic Logic Program, *where* $\mathcal{P}_D = \{P_v : v \in V\}$ *and* $D = (V, E)$, *such that* $\alpha \notin V$. *Let* S *be a set of states such that* $S \subseteq V$. *An interpretation* M_S *is a* stable model of $\mathcal{P}$ at the set of states S *iff* M_S *is a* stable model of $\mathcal{P}'$ at state α *where* $\mathcal{P}' = (\mathcal{P}_{D_\alpha}, D_\alpha)$ *is the* Multi-dimensional Dynamic Logic Program *such that* $\mathcal{P}_{D_\alpha} = \mathcal{P}_D \cup P_\alpha$ *and* $D_\alpha = (V_\alpha, E_\alpha)$ *where:*

$$P_\alpha = \{\} \tag{6.23}$$
$$V_\alpha = V \cup \{\alpha\} \tag{6.24}$$
$$E_\alpha = E \cup \{(i, \alpha) : i \in S\} \tag{6.25}$$

Proof. *From Prop.80 it follows that we can use Definition 106 both when determining the semantics at the set of states* S *and at the single state* α. *For the proof of the theorem it is sufficient to prove that for every interpretation* M_S *the following holds:* ∎

Proof.

1. $\rho(\mathcal{P})_S = \rho(\mathcal{P}')_{\{\alpha\}}$
2. $Reject(\mathcal{P}, S, M_S) = Reject(\mathcal{P}', \{\alpha\}, M_S)$
3. $Default(\rho(\mathcal{P})_S, M_S) = Default\left(\rho(\mathcal{P}')_{\{\alpha\}}, M_S\right)$

1. $\rho(\mathcal{P})_S$ contains all rules belonging to all programs indexed by a vertex of the relevancy DAG with respect to S, D_S. From the construction of D_α it follows that the relevancy DAG of D_α with respect to α contains precisely the same set of vertices as D_S, plus vertex α. Since the program indexed by α, P_α, is empty, it follows that $\rho(\mathcal{P}')_{\{\alpha\}}$ contains the same rules as $\rho(\mathcal{P})_S$.

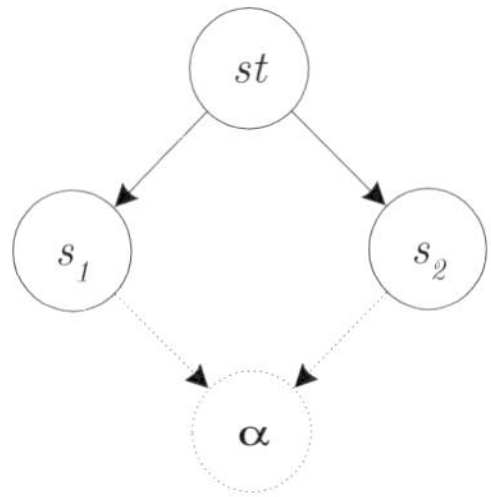

Figure 6.5: A DAG with one student, two supervisors and a sink

2. Let us start with

$$Reject\left(\mathcal{P}', \{\alpha\}, M_S\right) = \left\{ \begin{array}{c} r \in P_i \mid \exists s \in \{\alpha\}, \exists r' \in P_j, i <_{D_\alpha} j \leq_{D_\alpha} s, \\ r \bowtie r' \wedge M_s \vDash B(r') \end{array} \right\} \quad (6.26)$$

Since for all $v \in V, s \in S$ such that $v \leq_{D_\alpha} s$ we have that $v <_D \alpha$, we can rewrite the set $Reject\left(\mathcal{P}', \{\alpha\}, M_S\right)$ as:

$$Reject\left(\mathcal{P}', \{\alpha\}, M_S\right) = \left\{ \begin{array}{c} r \in P_i \mid \exists s \in S, \exists r' \in P_j, i <_D j \leq_D s, \\ r \bowtie r' \wedge M_s \vDash B(r') \end{array} \right\} \cup \quad (6.27)$$

$$\cup \left\{ \begin{array}{c} r \in P_i \mid \exists r' \in P_\alpha, i <_{D_\alpha} \alpha, \\ r \bowtie r' \wedge M_s \vDash B(r') \end{array} \right\} \quad (6.28)$$

Since $\nexists r' \in P_\alpha$, the set $Reject\left(\mathcal{P}', \{\alpha\}, M_S\right)$ can be reduced to

$$Reject\left(\mathcal{P}', \{\alpha\}, M_S\right) = \left\{ \begin{array}{c} r \in P_i \mid \exists s \in S, \exists r' \in P_j, i <_D j \leq_D s, \\ r \bowtie r' \wedge M_s \vDash B(r') \end{array} \right\} \quad (6.29)$$

i.e. $Reject\left(\mathcal{P}', \{\alpha\}, M_S\right) = Reject(\mathcal{P}, S, M_S)$.

3. According to Def.106,

$$Default\left(\rho\left(\mathcal{P}\right)_S, M_S\right) = \{not\ A \mid \nexists r \in \rho\left(\mathcal{P}\right)_S : (H(r) = A) \wedge M_S \vDash B(r)\} \quad (6.30)$$

Since $\rho\left(\mathcal{P}\right)_S = \rho\left(\mathcal{P}'\right)_{\{\alpha\}}$ then

$$Default\left(\rho\left(\mathcal{P}\right)_S, M_S\right) = \left\{not\ A \mid \nexists r \in \rho\left(\mathcal{P}'\right)_{\{\alpha\}} : (H(r) = A) \wedge M_S \vDash B(r)\right\} = \\ = Default\left(\rho\left(\mathcal{P}'\right)_{\{\alpha\}}, M_S\right)$$

which completes the proof. ■

Fig.6.5 depicts this construction for the student/supervisor example of Fig.6.4. Note that since P_α is empty, it does not contribute to the rejection of any rules. In the student/supervisors example, intuitively, it has the effect of joining the rules of s_2 and s_1.

Mark that the addition of state α does not affect the stable models at other states. This is so because α and the newly introduced edges do not belong to the relevancy DAG with respect to any other state. States such as α are usefully introduced as *observation*

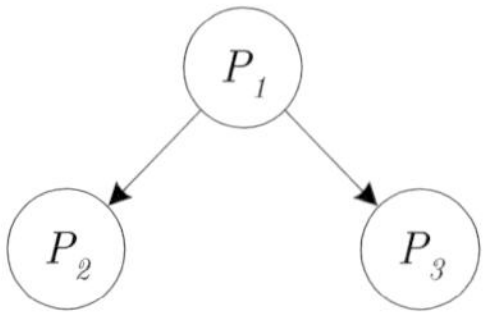

Figure 6.6: DAG of Example 58

nodes, because they provide *viewpoints* on the original DAG, without affecting the semantics at any of its original nodes.

Conceivably, this notion of observation node can be generalized to apply to a union of two (or more) Multi-dimensional Dynamic Logic Programs, $\mathcal{P}_1 = (\mathcal{P}_{D_1}, D_1)$ and $\mathcal{P}_2 = (\mathcal{P}_{D_2}, D_2)$, where the resulting DAG would be the union of both DAG's i.e., $D = D_1 \cup D_2 = \{V_1 \cup V_2, E_1 \cup E_2\}$.

In a subsequent Section, we provide some equivalence preserving simplifications to this definition, according to which, a subset of the new edges added in E_α can be removed whilst preserving the stable models.

6.3.3 Adding Strong Negation

The introduction of strong negation to the framework of Dynamic Logic Programming is, in all respects, similar to the case of DLP. The extended stable models are characterized as follows:

Definition 107 (Extended Stable Models at state s**)** *Let* $\mathcal{P} = (\mathcal{P}_D, D)$ *be a* Multi-dimensional Dynamic Logic Program, *where* $\mathcal{P}_D = \{P_v : v \in V\}$ *is an indexed set of extended logic programs in the language* $\mathcal{L}^*$ *and* $D = (V, E)$. *An extended interpretation* M_s *is an* extended stable model of $\mathcal{P}$ at state $s \in V$, *iff* M_s *is a* stable model of $\mathcal{P}^{exp}$ at state $s \in V$ *where* $\mathcal{P}^{exp}$ *is obtained from* $\mathcal{P}$ *by replacing each program* $P_s \in \mathcal{P}_D$ *by its expanded version* P_s^{exp}.

Again, in order to use strong negation in updates, one only needs to consider the expanded versions of each program and deal with complementary objective literals A and $-A$ as independent atoms.

The following example, adapted from [44][1], shows the use of strong negation:

Example 58 *Consider the set of security specifications, about a hierarchy of objects, represented by three programs indexed by the DAG of Fig.6.6:*

$$\begin{aligned} P_1 = \ & \{authorize(bob) \leftarrow not\, authorize(ann) \\ & authorize(ann) \leftarrow not\, authorize(tom), not\, \neg authorize(alice) \\ & authorize(tom) \leftarrow not\, authorize(ann), not\, \neg authorize(alice)\} \\ P_2 = \ & \{-authorize(alice) \leftarrow\} \\ P_3 = \ & \{-authorize(bob) \leftarrow\} \end{aligned}$$

The only extended stable models at state 2, *is:*

[1]The only difference from the original lies in the fact that, as usual, we encode exclusive disjunction as an even loop through default negation.

$$M_2 = \{-authorize(alice), authorize(bob)\}$$

At state 3 we obtain the following two extended stable models:

$$M_3 = \{authorize(ann), \neg authorize(bob)\}$$
$$M_3' = \{\neg authorize(tom), \neg authorize(bob)\}$$

6.4 Transformational Semantics for MDLP

Definition 105 above, establishes the semantics of *Multi-dimensional Dynamic Logic Programming* by characterizing its stable models at each state. Next we present an alternative definition, based on a purely syntactical transformation which, given a *Multi-dimensional Dynamic Logic Program,* $\mathcal{P} = (\mathcal{P}_D, D)$, produces a generalized logic program whose stable models are in a one-to-one equivalence relation with the stable models of the multi-dimensional dynamic logic program previously characterized. This transformation also provides a mechanism for implementing *Multi-dimensional Dynamic Logic Programming*: with a pre-processor performing the linear transformation, query answering is reduced to that over generalized logic programs.

Similar to *DLP*, and without loss of generality, we extend the DAG D with an initial state (s_0) and a set of directed edges (s_0, s') connecting the initial state to all the sources of D. Similarly, if we want to query a set of states, all needs doing is extending the *Multi-dimensional Dynamic Logic Program* with a new state α, as in Theorem 81, prior to the transformation. For our purposes, we extend $\overline{\mathcal{K}}$ with an ersatz new predicate *reject*/1. Therefore, from now on $\overline{\mathcal{K}}$ denotes the superset of the set $\mathcal{K}$ of propositional variables:

$$\overline{\mathcal{K}} = \mathcal{K} \cup \left\{A^-, A_s,\ A_s^-, A_{P_s},\ A_{P_s}^-, reject(A_s), reject(A_s^-) : A \in \mathcal{K},\ s \in V \cup \{s_0\}\right\} \tag{6.31}$$

Definition 108 (Multi-dimensional Dynamic Program Update) *Let* $\mathcal{P} = (\mathcal{P}_D, D)$ *be a* Multi-dimensional Dynamic Logic Program, *where* $\mathcal{P}_D = \{P_v : v \in V\}$ *and* $D = (V, E)$. *Given a fixed state* $s \in V$, *the multi-dimensional dynamic program update over* $\mathcal{P}$ *at state* s *is the generalized logic program* $\boxplus_s \mathcal{P}$, *which consists of the following clauses in the extended language* $\overline{\mathcal{L}}$, *where* $D_s = (V_s, E_s)$ *is relevancy DAG of* D *with respect to* s:

(RP) Rewritten program clauses:

$$A_{P_v} \leftarrow B_1, \ldots, B_m, C_1^-, \ldots, C_n^- \tag{6.32}$$

or

$$A_{P_v}^- \leftarrow B_1, \ldots, B_m, C_1^-, \ldots, C_n^- \tag{6.33}$$

for any clause:

$$A \leftarrow B_1,\ \ldots,\ B_m,\ \ not\, C_1,\ \ldots,\ not\, C_n \tag{6.34}$$

respectively, for any clause:

$$not\, A \leftarrow B_1,\ \ldots,\ B_m,\ not\, C_1,\ \ldots,\ not\, C_n \tag{6.35}$$

in the program P_v, *where* $v \in V_s$. *The rewritten clauses are obtained from the original ones by replacing atoms* A *(respectively, the default literals* $not\, A$*) occurring in their heads by the atoms* A_{P_v} *(respectively,* $A_{P_v}^-$*) and by replacing negative premises* $not\, C$ *by* C^-.

(IR) Inheritance rules:

$$A_v \leftarrow A_u, not\, reject(A_u) \tag{6.36}$$
$$A_v^- \leftarrow A_u^-, not\, reject(A_u^-) \tag{6.37}$$

for all atoms $A \in \mathcal{K}$ and all $(u, v) \in E_s$. The inheritance rules say that an atom A is true (respectively, false) in the state $v \in V_s$ if it is true (respectively, false) in any ancestor state u and it is not rejected, *i.e., forced to be false (respectively, true).*

(RR) Rejection Rules:

$$reject(A_u^-) \leftarrow A_{P_v} \tag{6.38}$$
$$reject(A_u) \leftarrow A_{P_v}^- \tag{6.39}$$

for all atoms $A \in \mathcal{K}$ and all $u, v \in V_s$ where $u <_{D_s} v$. The rejection rules say that if an atom A is true (respectively, false) in the program P_v, then it rejects inheritance of any false (respectively, true) atoms of any ancestor.

(UR) Update rules:

$$A_v \leftarrow A_{P_v} \tag{6.40}$$
$$A_v^- \leftarrow A_{P_v}^- \tag{6.41}$$

for all atoms $A \in \mathcal{K}$ and all $v \in V_s$. The update rules state that an atom A must be true (respectively, false) in the state $v \in V_s$ if it is true (respectively, false) in the program P_v.

(DR) Default Rules:

$$A_{s_0}^- \tag{6.42}$$

for all atoms $A \in \mathcal{K}$. Default rules describe the initial state s_0 by making all objective atoms initially false.

(CS$_s$) Current State Rules:

$$A \leftarrow A_s \tag{6.43}$$
$$A^- \leftarrow A_s^- \tag{6.44}$$
$$not\, A \leftarrow A_s^- \tag{6.45}$$

for all atoms $A \in \mathcal{K}$. Current state rules specify the current state s in which the program is being evaluated and determine the values of the atoms A and A^-, and the default literals not A.

Example 59 *Consider again the MDLP $\mathcal{P} = (\mathcal{P}_D, D)$ of Example 56, where*

$$\mathcal{P}_D = \{P_t, P_u, P_v, P_w\}$$

and

$$\begin{array}{ll} P_t = \{a \leftarrow not\, b\} & P_u = \{c \leftarrow\} \\ P_v = \{not\, a \leftarrow c\} & P_w = \{\} \end{array} \tag{6.46}$$

and $D = (V, E)$ where

$$V = \{s_0, t, u, v, w\} \tag{6.47}$$
$$E = \{(t,u), (t,v), (u,w), (v,w), (s_0,t)\} \tag{6.48}$$

The program $\boxplus_w \mathcal{P}$ contains the rules:

$$a_{P_t} \leftarrow b^- \tag{6.49}$$
$$c_{P_u} \leftarrow \tag{6.50}$$
$$a^-_{P_v} \leftarrow c \tag{6.51}$$
$$A_i \leftarrow A_j, not\, reject(A_j) \qquad \forall (j,i) \in E, \forall A \in \{a,b,c\} \tag{6.52}$$
$$A^-_i \leftarrow A^-_j, not\, reject(A^-_j) \qquad \forall (j,i) \in E, \forall A \in \{a,b,c\} \tag{6.53}$$
$$reject(A^-_i) \leftarrow A_{P_j} \qquad \forall i,j \in V : i <_D j, \forall A \in \{a,b,c\} \tag{6.54}$$
$$reject(A_i) \leftarrow A^-_{P_j} \qquad \forall i,j \in V : i <_D j, \forall A \in \{a,b,c\} \tag{6.55}$$
$$A_i \leftarrow A_{P_i} \qquad \forall i \in V, \forall A \in \{a,b,c\} \tag{6.56}$$
$$A^-_i \leftarrow A^-_{P_i} \qquad \forall i \in V, \forall A \in \{a,b,c\} \tag{6.57}$$
$$A^-_{s0} \qquad \forall A \in \{a,b,c\} \tag{6.58}$$
$$A \leftarrow A_w \qquad \forall A \in \{a,b,c\} \tag{6.59}$$
$$A^- \leftarrow A^-_w \qquad \forall A \in \{a,b,c\} \tag{6.60}$$
$$not\, A \leftarrow A^-_w \qquad \forall A \in \{a,b,c\} \tag{6.61}$$

whose only stable model, restricted to the initial language, is $M_w = \{not\, a, not\, b, c\}$, as expected.

As mentioned before, the stable models of the program obtained by the previous transformation coincide with those characterized in Def.105, as expressed in the following theorem:

Theorem 82 *Given a* Multi-dimensional Dynamic Logic Program $\mathcal{P} = (\mathcal{P}_D, D)$, *the generalized stable models of $\boxplus_s \mathcal{P}$, restricted to $\mathcal{L}$, coincide with the generalized stable models $\mathcal{P}$ at state s, according to Def.105.*

Proof. *According to Proposition 79 and that rules belonging to those programs indexed by the vertices that do not belong to the relevancy graph play no role in $\boxplus_s \mathcal{P}$, according to Def. 108, we can safely remove such rules from $\mathcal{P}$ and such vertices and corresponding edges from D, thus obtaining $\mathcal{P}_s = (\mathcal{P}_{D_s}, D_s)$ where $D_s = (V_s, E_s)$ is the relevancy DAG of D with respect to s. and $\mathcal{P}_{D_s} = \{P_v : v \in V_s\}$. Therefore, we need only prove the theorem for $\mathcal{P}_s$ or, alternatively, consider $D = D_s$ and, consequently, $\mathcal{P} = \mathcal{P}_s$.*

Let r^+ be a rule of the form:

$$A \leftarrow B_1, \ldots, B_m, not\, C_1, \ldots, not\, C_n \tag{6.62}$$

and let r^- be a rule of the form:

$$not\, A \leftarrow B_1, \ldots, B_m, not\, C_1, \ldots, not\, C_n \tag{6.63}$$

So $\boxplus_s\mathcal{P}$ contains the rules:

$$A_{P_v} \leftarrow B_1, \ldots, B_m, C_1^-, \ldots, C_n^- \qquad \forall r^+ \in P_v \tag{6.64}$$
$$A_{P_v}^- \leftarrow B_1, \ldots, B_m, C_1^-, \ldots, C_n^- \qquad \forall r^- \in P_v \tag{6.65}$$
$$A_v \leftarrow A_u, not\, reject(A_u) \qquad \forall (u,v) \in E, \forall A \in \mathcal{K} \tag{6.66}$$
$$A_v^- \leftarrow A_u^-, not\, reject(A_u^-) \qquad \forall (u,v) \in E, \forall A \in \mathcal{K} \tag{6.67}$$
$$reject(A_u^-) \leftarrow A_{P_v} \qquad \forall u,v \in V : u <_D v, \forall A \in \mathcal{K} \tag{6.68}$$
$$reject(A_u) \leftarrow A_{P_v}^- \qquad \forall u,v \in V : u <_D v, \forall A \in \mathcal{K} \tag{6.69}$$
$$A_v \leftarrow A_{P_v} \qquad \forall v \in V, \forall A \in \mathcal{K} \tag{6.70}$$
$$A_v^- \leftarrow A_{P_v}^- \qquad \forall v \in V, \forall A \in \mathcal{K} \tag{6.71}$$
$$A_{s0}^- \qquad \forall A \in \mathcal{K} \tag{6.72}$$
$$A \leftarrow A_s \qquad \forall A \in \mathcal{K} \tag{6.73}$$
$$A^- \leftarrow A_s^- \qquad \forall A \in \mathcal{K} \tag{6.74}$$
$$not\, A \leftarrow A_s^- \qquad \forall A \in \mathcal{K} \tag{6.75}$$

($\Rightarrow$)Suppose that N is a stable model of the program $\boxplus_s\mathcal{P}$ and let $R = \boxplus_s\mathcal{P} \cup N^-$. From Def.17 it follows that:

$$N = least\,(R) = least\,\left(\boxplus_s\mathcal{P} \cup N^-\right) \tag{6.76}$$

Let

$$T = \left[\rho\,(\mathcal{P})_s - Reject(\mathcal{P}, s, M)\right] \cup Default\,(\rho\,(\mathcal{P})_s\,, M) \tag{6.77}$$

and let

$$H = least\,(T) \tag{6.78}$$

be its least model (in the language $\mathcal{L}$). We will show that the restriction $M = N \mid \mathcal{L}$ of N to the language $\mathcal{L}$ coincides with H.

Denote by $\mathcal{S}$ the sub-language of $\widehat{\mathcal{L}}$ that includes only propositional symbols $\{A : A \in \mathcal{K}\} \cup \{A^- : A \in \mathcal{K}\}$. By means of several simple reductions we will transform the program $R = \boxplus_s\mathcal{P} \cup N^-$ in the language $\widehat{\mathcal{L}}$ into a simpler program Q in the language $\mathcal{S}$ so that:

- *The least model $J = least\,(Q)$ of Q is equal to the least model $N = least\,(R)$ of R when restricted to the language $\mathcal{S}$, i.e., $J = N \mid \mathcal{S}$;*
- *The program Q in the language $\mathcal{S}$ is syntactically identical to the program*

  $$T = \left[\rho\,(\mathcal{P})_s - Reject(\mathcal{P}, s, M)\right] \cup Default\,(\rho\,(\mathcal{P})_s\,, M)$$

  in the language $\mathcal{L}$, except that $not A$ is everywhere replaced by A^-.

First of all, according to Def.17, we observe that $not\, reject(A_u)$ belongs to N^-, iff $N \nvDash A_{P_v}^-, \forall u,v \in V : u <_D v$, since there are no rules for $not\, reject(A_u)$ (remember that $not A$ is treated as a propositional symbol). Similarly, $not\, reject(A_u^-)$ belongs to N^-, iff $N \nvDash A_{P_v}, \forall u,v \in V : u <_D v$. We can thus replace rules (6.66) and (6.67) with:

$$A_v \leftarrow A_u, not\, A_{P_w} \qquad \forall (u,v) \in E, w \in V, u <_D w \tag{6.79}$$
$$A_v^- \leftarrow A_u^-, not\, A_{P_w}^- \qquad \forall (u,v) \in E, w \in V, u <_D w \tag{6.80}$$

Since we are not interested in the truth value of the atoms of the form $reject(\_)$ *(they do not belong to* $\mathcal{S}$*) and they no longer appear in the body of any rules, we can eliminate rules (6.68) and (6.69). The transformed program,* R'*, now looks like:*

$$A_{P_v} \leftarrow B_1, \ldots, B_m, C_1^-, \ldots, C_n^- \qquad \forall r^+ \in P_v \tag{6.81}$$
$$A_{P_v}^- \leftarrow B_1, \ldots, B_m, C_1^-, \ldots, C_n^- \qquad \forall r^- \in P_v \tag{6.82}$$
$$A_v \leftarrow A_u, not\, A_{P_w} \qquad \forall (u,v) \in E, w \in V, u <_D w, \forall A \in \mathcal{K} \tag{6.83}$$
$$A_v^- \leftarrow A_u^-, not\, A_{P_w}^- \qquad \forall (u,v) \in E, w \in V, u <_D w, \forall A \in \mathcal{K} \tag{6.84}$$
$$A_v \leftarrow A_{P_v} \qquad \forall v \in V, \forall A \in \mathcal{K} \tag{6.85}$$
$$A_v^- \leftarrow A_{P_v}^- \qquad \forall v \in V, \forall A \in \mathcal{K} \tag{6.86}$$
$$A_{s0}^- \qquad \forall A \in \mathcal{K} \tag{6.87}$$
$$A \leftarrow A_s \qquad \forall A \in \mathcal{K} \tag{6.88}$$
$$A^- \leftarrow A_s^- \qquad \forall A \in \mathcal{K} \tag{6.89}$$
$$not\, A \leftarrow A_s^- \qquad \forall A \in \mathcal{K} \tag{6.90}$$
$$not\, A \qquad \forall A \in \overline{\mathcal{K}},\ not\, A \in N^- \tag{6.91}$$

If we partially evaluate rules (6.85) and (6.86), using rules (6.81) and (6.82), we obtain

$$A_v \leftarrow B_1, \ldots, B_m, C_1^-, \ldots, C_n^- \qquad \forall r^+ \in P_v \tag{6.92}$$
$$A_v^- \leftarrow B_1, \ldots, B_m, C_1^-, \ldots, C_n^- \qquad \forall r^- \in P_v \tag{6.93}$$

We can now simplify rules (6.83) and (6.84) by replacing them with the simpler rules

$$A_v \leftarrow A_u \qquad \forall (u,v) \in E, \forall A \in \mathcal{K} \tag{6.94}$$
$$A_v^- \leftarrow A_u^- \qquad \forall (u,v) \in E, \forall A \in \mathcal{K} \tag{6.95}$$

if we also remove from this new program the rules (6.92) such that

$$\exists (u,v) \in E, \exists w, v <_D w, \exists A_{P_v}^- \leftarrow Body \in R' : N \models Body \tag{6.96}$$

and the rules (6.93) such that

$$\exists (u,v) \in E, \exists w, v <_D w, \exists A_{P_v} \leftarrow Body \in R' : N \models Body \tag{6.97}$$

This is the same as saying one should remove rules (6.92) and (6.93) such that the original corresponding rules belong to $Reject(\mathcal{P}, s, M)$*. We also have to deal with the rules (6.87), which play no different role than rules (6.92) and (6.93), but with respect to the initial state. We should then eliminate all those rules such that*

$$\exists (s_0,v) \in E, \exists w, v <_D w, \exists A_{P_v} \leftarrow Body \in R' : N \models Body \tag{6.98}$$

which is the same as saying that we should preserve only those rules A_{s0}^- *if* $not\, A \in Default\,(\rho\,(\mathcal{P})_s\,, M)$*.*

In this proof, we can eliminate rules (6.81) and (6.82) since atoms of the form $A_{P_v}^-$ *and* A_{P_v} *do not belong to* $\mathcal{S}$ *and they no longer appear in the body of any clauses. The* *transformed program, R'', now looks like:*

$$A_v \leftarrow A_u \quad \forall (u,v) \in E, \forall A \in \mathcal{K} \tag{6.99}$$
$$A_v^- \leftarrow A_u^- \quad \forall (u,v) \in E, \forall A \in \mathcal{K} \tag{6.100}$$
$$A_v \leftarrow B_1, \ldots, B_m, C_1^-, \ldots, C_n^- \quad \forall r^+ \in \mathcal{P}_v, r^+ \notin Reject(\mathcal{P}, s, M) \tag{6.101}$$
$$A_v^- \leftarrow B_1, \ldots, B_m, C_1^-, \ldots, C_n^- \quad \forall r^- \in \mathcal{P}_v, r^- \notin Reject(\mathcal{P}, s, M) \tag{6.102}$$
$$A_{s0}^- \quad \forall not\, A \in Default\,(\rho\,(\mathcal{P})_s\,, M)\,. \tag{6.103}$$
$$A \leftarrow A_s \quad \forall A \in \mathcal{K} \tag{6.104}$$
$$A^- \leftarrow A_s^- \quad \forall A \in \mathcal{K} \tag{6.105}$$
$$not\, A \leftarrow A_s^- \quad \forall A \in \mathcal{K} \tag{6.106}$$
$$not\, A \quad \forall A \in \overline{\mathcal{K}},\ not\, A \in N^- \tag{6.107}$$

We can now remove all the negative facts in N^- and the default rule $not\, A \leftarrow A_s^-$ from R'' because they only involve propositional symbols not A which no longer appear in bodies of any other clauses from $R''$and thus do not affect the least model of R'' restricted to the language $\mathcal{S}$. Also, because there are edges $\forall (u,v) \in E$ from all states to state s (E is the relevancy graph of itself with respect to s), we can perform several partial evaluations and remove the rules for A_v and A_v^- until we are left only with rules for A and A^-. The result is the final program Q:

$$A \leftarrow B_1, \ldots, B_m, C_1^-, \ldots, C_n^- \quad \forall r^+ \in \mathcal{P}_s, r^+ \notin Reject(\mathcal{P}, s, M) \tag{6.108}$$
$$A^- \leftarrow B_1, \ldots, B_m, C_1^-, \ldots, C_n^- \quad \forall r^- \in \mathcal{P}_s, r^- \notin Reject(\mathcal{P}, s, M) \tag{6.109}$$
$$A^- \quad \forall not\, A \in Default\,(\rho\,(\mathcal{P})_s\,, M)\,. \tag{6.110}$$

Clearly, this program is entirely identical to the program

$$T = [\mathcal{P}_s - Reject(\mathcal{P}, s, M)] \cup Default\,(\rho\,(\mathcal{P})_s\,, M)$$

except that $notA$ is everywhere replaced by A^-. Consequently, the least model J of Q is identical to the least model H of T, except that $notA$ is everywhere replaced by A^-. Moreover, due to the way in which it was obtained, the least model $J = least(Q)$ of the program Q is equal to the least model $N = least(R)$ of R restricted to the language $\mathcal{S}$, i.e., $J = N \mid \mathcal{S}$. This entails that for any $A \in \mathcal{K}$:

$$A \in N \quad \textit{iff} \quad A \in J \quad \textit{iff} \quad A \in H \tag{6.111}$$
$$A^- \in N \quad \textit{iff} \quad A^- \in J \quad \textit{iff} \quad notA \in H. \tag{6.112}$$

We conclude that $M = N \mid \mathcal{L} = H$, because $notA \in N$ iff $A^- \in N$. This completes the proof in one direction. The converse implication is established in an analogous way. ■

The transformation of Definition 108 depends on the prior determination of the relevancy graph with respect to the given state. Our choice to make this so was based on criteria of clarity and readability. Nevertheless this needs not be so: one can also declaratively specify, by means of a logic program, the notion of relevancy graph, giving rise to the following transformation as the basis of an implementation:

Definition 109 (Multi-dimensional Dynamic Program Update) *(*Alternative Transformation*) Let $\mathcal{P} = (\mathcal{P}_D, D)$ be a* Multi-dimensional Dynamic Logic Program, *where* $\mathcal{P}_D = \{P_v : v \in V\}$ *and* $D = (V, E)$. *Given a fixed state* $s \in V$, *the alternative multi-dimensional dynamic program update over* $\mathcal{P}$ *at state* **s** *is the generalized logic program* $\boxplus_s^{'}\mathcal{P}$, *which consists of the following clauses in the extended language*

$$\overline{\mathcal{L}} \cup \{rel\_edge(u,v), rel\_path(u,v), rel\_vertex(u), edge(u,v) : u, v \in V\}$$

(RP) Rewritten program clauses:

$$A_{P_v} \leftarrow B_1, \ldots, B_m, C_1^-, \ldots, C_n^-$$
$$A_{P_v}^- \leftarrow B_1, \ldots, B_m, C_1^-, \ldots, C_n^-$$

for any clause:

$$A \leftarrow B_1,\ \ldots,\ B_m,\ not\, C_1,\ \ldots,\ not\, C_n$$

respectively, for any clause:

$$not\, A \leftarrow B_1,\ \ldots,\ B_m,\ not\, C_1,\ \ldots,\ not\, C_n$$

in the program P_v, where $v \in V$.

(IR) Inheritance rules:

$$A_v \leftarrow A_u, not\, reject(A_u), rel\_edge(u,v)$$
$$A_v^- \leftarrow A_u^-, not\, reject(A_u^-), rel\_edge(u,v)$$

for all atoms $A \in \mathcal{K}$ and all $u, v \in V$.

(RR) Rejection Rules:

$$reject(A_u^-) \leftarrow A_{P_v}, rel\_path(u,v)$$
$$reject(A_u) \leftarrow A_{P_v}^-, rel\_path(u,v)$$

for all atoms $A \in \mathcal{K}$ and all $u, v \in V$.

(UR) Update rules:

$$A_v \leftarrow A_{P_v}, rel\_vertex(v)$$
$$A_v^- \leftarrow A_{P_v}^-, rel\_vertex(v)$$

for all atoms $A \in \mathcal{K}$ and all $v \in V$.

(DR) Default Rules:

$$A_{s0}^-$$

for all atoms $A \in \mathcal{K}$.

(CS$_s$) Current State Rules:

$$A \leftarrow A_s \qquad A^- \leftarrow A_s^- \qquad not\, A \leftarrow A_s^-$$

for all atoms $A \in \mathcal{K}$.

(ER) Edge Rules

$$edge(u,v)$$

for all $(u,v) \in E$. Edge rules describe the edges in graph D.

(RER$_s$) Current State Relevancy Edge Rules

$$rel\_edge(X, s) \leftarrow edge(X, s)$$
$$rel\_edge(X, Y) \leftarrow edge(X, Y), rel\_path(Y, s)$$

Current State Relevancy Edge Rules define which edges are in the relevancy graph with respect to s.

(RPR) Relevancy Path Rules

$$rel\_path(X, Y) \leftarrow rel\_edge(X, Y)$$
$$rel\_path(X, Z) \leftarrow rel\_edge(X, Y), rel\_path(Y, Z)$$

Relevancy Path rules define the notion of relevancy path in a graph.

(RVR) Relevancy Vertex Rules

$$rel\_vertex(Y) \leftarrow rel\_edge(\_, Y)$$
$$rel\_vertex(Y) \leftarrow rel\_edge(Y, \_)$$
$$rel\_vertex(s_0) \leftarrow$$

Relevancy Vertex Rules define which vertices belong to the relevancy graph.

Proposition 83 *Let* $\mathcal{P} = (\mathcal{P}_D, D)$ *be a* Multi-dimensional Dynamic Logic Program. *Restricted to* $\mathcal{L}$, *the generalized stable models of* $\boxplus_s\mathcal{P}$ *coincide with the generalized stable models of* $\boxplus_s^{'}\mathcal{P}$.

This transformation of a *MDLP* into a single, equivalent, logic program directly provides us with a means to implement $\mathcal{MDLP}$. Via a preprocessor that, given a *MDLP* and a state s, produces the corresponding transformed logic program, the computation of the stable models at state s is reduced to the computation of the stable models of the logic program. For the latter purpose, a system that computes stable models of logic programs, such as the DLV-system [69] or SMODELS [176] can be used. A preprocessor, that translates $\mathcal{MDLP}$ programs into logic programs that can be run in the DLV-system, has been implemented [1] and is available.

6.5 Properties

In this section we study the basic properties of *Multi-dimensional Dynamic Logic Programming.*

The following theorem states that adding or removing edges from the DAG of a *Multi-dimensional Dynamic Logic Program* preserves the semantics if the transitive closure of the DAG is maintained. In particular, it allows the use of a transitive reduction of the original graph to determine the stable models.

Theorem 84 (DAG Simplification) *Let* $\mathcal{P} = (\mathcal{P}_D, D)$ *be a* Multi-dimensional Dynamic Logic Program, *where* $\mathcal{P}_D = \{P_v : v \in V\}$ *and* $D = (V, E)$. *Let* $\mathcal{P}_1 = (\mathcal{P}_D, D_1)$ *be a* Multi-dimensional Dynamic Logic Program, *where* $D_1 = (V, E_1)$ *such that* $D^+ = D_1^+$.*Then, for any state* $s \in V$, M *is a* stable model of $\mathcal{P}$ at state s *iff* M *is a* stable model of $\mathcal{P}_1$ at state s.

Proof. Since the relation $<_D$ (and $\leq_D$) is invariant with respect to the transitive closure of a DAG, we have that, $\forall u, v \in V$, the following holds:

$$u <_D v \iff u <_{D_1} v$$
$$u \leq_D v \iff u \leq_{D_1} v$$

therefore, according to Def.105, $\rho(\mathcal{P})_s$, $Reject(\mathcal{P}, s, M)$ and $Default(\rho(\mathcal{P})_s, M)$ coincide for both $\mathcal{P}$ and $\mathcal{P}_1$, and thus, their stable models coincide. ■

The following corollary says that to determine the stable models at a set of states we only need to connect the sinks of the relevancy DAG with respect to that set of states, to the new node α.

Corollary 85 *Let* $\mathcal{P} = (\mathcal{P}_D, D)$ *be a* Multi-dimensional Dynamic Logic Program, *where* $\mathcal{P}_D = \{P_v : v \in V\}$ *and* $D = (V, E)$. M_S *is a* stable model of $\mathcal{P}$ at states $S \subseteq V$ *iff* M_S *is a* stable model of $\mathcal{P}_\alpha$ at state α *where* $\mathcal{P}_\alpha = (\mathcal{P}_{D_\alpha}, D_\alpha)$ *is the* Multi-dimensional Dynamic Logic Program *such that* $\mathcal{P}_{D_\alpha} = \mathcal{P}_D \cup P_\alpha$ *and* $D_\alpha = (V_\alpha, E_\alpha)$ *where:*

$$P_\alpha = \{\} \tag{6.113}$$
$$V_\alpha = V \cup \{\alpha\} \tag{6.114}$$
$$E_\alpha = E \cup \{(i, \alpha) : i \in S \textit{ and } i \textit{ is a sink of } D_S\} \tag{6.115}$$

where D_S *is the relevancy DAG of* D *with respect to* S.

The following proposition relates the stable models of normal logic programs with the stable models of *MDLPs* whose set of programs only contains normal logic programs.

Proposition 86 *Let* $\mathcal{P} = (\mathcal{P}_D, D)$ *be a* Multi-dimensional Dynamic Logic Program, *where* $\mathcal{P}_D = \{P_v : v \in V\}$ *and* $D = (V, E)$. *Let* $S \subseteq V$ *be a set of states and* $D_S = (V_S, E_S)$ *the relevancy DAG of* D *with respect to* S. *If all* $P_v : v \in V_S$ *are normal logic programs, then* M *is a* stable model of $\mathcal{P}$ at states S *iff* M *is a* stable model *of the (normal) logic program*

$$\bigcup_{v \in V_S} P_v \tag{6.116}$$

Proof. The stable models of $\mathcal{P}$ at states S are the stable models at state α of $\mathcal{P}_\alpha$ where $\mathcal{P}_\alpha = (\mathcal{P}_{D_\alpha}, D_\alpha)$ is the *Multi-dimensional Dynamic Logic Program* such that $\mathcal{P}_{D_\alpha} = \mathcal{P}_D \cup P_\alpha$ and $D_\alpha = (V_\alpha, E_\alpha)$ where:

$$P_\alpha = \{\} \tag{6.117}$$
$$V_\alpha = V \cup \{\alpha\} \tag{6.118}$$
$$E_\alpha = E \cup \{(i, \alpha) : i \in S \text{ and } i \text{ is a sink of } D_S\} \tag{6.119}$$

Since the programs indexed by the vertices of the relevancy DAG with respect to α are normal logic programs (note that $P_\alpha = \{\}$), i.e. without default literals in the heads of clauses, from Def. 105 we conclude that for any interpretation M, $Reject(\mathcal{P}, \alpha, M) = \{\}$. Therefore, M is a stable model iff

$$M = least\left(\rho(\mathcal{P}_\alpha)_\alpha \cup Default\left(\rho(\mathcal{P}_\alpha)_\alpha, M\right)\right) \tag{6.120}$$

where

$$\rho(\mathcal{P}_\alpha)_\alpha = \bigcup_{v \in V_S} P_v \tag{6.121}$$

$$Default(\rho(\mathcal{P}_\alpha)_\alpha, M) = \{not\ A \mid \nexists r \in \rho(\mathcal{P}_\alpha)_\alpha : (H(r) = A) \wedge M \vDash B(r)\} \tag{6.122}$$

Since $Default(\rho(\mathcal{P}_\alpha)_\alpha, M)$ contains the same default literals as M^- in Def. 17, (6.120) reduces to the definition of the stable models of $\rho(\mathcal{P}_\alpha)_\alpha = \bigcup_{v \in V_S} P_v$, i.e.

$$M = least\left(\rho(\mathcal{P}_\alpha)_\alpha \cup M^-\right) = least\left(\bigcup_{v \in V_S} P_v \cup M^-\right) \tag{6.123}$$

■

We now explore some ways to simplify an MDLP. For simplicity, we assume that the semantics always refers to the set of all states.

Proposition 87 *Let* $\mathcal{P} = (\mathcal{P}_D, D)$ *be a* Multi-dimensional Dynamic Logic Program, *where* $\mathcal{P}_D = \{P_v : v \in V\}$ *and* $D = (V, E)$, *j and m two of its states such that* $j <_D m$. *Let r be a rule such that* $r \in P_m \in \mathcal{P}$ *and* $r \in P_j \in \mathcal{P}$. *Let* $\mathcal{P}' = (\mathcal{P}'_D, D)$ *be the multi-dimensional dynamic logic program obtained from* $\mathcal{P}$ *such that*

$$\forall P_k \in \mathcal{P}_D, k \neq j : P'_k = P_k \in \mathcal{P}'_D$$
$$P'_j = P_j - \{r\} \in \mathcal{P}'_D$$

Then an interpretation M_S *is a stable model of* $\mathcal{P}$ *iff* M_S *is a stable model of* $\mathcal{P}'$.

Proof. *An interpretation* M_S *is a stable model of* $\mathcal{P}$ *at the set of states* $S = V$ *iff:*

$$M_S = least\left([\rho(\mathcal{P}) - Reject(\mathcal{P}, S, M_S)] \cup Default(\rho(\mathcal{P}), M_S)\right)$$

Since every rule r' *in* $Reject(\mathcal{P}, S, M_S)$ *rejected by* $r \in P_j$ *is also rejected by* $r \in P_m$, *and if* $r \in P_m$ *belongs to* $Reject(\mathcal{P}, S, M_S)$ *then so does* $r \in P_j$, *and, in such case,* $r \in P'_m$ *also belongs to* $Reject(\mathcal{P}', S, M_S)$, *we have that* $Reject(\mathcal{P}, S, M_S) = Reject(\mathcal{P}', S, M_S)$. *Since* $\rho(\mathcal{P}) = \rho(\mathcal{P}')$ *and* $Default(\rho(\mathcal{P}), M_S) = Default(\rho(\mathcal{P}'), M_S)$, *it follows that* M_S *is a stable model of* $\mathcal{P}'$. *Similar reasoning applies in the opposite direction.* ■

Proposition 88 *Let* $\mathcal{P} = (\mathcal{P}_D, D)$ *be a* Multi-dimensional Dynamic Logic Program, *where* $\mathcal{P}_D = \{P_v : v \in V\}$ *and* $D = (V, E)$, *j and m two of its states such that* $j <_D m$. *Let r and r' be rules such that* $r \in P_m \in \mathcal{P}$, $r' \in P_j \in \mathcal{P}$, $H(r') = H(r)$ *and* $B(r) \subseteq B(r')$. *Let* $\mathcal{P}' = (\mathcal{P}'_D, D)$ *be the multi-dimensional dynamic logic program obtained from* $\mathcal{P}$ *such that*

$$\forall P_k \in \mathcal{P}, k \neq j : P'_k = P_k \in \mathcal{P}'_D$$
$$P'_j = P_j - \{r'\} \in \mathcal{P}'_D$$

Then an interpretation M_S *is a stable model of* $\mathcal{P}$ *iff* M_S *is a stable model of* $\mathcal{P}'$.

Proof. *An interpretation* M_S *is a stable model of* $\mathcal{P}$ *at the set of states* $S = V$ *iff:*

$$M_S = least\left([\rho(\mathcal{P}) - Reject(\mathcal{P}, S, M_S)] \cup Default(\rho(\mathcal{P}), M_S)\right)$$

Since every rule r'' *in* $Reject(\mathcal{P}, S, M_S)$ *rejected by* $r' \in P_j$ *is also rejected by* $r \in P_m$ *because if* $M_S \vDash B(r')$ *then* $M_S \vDash B(r)$. *If* $r \in P_m$ *belongs to* $Reject(\mathcal{P}, S, M_S)$ *then so does* $r' \in P_j$, *and, in such case,* $r \in P'_m$ *also belongs to* $Reject(\mathcal{P}', S, M_S)$, *we have one of the following two cases:*

1. *Reject*$(\mathcal{P}, S, M_S) =$ *Reject*$(\mathcal{P}', S, M_S)$ *if* r *is not rejected, in which case* $\rho(\mathcal{P}) = \rho(\mathcal{P}') \cup \{r'\}$ *and* $Default(\rho(\mathcal{P}), M_S) = Default(\rho(\mathcal{P}'), M_S)$. *But since* $r \in \rho(\mathcal{P}) -$ *Reject*$(\mathcal{P}, S, M_S)$ *it follows that* M_S *is a stable model of* $\mathcal{P}'$

2. *Reject*$(\mathcal{P}, S, M_S) =$ *Reject*$(\mathcal{P}', S, M_S) \cup \{r'\}$ *if* r *is rejected, in which case we have that* $\rho(\mathcal{P}) -$ *Reject*$(\mathcal{P}, S, M_S) = \rho(\mathcal{P}') -$ *Reject*$(\mathcal{P}', S, M_S)$. *Since* $Default(\rho(\mathcal{P}), M_S) = Default(\rho(\mathcal{P}'), M_S)$, *it follows that* M_S *is a stable model of* $\mathcal{P}'$.

Similar reasoning applies in the opposite direction. ■

Proposition 89 *Let* $\mathcal{P} = (\mathcal{P}_D, D)$ *be a* Multi-dimensional Dynamic Logic Program, *where* $\mathcal{P}_D = \{P_v : v \in V\}$ *and* $D = (V, E)$, j *and* m *two of its states such that* $j <_D m$. *Let* r *and* r' *be rules such that* $r \in P_m \in \mathcal{P}$, $r' \in P_j \in \mathcal{P}$, $r \bowtie r'$ *and* $B(r) = \emptyset$. *Let* $\mathcal{P}' = (\mathcal{P}'_D, D)$ *be the multi-dimensional dynamic logic program obtained from* $\mathcal{P}$ *such that*

$$\forall P_k \in \mathcal{P}, k \neq j : P'_k = P_k \in \mathcal{P}'$$
$$P'_j = P_j - \{r'\} \in \mathcal{P}'$$

Then an interpretation M_S *is a stable model of* $\mathcal{P}$ *iff* M_S *is a stable model of* $\mathcal{P}'$.

Proof. *First note that* r' *will always belong to the set* *Reject*$(\mathcal{P}, S, M_S)$ *from where we obtain that* $\rho(\mathcal{P}) -$ *Reject*$(\mathcal{P}, S, M_S) = \rho(\mathcal{P}') -$ *Reject*$(\mathcal{P}', S, M_S)$. *As to the set of defaults we have the following cases:*

1. $H(r') = not\, A$ *in which case we have* $Default(\rho(\mathcal{P}), M_S) = Default(\rho(\mathcal{P}'), M_S)$ *and the proposition follows;*

2. $H(r') = A$ *and* $M_S \not\vDash B(r')$ *in which case* $Default(\rho(\mathcal{P}), M_S) = Default(\rho(\mathcal{P}'), M_S)$ *and the proposition follows;*

3. $H(r') = A$ *and* $M_S \vDash B(r')$ *and* $\exists r'' \in \mathcal{P}'_S : H(r'') = A, M_S \vDash B(r'')$ *in which case* $not\, A \notin Default(\rho(\mathcal{P}'), M_S)$ *and* $Default(\rho(\mathcal{P}), M_S) = Default(\rho(\mathcal{P}'), M_S)$ *and the proposition follows;*

4. $H(r') = A$ *and* $M_S \vDash B(r')$ *and* $\nexists r'' \in \mathcal{P}'_S : H(r'') = A, M_S \vDash B(r'')$ *in which case* $not\, A \in Default(\rho(\mathcal{P}'), M_S)$ *and* $not\, A \notin Default(\rho(\mathcal{P}), M_S)$ *but since in this case* $r = not\, A$ *and* $r \in \mathcal{P}_S -$ *Reject*$(\mathcal{P}, S, M_S)$, *the proposition follows.*

Similar reasoning applies in the opposite direction. ■

Proposition 90 *Let* $\mathcal{P} = (\mathcal{P}_D, D)$ *be a* Multi-dimensional Dynamic Logic Program, *where* $\mathcal{P}_D = \{P_v : v \in V\}$ *and* $D = (V, E)$. *Let* j *be a state, i.e.* $j \in V$, *such that* $P_j = \{\}$. *Let* $\mathcal{P}' = (\mathcal{P}'_{D'}, D')$ *where* $D = (V', E')$ *be the multi-dimensional dynamic logic program obtained from* $\mathcal{P}$ *such that*

$$\mathcal{P}'_{D'} = \mathcal{P}_D - \{P_j\}$$
$$V' = V' - \{j\}$$
$$E' = E - \{(u, j), (j, v) : u, v \in V\} \cup \{(u, v) : (u, i) \in E, (i, v) \in E\}$$

Then an interpretation M_S *is a stable model of* $\mathcal{P}$ *iff* M_S *is a stable model of* $\mathcal{P}'$.

Proof. *Just note that an empty program does not affect any of* $\rho(\mathcal{P})$, *Reject*$(\mathcal{P}, S, M_S)$ *nor* $Default(\rho(\mathcal{P}), M_S)$, *and that the elimination of the state* j *does not affect the order relation among all other nodes, i.e. if* $u <_D v$ *then* $u <_{D'} v$, *for all* $u, v \neq j$. ■

The previous propositions were established for the semantics at the set of all states of the MDLP. Note, however, that if the simplifications mentioned are performed on the MDLP corresponding to the relevancy graph with respect to a set of nodes S, of an MDLP, the semantics at a set of nodes S', such that every state $s' \in S'$ is such that $s \leq_D s'$ for all states $s \in S$, also coincides. This is particularly important when we consider the evolution of MDLPs where the newly added states and programs prevail over previously existing ones. In such cases, we can simplify an MDLP with the guarantee that when we add such new states we obtain the same semantics as if no simplifications were performed at all. This amounts to a similar notion of update equivalence established for DLP. But, as shall be seen, the evolution (update) of an MDLP does not necessarily obey the condition that new states prevail over all existing ones, this being the reason for not establishing such a similar notion of update equivalence for MDLP.

6.5.1 Relationship to Dynamic Logic Programming

Since this work is rooted in *Dynamic Logic Programming*, it should properly extend it, i.e. *Multi-dimensional Dynamic Logic Programming* should be a generalization of *Dynamic Logic Programming.*

The next proposition states that MDLP properly extends DLP:

Proposition 91 *Let $\mathcal{P}_D = \{P_s : s \in S\}$ be a finite or infinite sequence of generalized logic programs in the language $\mathcal{L} = \mathcal{L}_K$, indexed by set of natural numbers $S = \{1, 2, 3, \ldots, n, ...\}$. Let $\mathcal{P} = (\mathcal{P}_D, D)$ be the* Multi-dimensional Dynamic Logic Program, *where $D = (S, E)$ is the acyclic digraph such that $E = \{(1,2), (2,3), ..., (n-1, n), ...\}$. Then, an interpretation M is a stable model of the dynamic logic program at state s, $\bigoplus_s \mathcal{P}_D$, if and only if M is a stable model of $\mathcal{P}$ at state s.*

Proof. *Simply observe that the relation induced by the graph D is the same as the order relation between the elements of S. Therefore both semantical characterizations coincide.* ■

In Chapter 3, to prove the soundness and completeness of the DLP transformational semantics with respect to the declarative semantics, we mentioned that it would immediately follow from the results in this chapter. Since we've proved soundness and completeness of the MDLP transformational semantics with respect to the declarative semantics, and we've proved the embedding of the DLP declarative semantics by the MDLP declarative semantics, to prove Theorem 40 in Chapter 3 we still need to establish that the transformational semantics for DLP is a particular case of the transformational for one MDLP. The following theorem states this result:

Theorem 92 (Embedding of DLP) *Let $\mathcal{P}_D = \{P_s : s \in S\}$ be a finite or infinite sequence of generalized logic programs in the language $\mathcal{L} = \mathcal{L}_K$, indexed by set of natural numbers $S = \{1, 2, 3, \ldots, n, ...\}$. Let $\mathcal{P} = (\mathcal{P}_D, D)$ be the* Multi-dimensional Dynamic Logic Program, *where $D = (S, E)$ is the acyclic digraph such that $E = \{(1,2), (2,3), ..., (n-1, n), ...\}$. Then, the generalized stable models of $\boxplus_s \mathcal{P}$, restricted to $\mathcal{L}$, coincide with the generalized stable models of $\biguplus_s \mathcal{P}_D$, restricted to $\mathcal{L}$.*

Proof. *Since the stable models of the multi-dimensional update at state s coincide with the stable models of the multi-dimensional dynamic logic program $\boxplus_s \mathcal{P}$, all we have to show is that:*

- *for every stable model* N_1 *of* $\bigoplus_s \mathcal{P}_D$*, there exists a stable model* N_2 *of* $\boxplus_s \mathcal{P}$ *such that* $N_1 \mid \mathcal{L} = N_2 \mid \mathcal{L}$*;*

- *for every stable model* N_2 *of* $\boxplus_s \mathcal{P}$*, there exists a stable model* N_1 *of* $\bigoplus_s \mathcal{P}_D$ *such that* $N_2 \mid \mathcal{L} = N_1 \mid \mathcal{L}$*.*

Because, as we've seen before, the programs indexed by states greater than s*, in a dynamic logic program, do not affect the semantics at state* s*, and the programs indexed by states that do not belong to the relevancy graph with respect to* s*, in a multi-dimensional dynamic logic program, do not affect the semantics at state* s*, we only need to prove the equivalence for* $s = n$*.*

Let r^+ *be a rule of the form:*

$$A \leftarrow B_1, \ \ldots, \ B_m, \ \ not\, C_1, \ \ldots, \ not\, C_n \tag{6.124}$$

and let r^- *be a rule of the form:*

$$not\, A \ \leftarrow B_1, \ \ldots, \ B_m, \ not\, C_1, \ \ldots, \ not\, C_n \tag{6.125}$$

The dynamic program update $\bigoplus_n \mathcal{P}_D$ *at state* n *contains the rules:*

$$A_{P_i} \leftarrow B_1, \ldots, B_m, C_1^-, \ldots, C_n^- \qquad \forall r^+ \in P_i \tag{6.126}$$
$$A_{P_i}^- \leftarrow B_1, \ldots, B_m, C_1^-, \ldots, C_n^- \qquad \forall r^- \in P_i \tag{6.127}$$
$$A_i \leftarrow A_{i-1}, not\, A_{P_i}^- \qquad \forall A \in \mathcal{K}, 1 \leq i \leq n \tag{6.128}$$
$$A_i^- \leftarrow A_{i-1}^-, not\, A_{P_i} \qquad \forall A \in \mathcal{K}, 1 \leq i \leq n \tag{6.129}$$
$$A_i \leftarrow A_{P_i} \qquad \forall A \in \mathcal{K}, 1 \leq i \leq n \tag{6.130}$$
$$A_i^- \leftarrow A_{P_i}^- \qquad \forall A \in \mathcal{K}, 1 \leq i \leq n \tag{6.131}$$
$$A_0^- \qquad \forall A \in \mathcal{K} \tag{6.132}$$
$$A \leftarrow A_n \qquad \forall A \in \mathcal{K} \tag{6.133}$$
$$A^- \leftarrow A_n^- \qquad \forall A \in \mathcal{K} \tag{6.134}$$
$$not\, A \leftarrow A_n^- \qquad \forall A \in \mathcal{K} \tag{6.135}$$

We can replace the relation $\leq$ *with* $\leq_D$*. We can transform this program, by introducing a predicate* reject*, with any* $A \neq$ reject*, without changing its models (in what concerns all other atoms), and replace rules (6.128) and (6.129) with the rules:*

$$A_i \leftarrow A_{i-1}, not\, reject(A_{i-1}) \qquad \forall A \in \mathcal{K}, 1 \leq_D i \leq_D n \tag{6.136}$$
$$A_i^- \leftarrow A_{i-1}^-, not\, reject(A_{i-1}^-) \qquad \forall A \in \mathcal{K}, 1 \leq_D i \leq_D n \tag{6.137}$$
$$reject(A_{i-1}^-) \leftarrow A_{P_i} \qquad \forall A \in \mathcal{K}, 1 \leq_D i \leq_D n \tag{6.138}$$
$$reject(A_{i-1}) \leftarrow A_{P_i}^- \qquad \forall A \in \mathcal{K}, 1 \leq_D i \leq_D n \tag{6.139}$$

The multi-dimensional dynamic logic program $\boxplus_n \mathcal{P}$ at state n contains the rules:

$$A_{P_v} \leftarrow B_1, \ldots, B_m, C_1^-, \ldots, C_n^- \qquad \forall r^+ \in P_i \tag{6.140}$$
$$A_{P_v}^- \leftarrow B_1, \ldots, B_m, C_1^-, \ldots, C_n^- \qquad \forall r^- \in P_i \tag{6.141}$$
$$A_i \leftarrow A_{i-1}, not\, reject(A_{i-1}) \qquad \forall A \in \mathcal{K}, 1 \leq_D i \leq_D n \tag{6.142}$$
$$A_i^- \leftarrow A_{i-1}^-, not\, reject(A_{i-1}^-) \qquad \forall A \in \mathcal{K}, 1 \leq_D i \leq_D n \tag{6.143}$$
$$reject(A_{i-1}^-) \leftarrow A_{P_j} \qquad \forall A \in \mathcal{K}, \forall i, j : 1 \leq_D i <_D j \leq_D n \tag{6.144}$$
$$reject(A_{i-1}) \leftarrow A_{P_j}^- \qquad \forall A \in \mathcal{K}, \forall i, j : 1 \leq_D i <_D j \leq_D n \tag{6.145}$$
$$A_i \leftarrow A_{P_i} \qquad \forall A \in \mathcal{K} \tag{6.146}$$
$$A_i^- \leftarrow A_{P_i}^- \qquad \forall A \in \mathcal{K} \tag{6.147}$$
$$A_0^- \qquad \forall A \in \mathcal{K} \tag{6.148}$$
$$A \leftarrow A_n \qquad \forall A \in \mathcal{K} \tag{6.149}$$
$$A^- \leftarrow A_n^- \qquad \forall A \in \mathcal{K} \tag{6.150}$$
$$not\, A \leftarrow A_n^- \qquad \forall A \in \mathcal{K} \tag{6.151}$$

In this program, rules (6.144) and (6.145) can be split into these:

$$reject(A_{i-1}^-) \leftarrow A_{P_i} \qquad \forall A \in \mathcal{K}, 1 \leq_D i \leq_D n \tag{6.152}$$
$$reject(A_{i-1}) \leftarrow A_{P_i}^- \qquad \forall A \in \mathcal{K}, 1 \leq_D i \leq_D n \tag{6.153}$$
$$reject(A_{i-1}^-) \leftarrow A_{P_{i+1}} \quad \ldots \quad reject(A_{i-1}^-) \leftarrow A_{P_n} \qquad \forall A \in \mathcal{K}, 1 \leq_D i <_D n-1 \tag{6.154}$$
$$reject(A_{i-1}) \leftarrow A_{P_{i+1}}^- \quad \ldots \quad reject(A_{i-1}) \leftarrow A_{P_n}^- \qquad \forall A \in \mathcal{K}, 1 \leq_D i <_D n-1 \tag{6.155}$$

Now we can see that the only difference between the modified (with the introduction of the reject predicate) dynamic program update $\bigoplus_n \mathcal{P}_D$ and the multi-dimensional dynamic logic program $\boxplus_n \mathcal{P}$ at state n is that the latter contains the extra sets of rules (6.154) and (6.155). We now have to show that these rules do not affect the models, when restricted to $\mathcal{L}$. In what concerns these rules, one of the following cases could occur:

- *none of the A_{P_j} and (resp. $A_{P_j}^-$) is true in the model, in which case both programs are trivially equivalent;*
- *one of the A_{P_j} (resp. $A_{P_j}^-$) is true in the model: in this case, in $\boxplus_n \mathcal{P}$, this will block all inertia rules from state $i-1$ forward until state j. At state j, an update rule will make A_j (resp. A_j^-) true. In $\bigoplus_n \mathcal{P}_D$, the truth of A_{P_j} (resp. $A_{P_j}^-$) only blocks inertia from state $j-1$ to state j, but the truth of A_j (resp. A_j^-) is the same due to an update rule. Since the current state rules have, as pre-conditions, the atoms A_n (resp. A_n^-), and the rules for the predicate $reject(A_{n-1})$ are the same in both $\boxplus_n \mathcal{P}$ and $\bigoplus_n \mathcal{P}_D$, inertia from state $n-1$ to n works the same way in both programs and thus, the truth value of the atoms A and $not\, A$ is the same;*
- *more than one of the A_{P_j} (resp. $A_{P_j}^-$) are true in the model: the reasoning is similar to the previous case.*

And this concludes the proof of this Theorem. ∎

As we've seen before, *interpretation updates*, originally introduced under the name *"revision programs"* by Marek and Truszczyński [157] constitute a special case of logic program updates. This result, together with the previous theorem, immediately imply that *Multi-dimensional Dynamic Logic Programming* embeds *Interpretation Updates* in the sense of [157]. Also follows that $\mathcal{MDLP}$ embeds *Logic Programs under the Stable Models Semantics*

6.5.2 Computational Complexity

The availability of a syntactical transformation into a logic program whose stable models are in a one-to-one correspondence with those of the original MDLP allow us, just as for DLP, to obtain the following complexity results:

Theorem 93 (Computational Complexity) *Given a dynamic logic program $\mathcal{P}$, and one of its states s, then:*

1. *deciding whether $\mathcal{P}$ has a stable model at state s is $NP-complete$;*
2. *deciding whether a given interpretation is a stable model of $\mathcal{P}$ at state s is P;*
3. *deciding whether a given atom is true in at least one stable model of $\mathcal{P}$ at state s is $NP-complete$;*
4. *deciding whether a given atom is true in all stable model of $\mathcal{P}$ at state s is $coNP-complete$.*

Proof. *The program $\boxplus_s\mathcal{P}$ can be obtained in polynomial time from $\mathcal{P}$, given s. All the results are therefore inherited from the results from the complexity of logic programs [155]. Note that even if we use the transformation that requires the transitive closure of the DAG, this can also be achieved in polynomial time.* ■

6.6 Illustrative Examples

In this section we discuss some domains where $\mathcal{MDLP}$ can be applied, illustrating each with a small example, all having been run and tested on the implementation of $\mathcal{MDLP}$.

6.6.1 Organizational Decision Making

By its very motivation and design, $\mathcal{MDLP}$ is well suited for combining knowledge from various sources, specially when some of these sources have priority over the others. More precisely, when rules from some sources are used to reject rules of other, less prior, sources. In particular, $\mathcal{MDLP}$ is well suited for combining knowledge originating within hierarchically organized sources, as the following schematic example illustrates by combining knowledge coming from divers sectors of such an organization.

Example 60 *Consider a company with a president, a board of directors and (at least) two departments: the quality management and the financial ones.*

To improve the quality of the products produced by the company, the quality management department has decided not to buy any product whose reliability is less than guaranteed. In other words, it has to adopted the rule:

$$not\,buy(X) \leftarrow not\,reliable(X)$$

On the other hand, to save money, the financial department has decided to buy products of a type in need if they are cheap, i.e.

$$buy(X) \leftarrow type(X,T), needed(T), cheap(X)$$

The board of directors, in order to keep production going, has decided that whenever there is still a need for a type of product, exactly one product of that type must be bought. This can be coded by the following logic programming rules, stating that if X is a product of a needed type, and if the need for that type of product has not been already satisfied by buying some other product of that type, then X must be bought; if the need is satisfied by buying some other product of that type, then X should not be bought:

$$\begin{array}{rcl} buy(X) & \leftarrow & type(X,T), needed(T), not\,satByOther(T,X) \\ not\,buy(X) & \leftarrow & type(X,T), needed(T), satByOther(T,X) \\ satByOther(T,X) & \leftarrow & type(Y,T), buy(Y), X \neq Y \end{array}$$

Finally, the president decided for the company never to buy products that have a cheap alternative. I.e. if two products are of the same type, and one of them is cheap, the company should not buy the other one:

$$not\,buy(X) \leftarrow type(X,T), type(Y,T), X \neq Y, cheap(Y), not\,cheap(X)$$

For this example, suppose that there are two products, a and b, the first being cheap and the latter reliable, both of type t and both of needed type t.

According to the company's organizational chart, the rules of the president can overrule those of all other sectors, and those established by the board can overrule those decided by the departments. No department has precedence over any other.

This situation can easily be modelled by the MDLP depicted in figure 6.7.

To know what would be the decision of each of the sectors, about which products to buy, not taking under consideration the deliberation of its superiors, all needs to be done is to determine the stable models at the state corresponding to that sector. For example, the reader can check that at state QMD there is a single stable model in which both $not\,buy(a)$ and $not\,buy(b)$ are true. At the state BD there are two stable models: one in which $buy(a)$ and $not\,buy(b)$ are true; another where $not\,buy(a)$ and $buy(b)$ are true instead.

More interesting would be to know what is the decision of the company as a whole, when taking into account the rules of all sectors and their hierarchical organization. This is reflected by the stable models of the whole MDLP, *i.e. the stable models at the set of all states of the* MDLP. *The reader can check that, in this instance, there is a single stable model in which $buy(a)$ and $not\,buy(b)$ are true. It coincides with the single stable model at state president because all other states belong to its relevancy graph.*

6.6.2 Multiple Inheritance

Multi-dimensional Dynamic Logic Programming can be used to represent and reason about complex taxonomies, as exemplified in the next two examples:

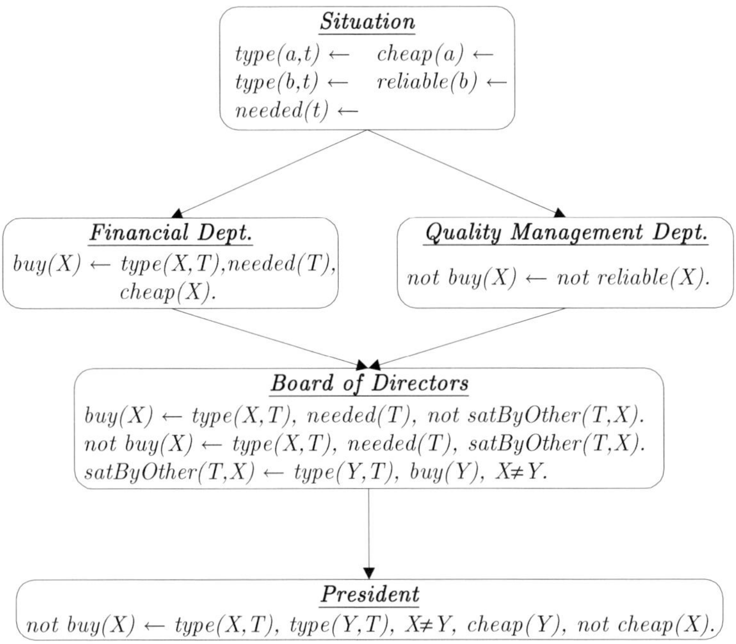

Figure 6.7: An *MDLP* representing a company

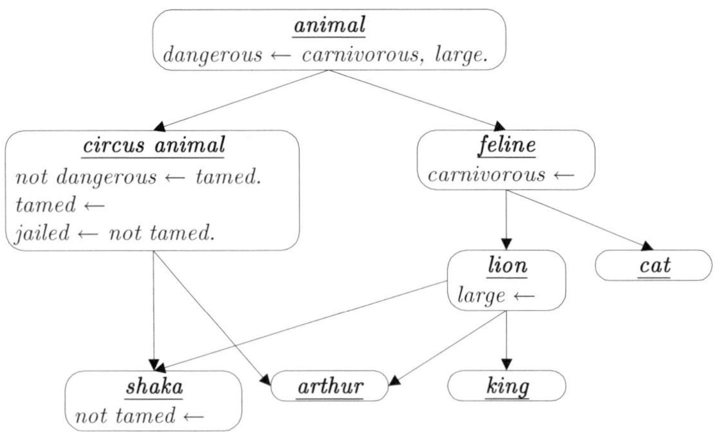

Figure 6.8: A Taxonomy

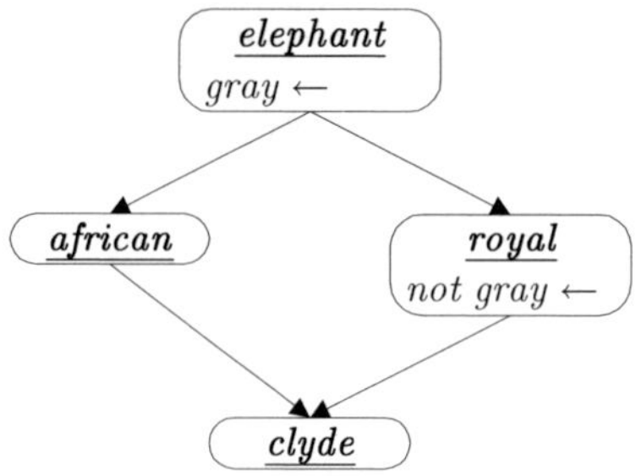

Figure 6.9: Clyde - The Royal Elephant

Example 61 *Consider the taxonomy with multiple inheritance, as per Fig. 6.8 (adapted from [54]). The reader can easily verify that the stable models at states* shaka, arthur *and* king *are, as expected:*

$$\begin{aligned} M_{shaka} &= \{large, carnivorous, dangerous, jailed\} \\ M_{arthur} &= \{large, carnivorous, tamed\} \\ M_{king} &= \{large, carnivorous, dangerous\} \end{aligned}$$

The next example shows how the well known *royal-elephant* scenario (adapted from [213]) can be easily encoded in $\mathcal{MDLP}$.

Example 62 *The* royal-elephant *scenario is described by the sentences: Elephants are gray; African elephants are elephants; Royal elephants are elephants; Clyde is a royal elephant; Clyde is an african elephant; Royal elephants aren't gray.*

This can be encoded by the MDLP *with* $\mathcal{P} = (\mathcal{P}_D, D)$ *such that*

$$\mathcal{P}_D = \{P_{elephant}, P_{african}, P_{royal}, P_{clyde}\}$$

where:

$$\begin{array}{ll} P_{elephant} = \{gray \leftarrow\} & P_{african} = \{\} \\ P_{royal} = \{not\ gray \leftarrow\} & P_{clyde} = \{\} \end{array} \tag{6.156}$$

and $D = (V, E)$ *where*

$$V = \{elephant, african, royal, clyde\} \tag{6.157}$$

$$E = \{(elephant, african), (elephant, royal), (african, clyde), (royal, clyde)\} \tag{6.158}$$

as depicted in Fig.6.9. The only stable model at state clyde *is* $M_{clyde} = \{not\ gray\}$*. In fact, we have that:*

$$Reject(\mathcal{P}_{clyde}, clyde, M_{clyde}) = \{gray \leftarrow\} \qquad Default(\mathcal{P}_{clyde}, M_{clyde}) = \{not\ gray\} \tag{6.159}$$

and, finally,

$$[\mathcal{P}_{clyde} - Reject(\mathcal{P}_{clyde}, s, M_{clyde})] \cup Default(\mathcal{P}_{clyde}, M_{clyde}) = \{not\ gray \leftarrow; not\ gray\} \tag{6.160}$$

whose least model is M_{clyde}*. Note that at state* african *the only stable model is* $M_{african} = \{gray\}$ *because the rule not gray ← only rejects the rule gray ← at state* clyde*, that is, when both the rules not gray ← and gray ← are present in the relevancy graph.*

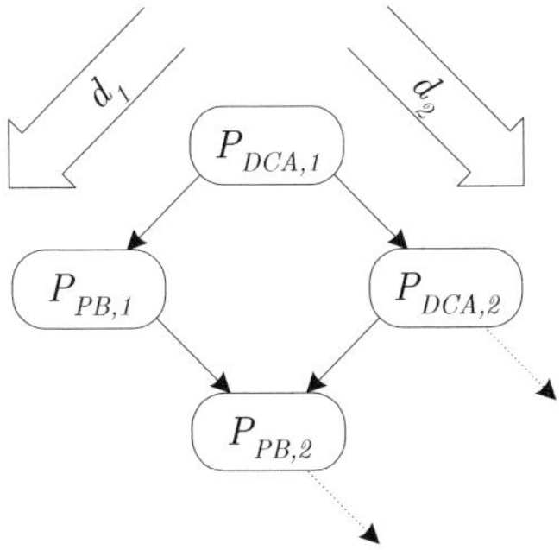

Figure 6.10: DAG of Example 63

6.6.3 Legal Reasoning

This example describes how $\mathcal{MDLP}$ can deal with collision principles, found in legal reasoning, such as *Lex Superior (Lex Superior Derogat Legi Inferiori)* according to which the rule issued by a higher hierarchical authority overrides the one issued by a lower one, and *Lex Posterior (Lex Posterior Derogat Legi Priori)* according to which the rule enacted at a later point in time overrides the earlier one, i.e how the combination of a temporal and an hierarchical dimensions can be combined into a single $\mathcal{MDLP}$.

Example 63 *In February 97, the President of Brazil (PB) passed a law determining that, in order to guarantee the safety aboard public transportation airplanes, all weapons were forbidden. Furthermore, all exceptional situations that, due to public interest, require an armed law enforcement or military agent are to be the subject of specific regulation by the Military and Justice Ministries. We will refer to this as rule 1. At the time of this event, there was in force an internal norm of the Department of Civil Aviation (DCA) stating that "Armed Forces Officials and Police Officers can board with their weapons if their destination is a national airport". We will refer to this as rule 2. Restricting ourselves to the essential parts of these regulations, they can be encoded by generalized logic program clauses:*

$$\begin{aligned} rule1: &\ not\, carry\_weapon \leftarrow not\, exception \\ rule2: &\ carry\_weapon \leftarrow armed\_officer \end{aligned}$$

Let us consider a lattice with two distinct dimensions, corresponding to the two principles governing this situation: Lex Superior (d_1) *and* Lex Posterior (d_2). *Besides the two agencies involved in this situation (PB and DCA), we will consider two time points representing the time when the two regulations were enacted. We have then a graph whose vertices are* $\{(PB,1),(PB,2),(DCA,1),(DCA,2)\}$ *(in the form (agency,time)) as portrayed in Fig.6.10. We have that* $P_{DCA,1}$ *contains rule 2,* $P_{PB,2}$ *contains rule 1 and the other two programs are empty. Let us further assume that there is an armed_officer represented by a fact in* $P_{DCA,1}$. *Applying Def.105, for* $M_{PB,2} = \{not\, carry\_weapon,\ not\, exception,\ armed\_officer\}$ *at state* $(PB,2)$ *we have that:*

$$Reject(\mathcal{P},(PB,2),M_{PB,2}) = \{carry\_weapon \leftarrow armed\_officer\}$$
$$Default\left(\rho\left(\mathcal{P}\right)_{PB,2}, M_{PB,2}\right) = \{not\, exception\}$$

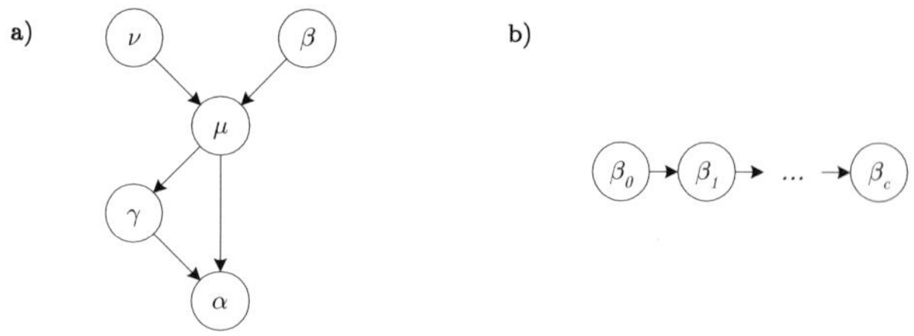

Figure 6.11: Two Dimensions of a Multi-Agent System

it is trivial to see that

$$M_{PB,2} = least \left(\begin{array}{c} \left[\rho\left(\mathcal{P}\right)_{PB,2} - Reject(\mathcal{P},(PB,2),M_{PB,2})\right] \cup \\ \cup Default\left(\rho\left(\mathcal{P}\right)_{PB,2}, M_{PB,2}\right) \end{array} \right)$$

which means that in spite of rule 2, since the exceptions have not been regulated yet, rule 1 prevails for all situations, and no one can carry a weapon aboard an airplane. This would correspond to the only stable model of $\boxplus_{PB,2}\mathcal{P}$.

6.6.4 Representing Inter- and Intra-Agent Social Viewpoints

The previous section contains the definition of the notion of *Multi-dimensional Dynamic Logic Programming*, $\mathcal{MDLP}$, as an extension of *DLP* to allow for states to be related by an arbitrary DAG. The stable models of $\mathcal{MDLP}$ have been characterized but nothing has been yet explained as how to use such DAGs to represent real problems. In particular, we have not shown how DAGs allow for the combination of more than one representational dimension, the very motivation to introduce $\mathcal{MDLP}$. Here, we explore some particular classes of DAGs suitable in the context of multi-agent systems.

Agents are situated and therefore need to represent and reason about information they obtain directly by sensing the environment or communicated by other agents. These agents, as well as the environment, evolve in time, i.e. the incoming information is to be used as an update over existing knowledge. Moreover these agents do not have the same credibility, this being represented via a hierarchy of predominance. In this section we explore DAGs that provide a way to represent the evolution in time of knowledge with provenance in a community of hierarchically related agents.

We start with an agent α, situated in a community of agents represented by the greek letters β, γ, μ, ν. The multi-agent system is $\mathcal{A} = \{\alpha, \beta, \gamma, \mu, \nu\}$. According to agent's α hierarchical view of the world, and its position within the community, all agents are related according to the DAG $D_h = (\mathcal{A}, E_h)$ where $E_h = \{(\nu, \mu), (\beta, \mu), (\mu, \gamma), (\mu, \alpha), (\gamma, \alpha)\}$, depicted in Fig. 6.11 a).

According to this DAG, agent α's opinions prevail over those of every other agent. However this need not be so. If, for example, one of these agent's role was to coordinate the community, it would be natural to exist an edge connecting α to this agent.

In a static environment, this representation would be sufficient to determine the semantics of α's view of the community. In such a situation, the rules asserted by each agent would constitute programs indexed by the DAG of Fig. 6.11 a), i.e. $P_\beta, P_\gamma, P_\mu, ...$

In a realistic scenario, where the dynamics of the system cannot be ignored, there is no single program representing each agent. Rather, there is a sequence of programs

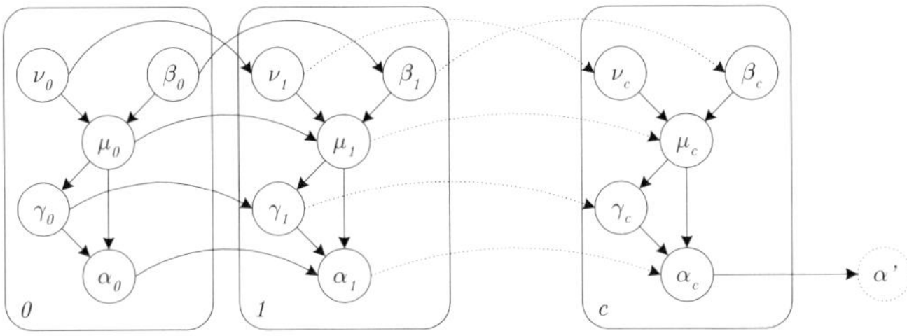

Figure 6.12: Equal Role Representation

representing the knowledge of each agent at each time point. Suppose these time points were represented by the set $T = \{0, 1, ..., c\}$ (where by c we mean the current time state), then, for example, the knowledge of agent β would be represented by the set of programs $\{P_{\beta_0}, P_{\beta_1}, ..., P_{\beta_c}\}$, indexed according to the DAG $D_{\beta_t} = (B_t, E_t)$ where $B_t = \{\beta_t : t \in S\}$ and $E_t = \{(0,1), ..., (c-1, c)\}$ as depicted in Fig. 6.11 b).

The full dynamic hierarchical scenario, comprising all agents, is then represented by the set of programs $\mathcal{P}_D = \{P_{a_t} : a \in \mathcal{A}, t \in T\}$ indexed by the DAG $D = (\mathcal{A}_T, E)$ where $\mathcal{A}_T = \{a_t : a \in \mathcal{A}, t \in T\}$.

There still remains to be defined the relationships between all these programs, i.e. the edges belonging to E. To this purpose, we will propose three basic ways to systematically relate these programs.

Equal Role Representation

The first approach to combining the hierarchical and temporal dimensions is accomplished by assigning equal roles to both precedence relations. In this scenario, we maintain the temporal precedence relation within each agent, and the hierarchical one within each time state, and we do not relate any two programs that fall outside this scope, i.e. there is no precedence between a higher ranked older program and a lower ranked newer one. Accordingly, the set of edges E, of the DAG D contains the union of the following two sets of edges:

Time Dependence Edges (TDE) : $\{(a_{t_1}, a_{t_2}) : a \in \mathcal{A}, t_1, t_2 \in T, t_1 < t_2\}$.

Hierarchy Dependence Edges (HDE) : $\{(a_t, b_t) : a, b \in \mathcal{A}, t \in T, a <_{D_h} b\}$.

Intuitively, each rule can be used to reject any rule of a lower ranked agent indexed by a time state equal or lower than its own. This situation is depicted in Fig. 6.12.

Remark 94 *Throughout this section, we have chosen a simplified representation of the DAGs to make their interpretation easier. For this purpose, we introduce new nodes (meta-nodes) encapsulating part of the DAG (detail). To obtain the complete DAG from this simplification one needs to replace the meta-node with the detail while replacing the edges entering the meta-node with a set of edges entering each source node of the detail. Similarly, one needs to replace each node departing from the meta-node with a set of edges departing from each sink of the detail. In every DAG, we have added a new node labelled α', which becomes its single sink, and an empty program associated with it, indicating where the semantics corresponding to agent α's view of the overall system at time state c can be determined. Also, since the semantics of MDLP is invariant with*

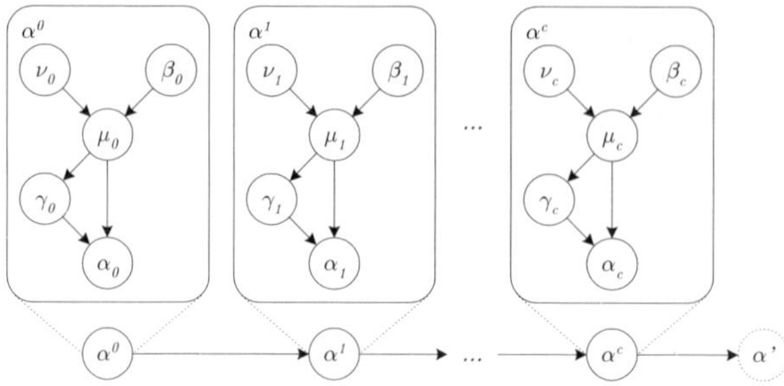

Figure 6.13: Time Prevailing Representation

respect to the transitive closure of the DAG, we will often be omitting some edges that do not affect such transitive closure.

Such a scenario can be found in legal reasoning, where the legislative agency is divided conforming to a hierarchy of power, governed by the principle *Lex Superior (Lex Superior Derogat Legi Inferiori)* according to which the rule issued by a higher hierarchical authority overrides the one issued by a lower one, and the evolution of law in time is governed by the principle *Lex Posterior (Lex Posterior Derogat Legi Priori)* according to which the rule enacted at a later point in time overrides the earlier one. *Lex Superior* is encoded by the Hierarchy Dependence Edges and *Lex Posterior* is encoded the Time Dependence Edges.

Allowing rejection governed by time and hierarchy alone, potentiates contradiction inasmuch as there are many pairs of programs not related according to this graph. If the purpose of our agency system were to perform some sort of paraconsistent reasoning, such as in an agent based negotiation system trying to reach an agreement, this would be the ideal scenario: contradiction would generate messages to the responsible agents to possibly review their positions. But often this is not the case and we may want to reduce the amount of contradiction, namely by establishing a skewed relation between the temporal and hierarchical dimensions. Two approaches will be explored in the following subsections.

Time Prevailing Representation

According to this representation, the DAG D contains, besides the Time and Hierarchy Dependence Edges, the following edges:

Time Prevailing Edges (TPE) : $\{(a_{t_1}, b_{t_2}) : a, b \in \mathcal{A}, t_1, t_2 \in T, t_1 < t_2\}$.

The intuitive reading is that any rule indexed by a more recent time state overrides any older rule, independently of which agents these rules belong to. This situation is depicted in Fig. 6.13.

This representation is particularly useful in very dynamic situations where competence is distributed, i.e. when knowledge changes rapidly and different agents will typically provide rules about different literals. This is so mainly because any newer rule always overrides any older one. It means that if a situation is completely defined by the rules issued by the community at a given time state, one can simply ignore older rules.

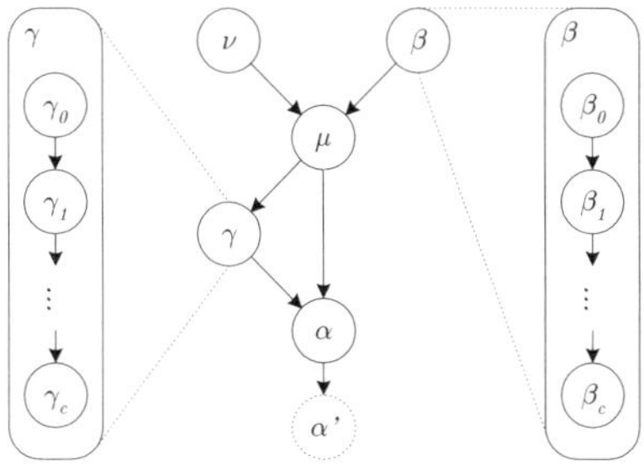

Figure 6.14: Hierarchy Prevailing Representation

The main drawback of this representation relates to the trustfulness of agents in the community. It requires all agents to be fully trusted because, in allowing all new rules to override all old ones, irrespective of their hierarchical position, any untrustworthy lower ranked agent can override any higher ranked agent just by issuing a rule at a later time state. This leads us to the next, alternative, representation.

Hierarchy Prevailing Representation

According to this representation, the DAG D contains, besides the Time and Hierarchy Dependence Edges, the following edges:

Hierarchy Prevailing Edges (HPE) : $\{(a_{t_1}, b_{t_2}) : a, b \in \mathcal{A}, t_1, t_2 \in T, a <_{D_h} b\}$.

The intuitive reading is that any rule indexed by a higher ranked agent overrides any lower ranked agent's rule, independently of the time state it is indexed by. This situation is depicted in Fig. 6.14.

This situation is useful, in contrast with the previous one, when some of the agents are untrustworthy because a lower ranked agent rule, to be used, may not be contradicted by any (even if older) higher ranked agent rule. The main drawback is that one has to consider the entire history of all higher ranked agents in order to accept/reject a rule provided by a lower ranked agent. However, a number of techniques to reduce the size of a dynamic logic program are being developed, useful for simplifying the time sequence of programs of each individual agent. These are outside the scope of this Chapter.

Again in the context of Legal Reasoning, this scenario corresponds to the one used in many Legislatures, where collisions between rules are governed by the principle *Lex Superior Priori Derogat Legi Inferiori Posterior*, i.e. the rule issued by a higher hierarchical authority at an earlier point overrides the one issued by a lower hierarchical authority at a later point.

Representing Inter- and Intra-Agent Relationships

The representations set forth in the previous sub-sections refer to a community of agents. Nevertheless, they can be used at different levels of abstraction to represent macro and micro aspects of a multi-agent system, in a unified manner. Let us suppose that agent α is composed of several sub-agents concurrently performing dedicated tasks while reading and writing onto a common knowledge structure. According to this view,

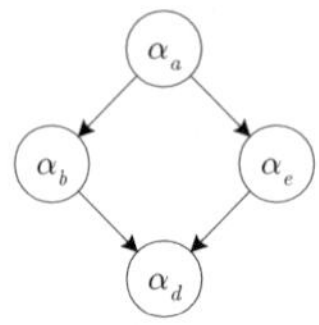

Figure 6.15: Sub-agent Hierarchy

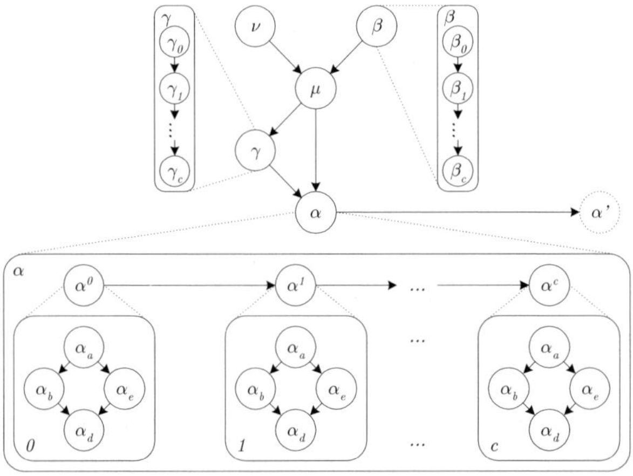

Figure 6.16: Inter- and Intra-Agent Relationship Representation

agent α can now be seen as a community of sub-agents $\mathcal{A}_\alpha = \{\alpha_a, \alpha_b, \alpha_d, \alpha_e\}$, related, for example, according to the DAG $D_\alpha = (\mathcal{A}_\alpha, E_\alpha)$ where $E_\alpha = \{(\alpha_a, \alpha_b), (\alpha_a, \alpha_e), (\alpha_b, \alpha_d), (\alpha_e, \alpha_d)\}$ as in Fig. 6.15. The overall dynamic system, comprising all agents and sub-agents, is now represented by the set of programs $\mathcal{P}_D = \{P_{a_t} : a_t \in \mathcal{A}_T\}$ indexed by the DAG $D = (\mathcal{A}_T, E)$ where $\mathcal{A}_T = \{a_t : a \in \mathcal{A} \diagdown \{\alpha\}, t \in T\} \cup \{a_t : a \in \mathcal{A}_\alpha, t \in T\}$.

As for the relations between the programs, we propose a combination of the time and hierarchy prevailing representations to relate the sub-agents and agents respectively. As mentioned before, the time prevailing representation is the most efficient but requires all agents to be trusted. One would expect an agent to trust its component sub-agents. As for the representation of other agents, we will opt for the hierarchy prevailing relation. Formally, the set of edges in the DAG contains:

Time Prevailing Edges (TPE) : $\{(a_{t_1}, b_{t_2}) : a, b \in \mathcal{A}_\alpha, t_1, t_2 \in T, t_1 < t_2\}$, to model the relationships between the sub-agents of α.

Hierarchy Prevailing Edges (HPE) : $\{(a_{t_1}, b_{t_2}) : a, b \in \mathcal{A}, t_1, t_2 \in T, a <_{D_h} b\}$, to model the relationships between the agents of the system. Note that each edge entering (resp. departing from) α_t should be interpreted as a set of edges entering (resp. departing from) each of $\{\alpha_{a_t}, \alpha_{b_t}, \alpha_{d_t}, \alpha_{e_t}\}$.

This situation is depicted in Fig. 6.16. Note however that this is just one proposal of the many possible existing combinations to represent such relations.

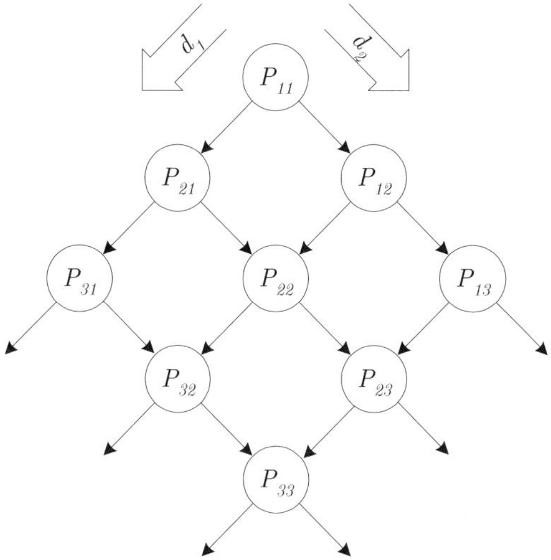

Figure 6.17: A Lattice with two dimensions

6.6.5 $\mathcal{MDLP}$ and Multi-agent Systems

The previous example is a particular case suggesting that some particular acyclic digraphs are especially useful to model several aspects of multi-agent systems. We have in mind n-dimensional lattices, where each dimension represents one particular characteristic to be modelled. Suppose a linear hierarchically related society of agents situated in a dynamic environment. Fig.6.17 represents the lattice that encodes this situation. It has two dimensions, one representing the linearly arranged agents, and the other representing time. If d_1 represents time and d_2 represents the hierarchy, P_{11} contains the new knowledge of agent 1 at time 1. P_{32} contains the knowledge of agent 2 (who is hierarchically superior to agent 1) at time 3, and so on... The overall semantics of a system consisting of n agents at time t is given by $\boxplus_{t,n}\mathcal{P}$.

The applicability of $\mathcal{MDLP}$ in a multi-agent context is not limited to the assignment of a single semantics to the overall system, i.e., the multi-agent system does not have to be described by a single *DAG*. Instead we could determine each agent's view of the world by associating a *DAG* with each agent, representing its own view of its relationships to other agents and of these amongst themselves. The stable models over a set of states from *DAG*s of different agents can provide us with interagent views.

Example 64 *Consider a society of agents representing a hierarchically structured research group. We have the Senior Researcher (A_{sr}), two Researchers (A_{r1} and A_{r2}) and two students (A_{s1} and A_{s2}) supervised by the two Researchers. The hierarchy is deployed in Fig.6.18, which also represents the view of the Senior Researcher. Typically, students think they are always right and do not like hierarchies, so their view of the community is quite different. Fig.6.19 manifests one possible view by A_{s1}. In this scenario, we could use $\mathcal{MDLP}$ to determine and eventually compare A_{sr}'s view, given by $\boxplus_{sr}\mathcal{P}$ in Fig.6.18, with A_{s1}'s view, given by $\boxplus_{s1}\mathcal{P}$ in Fig.6.19. If we assign the*

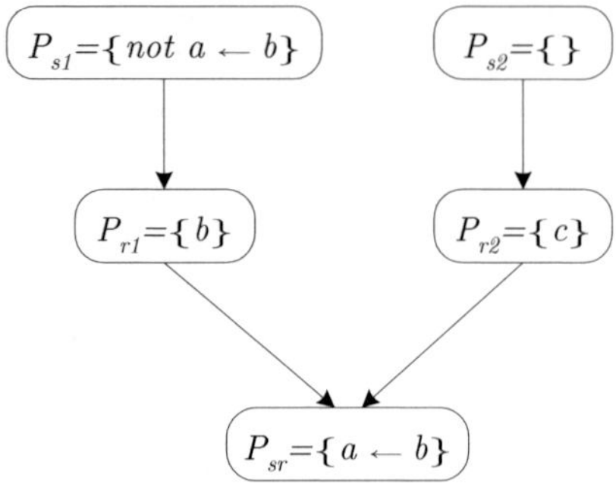

Figure 6.18: The view of the Senior Researcher

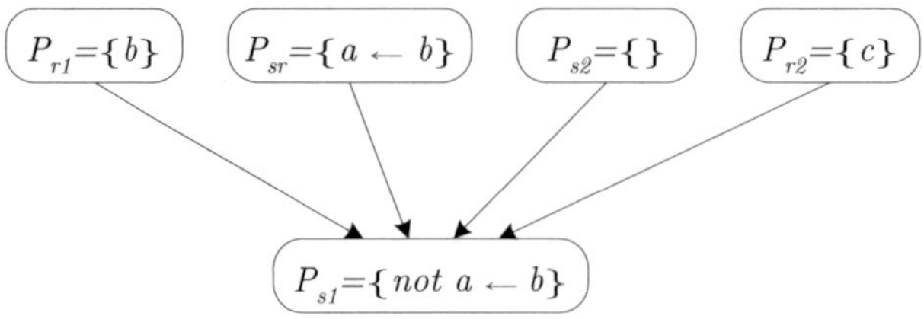

Figure 6.19: The view of the Student

following simple logic programs to the five agents:

$$\begin{array}{ll} P_{sr} = \{a \leftarrow b\} & P_{r1} = \{b\} \\ P_{s1} = \{not\, a \leftarrow c\} & P_{r2} = \{c\} \\ P_{s2} = \{\} & \end{array}$$

we have that $\boxplus_{sr}\mathcal{P}$ in Fig.6.18 has $M_{sr} = \{a, b, c\}$ as the only stable model, and $\boxplus_{s1}\mathcal{P}$ in Fig.6.19 has $M_{s1} = \{not\, a, b, c\}$ as its only stable model. That is, according to student A_{s1}'s view of the world a is false, while according to the senior researcher A_{sr}'s view of the world a is true.

This example suggests $\mathcal{MDLP}$ to be a useful practical framework to study changes in behaviour of such multi-agent systems and how they hinge on the relationships amongst the agents i.e., on the current DAG that represents them. $\mathcal{MDLP}$ offers an important basic tool in the formal study of the social behaviour in multi-agent communities. In the final section, we elaborate on extensions to $\mathcal{MDLP}$ to enhance this tool.

6.7 Comparison with other work

In Chapter 3 we overviewed DLP$^<$, a language that extends LP with inheritance, relating programs according to a strict partial order "<". For the case where the partial order induces a sequence of logic programs, we have established the relationship with DLP. We now present several results, whose proofs are similar to the ones for the DLP case and thus omitted, that establish the relationship between $\mathcal{MDLP}$ and DLP$^<$.

Theorem 95 *Let* $P^{<} = \{\langle o_1, P_1\rangle, ..., \langle o_n, P_n\rangle\}$ *be an inheritance program (without disjunction) and* $<$ *a strict partial order between object identifiers. Let* $\mathcal{P} = (\mathcal{P}_D, D)$ *be a* Multi-dimensional Dynamic Logic Program, *where* $\mathcal{P}_D = \{P_{o_i} : o_i \in V\}$, $D = (V, E)$, $V = \{o_1, ..., o_n\}$ *and* $E = \{(o_i, o_j) : o_i, o_j \in V, o_i < o_j\}$. *Then, an (extended)* Stable Model of $\mathcal{P}$ *is an* answer set *of* $P^{<}$.

Although $\mathcal{P}$-Justified Updates were never extended to the multi-dimensional case, such extension can be accomplished in a very natural way, according to the following definition:

Definition 110 ($\mathcal{P}$-Justified Updates at the set of states S) *Let* $\mathcal{P} = (\mathcal{P}_D, D)$ *be a* Multi-dimensional Dynamic Logic Program, *where* $\mathcal{P}_D = \{P_v : v \in V\}$ *and* $D = (V, E)$ *and each* P_v *is a* Generalized Extended Logic Program. *An (extended) interpretation* M *is a* $\mathcal{P}$-Justified Update *at the set of states* S, *iff* M *is a (extended) stable model of:*

$$\rho(\mathcal{P})_S - Reject(\mathcal{P}, S, M) \tag{6.161}$$

where

$$\rho(\mathcal{P})_S = \bigcup_{s \in S} \left(\bigcup_{i \leq_D s} P_i \right) \tag{6.162}$$

$$Reject(\mathcal{P}, S, M) = \{r \in P_i \mid \exists s \in S, \exists r' \in P_j, i <_D j \leq_D s, r \bar{\bowtie} r' \wedge M \vDash B(r')\} \tag{6.163}$$

and $r \bar{\bowtie} r'$ *iff* $H(r) = not\ H(r')$ *or* $H(r) = -H(r')$.

Similarly, we can extend the notion of U-Models to the multi-dimensional case:

Definition 111 (U-Models at the set of states S) *Let* $\mathcal{P} = (\mathcal{P}_D, D)$ *be a* Multi-dimensional Dynamic Logic Program, *where* $\mathcal{P}_D = \{P_v : v \in V\}$ *and* $D = (V, E)$ *and each* P_v *is a* Generalized Extended Logic Program. *An (extended) interpretation* M *is a* U-model *at the set of states* S *iff:*

$$M = least\left([\rho(\mathcal{P})_S - Rej^*(M, S, \mathcal{P})] \cup Default(\rho(\mathcal{P})_S, M)\right) \tag{6.164}$$

where

$$Rej^*(M, S, \mathcal{P}) = \left\{ \begin{array}{c} r \in P_i \mid \exists s \in S, \exists r' \in P_j \setminus Rej^*(M, S, \mathcal{P}), \\ i <_D j \leq_D s, r \bar{\bowtie} r' \wedge M \vDash B(r') \cup B(r) \end{array} \right\}$$

$$Default(\rho(\mathcal{P})_S, M) = \{not\ A \mid \nexists r \in \rho(\mathcal{P})_S : (H(r) = A) \wedge M \vDash B(r)\}$$

$\rho(\mathcal{P})_S$ *and* $\bar{\bowtie}$ *are defined as before.*

And finally we can extend the generalized update answer-set semantics to deal with multiple dimensions, as follows:

Definition 112 (Update Answer-Sets at the set of states S) *Let* $\mathcal{P} = (\mathcal{P}_D, D)$ *be a* Multi-dimensional Dynamic Logic Program, *where* $\mathcal{P}_D = \{P_v : v \in V\}$ *and* $D = (V, E)$ *and each* P_v *is a* Generalized Extended Logic Program. *An (extended) interpretation* M *is an* Update Answer-set *at the set of states* S, *iff* M *is a (extended) stable model of:*

$$\rho(\mathcal{P})_S - Rej^*(M, S, \mathcal{P}) \tag{6.165}$$

where $\rho(\mathcal{P})_S$ *and* $Rej^*(M, S, \mathcal{P})$ *are defined as before.*

As before, if we do not make explicit mention to the state being considered, we assume the set of all states.

Immediately, as for the single dimensional case, we obtain that for the case of an MDLP consisting only if extended logic programs, the semantics of inheritance programs coincides with that of multi-dimensional Update Answer-sets:

Theorem 96 *$\mathcal{P} = (\mathcal{P}_D, D)$ be a* Multi-dimensional Dynamic Logic Program *over a language $\mathcal{L}^*$ generated by $\mathcal{K}^*$, where $\mathcal{P}_D = \{P_{o_i} : o_i \in V\}$, $D = (V, E)$ and each P_{o_i} is an* extended logic program. *Let $P^< = \{\langle o_v, P_v\rangle : v \in V\}$ with inheritance order equal to the partial order induced by D. Then, an extended interpretation M is an* Update Answer-set *of $\mathcal{P}$ iff M is an* answer set *of $P^<$.*

The four existing multi-dimensional semantics are related just as for their single dimension counterparts. The following Theorem summarize the results, where we consider $\mathcal{P} = (\mathcal{P}_D, D)$, where $\mathcal{P}_D = \{P_{o_i} : o_i \in V\}$, $D = (V, E)$, to be an (extended) *Multi-dimensional Dynamic Logic Program* over a language $\mathcal{L}^*$ generated by $\mathcal{K}^*$, and $S \subseteq V$ a set of its states.

Theorem 97 *Let $MDLP(\mathcal{P})_S$ denote the set of (extended) stable models of $\mathcal{P}$ at states S; $MJU(\mathcal{P})_S$ denote the set of $\mathcal{P}$-*Justified Update *at states S; $MAS(\mathcal{P})_S$ denote the set of* Update Answer-Set *at states S; and $MU(\mathcal{P})_S$ denote the set of* U-models *at states S. Then:*

$$MDLP(\mathcal{P})_S \subseteq MJU(\mathcal{P})_S \subseteq MAS(\mathcal{P})_S$$
$$MDLP(\mathcal{P})_S \subseteq MU(\mathcal{P})_S \subseteq MAS(\mathcal{P})_S$$

Conditions such as the chain and the graph conditions set forth for DLP could also be tested on the multi-dimensional case to obtain situations where the semantics coincide, although we will not explore them here.

6.8 Conclusions and Future Work

We have shown how $\mathcal{MDLP}$ generalizes *DLP* in allowing for collections of states organized by arbitrary acyclic digraphs, and not just linear sequences of states. Indeed, $\mathcal{MDLP}$ assigns semantics to sets and subsets of logic programs, on the basis of how they stand in relation amongst each other, as defined by an acyclic digraph. Such a natural generalization imparts added expressiveness to updating, thereby amplifying the coverage of its application domains. The flexibility provided by a *DAG* accrues to the scope and variety of the new possibilities. The new characteristics of multiplicity and composition of $\mathcal{MDLP}$ impart an innovative "societal" viewpoint to *Logic Programming.*

Much remains to be done. Some of the more immediate themes of ongoing work regarding the further development of multi-dimensional updates comprise:

- Studying the conditions for and uses of dropping the acyclicity condition.
- Capturing with $\mathcal{MDLP}$ assorted program composition operators [41].
- Establishing a paraconsistent $\mathcal{MDLP}$ semantics and defining contradiction removal over DAGs.

Inevitably, updating raises other issues, such as about revising and preferring, and work is emerging on the articulation of these distinct but highly complementary aspects [13]. Learning is usefully seen as successive approximate change, as opposed to exact change, and combining the results of learning by multiple agents, multiple strategies, or multiple data sets, inevitably poses problems within the province of updating, cf. [127]. Also, other domains can use $\mathcal{MDLP}$ to their advantage, such as: software development, distributed heterogeneous knowledge bases, model-based diagnosis, agent architectures. Some are currently being actively pursued by others.

In the next Chapter, we enhance *KABUL* to allow for knowledge organized as an $\mathcal{MDLP}$ and extend its syntax to deal with such an $\mathcal{MDLP}$ based knowledge representation.

Chapter 7

Multi-dimensional Knowledge and Behaviour Update Language

In this Chapter, we extend KABUL to allow for the specification and updating of MDLP based evolving knowledge bases, therefore increasing their expressive power. This is attained incrementally, first by extending the basic commands to allow the update of specific nodes in an MDLP which builds up according to a fixed evolution mode. Subsequently we introduce commands to allow the dynamic specification of the hierarchy relating different nodes, and the prevalence modes that govern the MDLP's evolution. Finally, we introduce the notion of multiple update programs each of them partially encoding the internal behaviour of the evolving knowledge base, thus concurrently specifying its evolution. Parts of this Chapter appeared in [139].

7.1 Introduction

In Chapter 3 the paradigm of *Dynamic Logic Programming* was introduced. Based on rule updates instead of model updates, DLP allows knowledge to be given by a linearly ordered sequence of theories (encoded as generalized logic programs) that represent distinct and dynamically changing states of the world. These different states can represent different time periods, different agents, different hierarchical instances, or even different domains of knowledge. Consequently, individual theories may comprise mutually contradictory as well as overlapping information. The role of *DLP* is to employ the mutual relationships existing between different knowledge states to precisely determine the declarative as well as the procedural semantics of the combined (updated) theory comprised of all individual theories at each state.

Whereas *DLP* provides a declarative and procedural semantics for a sequence of program updates, it does not provide any natural or practical language for the specification of such updates, which typically depend on the knowledge acquired in the intervening states. In order to overcome this drawback, in [15], the so-called *Language for Dynamic Updates* (*LUPS*) was established and investigated. *LUPS* allows us to associate with any given knowledge state a set of transition or update rules, which determine what updates should be applied to the current knowledge state. In Chapter 4 we have extended the *LUPS* language with new commands and changed its semantics to correct an undesirable behaviour when dealing with non-inertial commands, introducing *KUL*. Whereas *KUL* provides a declarative way to specify the behaviours of agents when dealing with updates of knowledge bases, it does not provide a way to update such behaviour specifications. In Chapter 5 we have introduced *KABUL* as a language to allow the specification of both the updates of knowledge bases and also the update of the behaviours that specify such updates, to support the notion of *Evolving Knowledge Bases.*

Although well-suited to encode a single update dimension (e.g. time, hierarchies, or other priorities), *DLP* (*KUL* and *KABUL*) cannot deal with more than one update dimension at a time. For example, *DLP* can be used to model the relationship of a group of agents linked according to a linear hierarchy, and *DLP* can be used to model the evolution of the knowledge of a single agent over time. But *DLP*, as it stands, cannot deal with both dimensions of dynamic change simultaneously. Nor can it model hierarchical relations amongst agents who have more than one superior (and thus require multiple inheritance). This is, of course, due to that *DLP* is only defined for linear sequences of knowledge states. In order to overcome this limitation, *Multi-dimensional Dynamic Logic Programming* ($\mathcal{MDLP}$) was introduced in Chapter 6. According to $\mathcal{MDLP}$, a generalization of DLP, knowledge is given by a set of logic programs, indexed by collections of states organized into arbitrary acyclic directed graphs (*DAG*s) representing precedence relations. The extra flexibility afforded by the *DAG* allows $\mathcal{MDLP}$ to provide a semantic framework for the representation, in a unified manner and with precise declarative and procedural semantics, to not only knowledge represented by logic programs related according to some hierarchy (possibly involving multiple inheritance), but also to represent its inner dynamics, i.e. its evolution in time.

Whereas $\mathcal{MDLP}$ provides a declarative and procedural semantics of a sequence of program updates, based on a hierarchy determined by a *DAG*, as it was the case with *DLP*, it does not provide any language for the specification of such multi-dimensional updates, which depend on the knowledge acquired in the intervening states and on the topology of the *DAG*. It also does not provide any language for the specification (and possible updating) of the precedence topology itself.

In order to address this issue, in this Chapter, we extend *KABUL* with the powerful capability of expressing simultaneous (in time) updates of a number of separate knowledge bases (KBs), represented by sequences of generalized logic programs. We dub this extension $KABUL^m$ Intuitively, update commands (such as asserts, retracts, persistent asserts, etc) are given to such separate KBs. As a result of the commands each KB evolves as a linearly ordered sequence of programs, each program containing the rules added to that KB at each time point. In these time lines, rules from later programs may be used to reject rules from previous ones. Additionally, these KBs can be hierarchically organized as nodes of a directed precedence graph, so that rules from preferred KBs prevail over rules from less preferred ones. The KBs' hierarchy imposes an organization among the programs that constitute the KBs time lines. Different policies of imposing organizations over the programs are possible. E.g.: by KB_1 being preferred over KB_2 one may simply want to state that rules given at a time point t to KB_1 may be used to reject rules given to KB_2 at t (as we've seen before, we dub this policy *"equal role representation"*). But one may want to impose more. Namely, that any rule of KB_1, even if given before t, may be used to reject rules given to KB_2 at t (*"hierarchy prevalence representation"*). The update commands of $KABUL^m$ can be made conditional on the present state of a collection of KBs and thus dynamically change with the changes in individual KBs or changed in their mutual relationships. Moreover, the edges of the directed graph may be subjected to update commands as well, thereby catering for a dynamic reconfiguration of the topology of the preference relation among nodes. Sequences of sets of $KABUL^m$ statements applied to the initial state of the graph result in a sequence of graphs whose semantics of intermediate and final nodes precisely coincides with the semantics of the *multi-dimensional dynamic logic program* generated by those commands.

Throughout this Chapter *KABUL* will be extended in an incremental fashion. We start with a simple version comprising a set of commands that permit the specification of the next temporal state of a knowledge base, but whose organizing *DAG* evolves according to a fixed preference policy. Namely, according to *equal role representation.*

Subsequently, we introduce a new set of commands, augmenting the previous ones, that allow the hierarchy among the knowledge bases itself to evolve from state to state, by adding or removing edges. Then we include yet another set of commands with the purpose of changing the policy of connecting the various time lines of the KBs. These commands foresee the specification of precedence relations between otherwise unrelated states of different knowledge bases, such as precedence relations between older hierarchically superior knowledge states and newer hierarchically inferior ones. In other words, these commands allow for the specification of prevalence relations between the already existing temporal and hierarchical equal role relations. Finally, we introduce the notion of multiple update programs each of them partially encoding the internal behaviour of the evolving knowledge base, thus concurrently specifying its evolution. This notion of multiple update programs opens the ground for the specification of what can be seen as specialized sub-agents concurrently carrying out independent tasks within an evolving knowledge base. In the next Chapter, we will present two illustrative examples on the use of this extended version of *KABUL*.

7.2 Core Language

In this section we set forth the *core* language of $KABUL^m$. We start with a fixed set of agents[1] $\mathcal{A} = \{\alpha^0, \alpha^1, \alpha^2, ..., \alpha^m\}$ represented by nodes linked according to a fixed hierarchy encoded by the (labelled) *hierarchy DAG* $\mathcal{H} = (\mathcal{A}, HE)$ where HE is a set of labelled edges of the form (α^i, α^j, t) where $\alpha^i, \alpha^j \in \mathcal{A}$ and $t \in \mathcal{T}$, where $\mathcal{T} = \{0, 1, ..., n, ...\}$ is a set of (time) states. We call it *core* because the evolution of the topology of the DAG is fixed, in the sense that the edges linking the various nodes are determined as per an initial hierarchy, plus the sequence of time states. At each time state a new node for each agent in $\mathcal{A}$ is created, linked to its previous instance. Such new nodes are linked amongst themselves according to the hierarchy $\mathcal{H}$. Subsequently, we extend *KABUL* to cater for the specification of the evolution of $\mathcal{H}$. Because each new node is also linked to its predecessor, i.e. the node corresponding to the same agent at the previous time state, there is created a time state line in each agent. In this scenario, which gives rise to the "*equal role representation*" introduced in Section 6.6.4, a rule given to an agent α^i at time t may be rejected by a rule given to the same α^i at any later time $t_l > t$, or by a rule given to a preferred agent α^j at the same t. No precedence exists over a higher ranked older program by a lower ranked but newer one. Subsequently, we also extend *KABUL* to allow other evolution modes. The label in the

[1]To be more precise, we should refer to these entities as knowledge sources. For simplicity we refer to them as agents, but agency is just one of the possible applications of $KABUL^m$.

hierarchy DAG will not be used in the core version and, therefore, the element t in the edges of the form (α^i, α^j, t) can be ignored for the time being. We will come back to this issue in Section 7.3.

In this extended framework, each knowledge state will consist of an MDLP, $\mathcal{P}_s = (\mathcal{P}_{D_s}, D_s)$ where $D_s = (V_s, E_s)$ is a *DAG* (referred to as the *MDLP DAG*) and $\mathcal{P}_{D_s} = \{P_v : v \in V_s\}$, instead of the DLP of *KABUL*, a set of statements corresponding to the self updates, SU_s, the current hierarchy $\mathcal{H}_s = (\mathcal{A}, HE_s)$, and the necessary knowledge about the evolution mode, $\mathcal{M}_s$, i.e. each knowledge state will be a tuple of the form $\langle \mathcal{P}_s, SU_s, \mathcal{H}_s, \mathcal{M}_s \rangle$. Since in the core version we have a fixed hierarchy, we have that $\mathcal{H}_s = \mathcal{H}$ for all states. The form and content of $\mathcal{M}_s$ will only be explained in a subsequent section when we extend this core version to cater for other evolution modes, other than the equal representation one. Until then, it can simply be ignored.

As before, there is a cycle that drives state transitions which have the generic form:

$$\langle \mathcal{P}_s, SU_s, \mathcal{H}_s, \mathcal{M}_s \rangle \overset{\langle EU_{s+1}, EO_{s+1} \rangle}{\longrightarrow} \langle \mathcal{P}_{s+1}, SU_{s+1}, \mathcal{H}_{s+1}, \mathcal{M}_{s+1} \rangle$$

Again, we use the notation $\langle \mathcal{P}_0, SU_0, \mathcal{H}_0, \mathcal{M}_0 \rangle \otimes \langle EU_1, EO_1 \rangle \otimes \langle EU_2, EO_2 \rangle \otimes ... \otimes \langle EU_s, EO_s \rangle$ to denote the knowledge state produced by such sequence, starting from the initial knowledge state (defined below), i.e. the knowledge state $\langle \mathcal{P}_s, SU_s, \mathcal{H}_s, \mathcal{M}_s \rangle$.

7.2.1 *KABUL*^{m} - Syntax

For *KABUL*^{m}, the syntax must be modified to allow the statement conditions to refer to particular nodes in the *MDLP*, where their truth value should be determined. For this purpose, each literal L, **in**(R) and **out**(R) in such conditions, is to be evaluated at the most recent nodes of the set of agents Θ, and will be represented by $L@\Theta$, **in**$(R)@\Theta$ and **out**$(R)@\Theta$. Moreover, the commands should include a reference to indicate where (in the *MDLP*) the commands should be executed, i.e. where the rules should be asserted and retracted. For example, to express that some rule R should be asserted at the new node of agent α, we use the convention **assert** $(R@\alpha)$. This convention is also used with the command conditions where, for example, one such condition of the form **retract_event** $(R@\alpha)$ means that whichever command is specified by the statement should only be executed if rule R is non-inertially retracted at the new node of agent α. Except for these changes, the syntax of *KABUL*^{m} is similar to the one of *KABUL*.

Definition 113 (*KABUL*^{m} - Syntax) *Let $\mathcal{A} = \{\alpha^0, \alpha^1, \alpha^2, ..., \alpha^m\}$ be a set of agents. Let $\mathcal{L}$ be a propositional language. Let $\mathcal{R}$ be the set of rules generated by $\mathcal{L}$. Let $\mathcal{E}$ be a language of observations*[2]*. A* statement *is a propositional expression of the form*

$$\begin{aligned} C_0 \left(\rho_0 \left[@\alpha^0\right]\right) \Leftarrow C_1 \left(\rho_1 \left[@\alpha^1\right]\right), ..., C_n \left(\rho_n \left[@\alpha^n\right]\right), L_1@\Theta^{n+1}, \ldots, L_k@\Theta^{n+k}, \\ \mathbf{R} : \mathbf{in}\left(R_1@\Theta^1\right), ..., \mathbf{in}\left(R_m@\Theta^m\right), \mathbf{out}\left(R_{m+1}@\Theta^{m+1}\right), ..., \mathbf{out}\left(R_n@\Theta^n\right), \\ \mathbf{E} : \mathbf{in}\left(E_1\right), ..., \mathbf{in}\left(E_p\right), \mathbf{out}\left(E_{p+1}\right), ..., \mathbf{out}\left(E_q\right) \end{aligned}$$

where:

- *$C_0(\rho_0 \left[@\alpha^0\right])$ is either a persistent command, a non-persistent command or an inhibition command;*

[2]We include agents in $\mathcal{A}$ in the set of terms used to generate $\mathcal{E}$.

- *each* $C_1(\rho_1\,[@\alpha^1]), ..., C_n(\rho_n\,[@\alpha^n])$ $(n \geq 0)$ *is either a non-persistent command or an inhibition command.*

- *each* $L_1, ..., L_k$ $(k \geq 0)$ *is a literal from* $\mathcal{L}$*;*

- *each* $\Theta^1, ..., \Theta^{n+k}$ $(n, k \geq 0)$ *is a set of agents from* $\mathcal{A}$*, i.e.* $\Theta^{n+k} \subseteq \mathcal{A}$*;*

- *each* $R_1, ..., R_n$ $(n \geq 0)$ *is a rule from* $\mathcal{R}$*;*

- *each* $E_1, ..., E_q$ $(m \geq 0)$ *is an observation from* $\mathcal{E}$*.*

Let $\mathcal{S}$ *denote the set of all statements.*

A command *is a propositional expression of any of the forms*[3]*:*

$$[\textbf{always\_} \mid \textbf{once\_}]\,\textbf{assert}\,[\textbf{\_event}]\,(R@\alpha) \tag{7.1}$$
$$[\textbf{always\_} \mid \textbf{once\_}]\,\textbf{retract}\,[\textbf{\_event}]\,(R@\alpha) \tag{7.2}$$
$$[\textbf{always\_} \mid \textbf{once\_}]\,\textbf{assert}\,(S) \tag{7.3}$$
$$[\textbf{always\_} \mid \textbf{once\_}]\,\textbf{retract}\,(S) \tag{7.4}$$

where $R \in \mathcal{R}$ *is a rule,* $S \in \mathcal{S}$ *is a statement and* $\alpha \in \mathcal{A}$ *is an agent. A* persistent command *is a command containing one of the keywords* **always** *or* **once**. *A* non-persistent command *is a command that is not persistent.*

An inhibition command *is a propositional expression of any of the forms:*

$$not\,\textbf{assert}\,[\textbf{\_event}]\,(R@\alpha) \tag{7.5}$$
$$not\,\textbf{retract}\,[\textbf{\_event}]\,(R@\alpha) \tag{7.6}$$
$$not\,\textbf{assert}\,(S) \tag{7.7}$$
$$not\,\textbf{retract}\,(S) \tag{7.8}$$

where $R \in \mathcal{R}$ *is a rule,* $S \in \mathcal{S}$ *is a statement and* $\alpha \in \mathcal{A}$ *is an agent.*

We call commands of form (7.1) and (7.2) rule commands, *and those of form (7.3) and (7.4)* statement commands.

Given a rule command or inhibition rule command $c = [not]\,C(R@\alpha)$*, by the destination of* c*, denoted by* $Dest\,(c)$*, we mean* α*.*

If S *is a statement as above, then:*

$$\begin{aligned}
&\mathbf{H}\,(S) = C_0(\rho_0\,[@\alpha^0]) \\
&\mathbf{D}\,(S) = Dest\,(C_0(\rho_0\,[@\alpha^0]))\ \textit{if } \rho_0 \textit{ is a rule, otherwise it is not defined.} \\
&\mathbf{C}\,(S) = C_1(\rho_1\,[@\alpha^1]), ..., C_n(\rho_n\,[@\alpha^n]) \\
&\mathbf{L}\,(S) = L_1@\Theta^1, \ldots, L_k@\Theta^k \\
&\mathbf{R}\,(S) = \mathbf{in}(R_1@\Theta^1), ..., \mathbf{in}(R_m@\Theta^m), \mathbf{out}(R_{m+1}@\Theta^{m+1}), ..., \mathbf{out}(R_n@\Theta^n) \\
&\mathbf{E}\,(S) = \mathbf{in}\,(E_1)\,, ..., \mathbf{in}\,(E_p)\,, \mathbf{out}\,(E_{p+1})\,, ..., \mathbf{out}\,(E_q)
\end{aligned}$$

If we omit the $@\Theta^i$ reference in an element of either $\mathbf{L}\,(S)$ or $\mathbf{R}\,(S)$, then $@\mathcal{A}$ should be assumed. There follow some examples of statements in $KABUL^m$:

[3] Where $[\mathbf{a} \mid \mathbf{b}]$ will be used for notational convenience denoting the presence of either **a**, or **b**, or absence of both.

Example 65 *A statement specifying that every rule R sent by agent agent should be asserted in the corresponding agent's node if such rule was not present at agent's node would be encoded as:*

$$\mathbf{always\_assert}\,(R@agent) \Leftarrow \mathbf{R}:\mathbf{out}(R@agent), \mathbf{E}:\mathbf{in}\,(message\,(agent, R))$$

Example 66 *Suppose we have a scenario where one of the system agents represents information incoming from the stock market, namely characteristics of stocks. When we receive the latest value for such characteristics, the previous value should be replaced. This could be achieved with the following two statements:*

$$\begin{aligned}\mathbf{always\_assert}\,(char\,(N,S,V)\,@mrkt) &\Leftarrow \mathbf{E}:char\,(N,S,V)\\ \mathbf{always\_retract}\,(char\,(N,S,V')\,@mrkt) &\Leftarrow \mathbf{assert}\,(char\,(N,S,V)\,@mrkt)\,,\\ &\qquad \mathbf{R}:\mathbf{in}\,(char\,(N,S,V')\,@mrkt)\end{aligned}$$

Further suppose that there are two financial advisors (adv1 and adv2). If adv1 tells us that if we are willing to take risks then we should buy yahoo stocks, we would update the knowledge base with the statement:

$$\mathbf{assert}\,(buy\,(yahoo) \leftarrow risk@adv1) \Leftarrow$$

If adv2 tells us that under no circumstances should we buy yahoo stock if the market is bear, *we would update the knowledge base with the statement:*

$$\mathbf{assert}\,(not\,buy\,(yahoo) \leftarrow bear@adv2) \Leftarrow$$

Suppose that there is an agent (ii) that obtains insider information and has just received a tip according to which there was going to be a major takeover and the share price for Altitude would rise above 28 to then drop back again. The order would then be to buy until that value and, once the price rises above 28, sell it all. This can be encoded as follows: a statement immediately asserting that we should buy Altitude stock (of course that all the statements are executed at the corresponding ii agent, and the final result will depend on the information provided by other agents and the hierarchy relating them):

$$\mathbf{assert}\,(buy\,(alt)\,@ii) \Leftarrow$$

Then, we also need two statements changing the recommendation from buy to sell once the correct price is reached:

$$\begin{aligned}\mathbf{once\_retract}\,(buy\,(alt)\,@ii) &\Leftarrow price\,(alt,V)\,@mrkt, V > 28\\ \mathbf{once\_assert}\,(sell\,(alt)\,@ii) &\Leftarrow price\,(alt,V)\,@mrkt, V > 28\end{aligned}$$

Finally, once the price of 28 is reached, we need to "activate" a statement that will wait until the price drops back to 24, to retract the sell recommendation, specified as follows:

$$\begin{aligned}\mathbf{once\_assert}\,(\mathbf{once\_retract}\,(sell\,(alt)\,@ii) \Leftarrow price\,(alt,V)\,@mrkt, V < 24) \Leftarrow\\ price\,(alt,V)\,@mrkt, V > 28\end{aligned}$$

In the following Chapter, we will explore in greater detail an example based on such financial scenario.

The following table summarizes the syntax of the update language, in BNF.

$$
\begin{array}{lll}
\langle statement\rangle & ::= & \langle command\rangle\ [\Leftarrow \langle conditions\rangle]\ ; \\
\langle base\_comm\rangle & ::= & \textbf{assert}\ [\textbf{\_event}]\ (\langle rule\rangle\ @\ \langle agent\rangle) \mid \\
 & & \mid \textbf{retract}\ [\textbf{\_event}]\ (\langle rule\rangle\ @\ \langle agent\rangle) \mid \\
 & & \mid \textbf{assert}\ (\langle statement\rangle) \mid \textbf{retract}\ (\langle statement\rangle)\ ; \\
\langle per\_comm\rangle & ::= & \textbf{always\_}\ \langle base\_comm\rangle \mid \textbf{once\_}\ \langle base\_comm\rangle\ ; \\
\langle inhib\_comm\rangle & ::= & not\ \langle base\_comm\rangle\ ; \\
\langle command\rangle & ::= & \langle base\_comm\rangle \mid \langle per\_comm\rangle \mid \langle inhib\_comm\rangle\ ; \\
\langle conditions\rangle & ::= & [\langle comm\_conds\rangle\ ,]\ [\langle lit\_conds\rangle\ ,] \\
 & & [\mathbf{R} : \langle rule\_conds\rangle\ ,]\ [\mathbf{E} : \langle env\_conds\rangle]\ ; \\
\langle comm\_conds\rangle & ::= & \langle base\_comm\rangle\ [, \langle comm\_conds\rangle] \mid \\
 & & \mid \langle inhib\_comm\rangle\ [, \langle comm\_conds\rangle]\ ; \\
\langle lit\_conds\rangle & ::= & \langle literal\rangle\ @\ \langle agents\rangle\ [, \langle lit\_conds\rangle]\ ; \\
\langle rule\_conds\rangle & ::= & \textbf{in}\ (\langle rule\rangle\ @\ \langle agents\rangle)\ [, \langle rule\_conds\rangle] \mid \\
 & & \mid \textbf{out}\ (\langle rule\rangle\ @\ \langle agents\rangle)\ [, \langle rule\_conds\rangle]\ ; \\
\langle env\_conds\rangle & ::= & \textbf{in}\ (\langle observ\rangle)\ [, \langle env\_conds\rangle] \mid \\
 & & \mid \textbf{out}\ (\langle observ\rangle)\ [, \langle env\_conds\rangle]\ ; \\
\langle agents\rangle & ::= & \{\langle agent\rangle\ [, \langle agents\rangle]\}
\end{array}
$$

Definition 114 (Update Program) *An* update program *in language* KABUL^m *is a set of statements.*

We will extend the notion of query to include references to the sets of agents where evaluation is to be accomplished:

Definition 115 (Query) *A query to the knowledge base is a propositional expression of the form:*

$$
\textbf{holds}\left(\begin{array}{c} L_1@\Theta^1, \ldots, L_k@\Theta^k, \textbf{in}(R_1@\Theta^1), ..., \textbf{in}(R_m@\Theta^m), \\ \textbf{out}(R_{m+1}@\Theta^{m+1}), ..., \textbf{out}(R_n@\Theta^n) \end{array}\right) \textbf{ at } q\ ?
$$

where $L_1, ..., L_k$ are literals and $R_1, ..., R_n$ are rules, and q is a state such that $q \leq s$ where s is the current state and $\Theta^1, ..., \Theta^n$ are sets of agents.

7.2.2 *KABUL^m* - Semantics

The semantics of *KABUL^m* is determined in a way similar to that of *KABUL*. Given a KB state $\langle \mathcal{P}_s, SU_s, \mathcal{H}_s, \mathcal{M}_s \rangle$, where $\mathcal{P}_s = (\mathcal{P}_{D_s}, D_s)$ is an MDLP, an external update program EU_{s+1} and a set of external observations EO_{s+1}, we want to characterize the successor KB state $\langle \mathcal{P}_{s+1}, SU_{s+1}, \mathcal{H}_{s+1}, \mathcal{M}_{s+1} \rangle$, where $\mathcal{P}_s = \left(\mathcal{P}_{D_{s+1}}, D_{s+1}\right)$, i.e. we want to characterize P_{s+1} and SU_{s+1}, which will depend on a suitable combination of both update programs (self and external), as well as EO_{s+1} and $\mathcal{P}_s$. This will be achieved, as before, in three steps: first we partially evaluate the statements in SU_s and EU_{s+1} with respect to the external set of observations and current object level KB to determine two update program reducts; then based on these reducts, we determine a set of commands to be executed; finally we determine the next state knowledge base.

We begin by defining the initial knowledge state:

Definition 116 (Initial Knowledge State) *The* initial knowledge state *is the knowledge state at state* 0, $\langle \mathcal{P}_0, SU_0, \mathcal{H}_0, \mathcal{M}_0 \rangle$ *where (assuming a fixed hierarchy* $\mathcal{H}$*):*

$$\begin{array}{ll} \mathcal{P}_0 = (\mathcal{P}_{D_0}, D_0) & D_0 = (V_0, E_0) \\ SU_0 = \{\} & V_0 = \{\alpha_0 : \alpha \in \mathcal{A}\} \\ \mathcal{H}_0 = (\mathcal{A}, HE_0) = \mathcal{H} & E_0 = \{(\alpha_0^j, \alpha_0^k) : (\alpha^j, \alpha^k, t) \in HE_0\} \\ \mathcal{M}_0 = \{\} & P_{\alpha_0} = \{\} \\ \mathcal{P}_{D_0} = \{P_{\alpha_0} : \alpha_0 \in V_0\} & \end{array}$$

Before we continue, let us introduce the notion of *transition frame* for this extended framework. A transition frame is now a tuple $\langle \mathcal{P}_s, \models, SU_s, \mathcal{H}_s, \mathcal{M}_s, EU_{s+1}, EO_{s+1}, <, Sel(.) \rangle$ where every element has been introduced before. As before, with the two updates, SU_s and EU_{s+1}, we obtain the four sets of statements $SU_s^+, SU_s^-, EU_{s+1}^+$ and EU_{s+1}^-, corresponding to the positive and inhibition updates of both the self and external updates.

7.2.3 Update Program Reduct

The partial evaluation of statements to is similar to the one presented in a previous Chapter, except that we are now using a consequence operator on a MDLP rather than a DLP as before. Again, the semantics for such partial evaluation depends on the type of conditions and is as follows:

Literals In this case, a conjunction of literals $\mathbf{L}(S) = L_1@\Theta^1, \ldots, L_k@\Theta^k$ is evaluated to true, denoted by $\bigoplus \mathcal{P}_s \models_{sm} L_1@\Theta^1, \ldots, L_k@\Theta^k$, or $\bigoplus \mathcal{P}_s \models_{sm} \mathbf{L}(S)$ for short, iff

$$\bigoplus_{\{\alpha_s^j : \alpha^j \in \Theta^1\}} \mathcal{P}_s \models_{sm} L_1 \wedge \ldots \wedge \bigoplus_{\{\alpha_s^j : \alpha^j \in \Theta^k\}} \mathcal{P}_s \models_{sm} L_k$$

Rules A rule condition

$$\mathbf{R}(S) = \mathbf{in}(R_1@\Theta^l), ..., \mathbf{in}(R_m@\Theta^m), \mathbf{out}(R_{m+1}@\Theta^{m+1}), ..., \mathbf{out}(R_n)@\Theta^n$$

evaluates to true, denoted by $\bigoplus \mathcal{P}_s \models_{rule} \mathbf{R}(S)$ iff

$$\bigoplus_{\{\alpha_s^j : \alpha^j \in \Theta^l\}} \mathcal{P}_s \models_{sm} N(R_1) \wedge \ldots \wedge \bigoplus_{\{\alpha_s^j : \alpha^j \in \Theta^m\}} \mathcal{P}_s \models_{sm} N(R_1) \wedge$$
$$\wedge \bigoplus_{\{\alpha_s^j : \alpha^j \in \Theta^{m+1}\}} \mathcal{P}_s \models_{sm} not\, N(R_{m+1}) \wedge \ldots \wedge \bigoplus_{\{\alpha_s^j : \alpha^j \in \Theta^n\}} \mathcal{P}_s \models_{sm} not\, N(R_n)$$

Observations The evaluation of conditions on external observations, $\mathbf{E}(S)$, of a statement S, is exactly as before, i.e. will be done simply by checking for their presence or absence in the set EO_{s+1}. Accordingly, $\mathbf{E}(S) = \mathbf{in}(E_1), ..., \mathbf{in}(E_p), \mathbf{out}(E_{p+1}), ..., \mathbf{out}(E_q)$ evaluates to true, denoted by $EO_{s+1} \models_{obs} \mathbf{E}(S)$, iff $\{E_1, ..., E_p\} \subseteq EO_{s+1}$ and $E_{p+1} \notin EO_{s+1}, ..., E_q \notin EO_{s+1}$.

For a statement of the form:

$$\begin{array}{l} C_0(\rho_0 [@\alpha^0]) \Leftarrow C_1(\rho_1 [@\alpha^1]), ..., C_n(\rho_n [@\alpha^n]), L_1@\Theta^{n+1}, \ldots, L_k@\Theta^{n+k}, \\ \qquad \mathbf{R} : \mathbf{in}(R_1)@\Theta^1, ..., \mathbf{in}(R_m)@\Theta^m, \mathbf{out}(R_{m+1})@\Theta^{m+1}, ..., \mathbf{out}(R_n)@\Theta^n, \\ \qquad \mathbf{E} : \mathbf{in}(E_1), ..., \mathbf{in}(E_p), \mathbf{out}(E_{p+1}), ..., \mathbf{out}(E_q) \end{array}$$

a partially evaluated statement has the form:

$$C_0(\rho_0 [@\alpha^0]) \Leftarrow C_1(\rho_1 [@\alpha^1]), ..., C_n(\rho_n [@\alpha^n])$$

Each update program is reduced as per the following definition:

Definition 117 (Update Program Reduct) *The reduct of an update program U, with respect to a set of external observations EO and a dynamic logic program $\mathcal{P}_s$ at state s, is the set of (reduced) statements U^r, defined as follows:*

$$U^r = \{\mathbf{H}(S) \Leftarrow \mathbf{C}(S) : (\mathbf{H}(S) \Leftarrow \mathbf{C}(S), \mathbf{L}(S), \mathbf{R} : \mathbf{R}(S), \mathbf{E} : \mathbf{E}(S)) \in U \wedge \\ \bigoplus \mathcal{P}_s \models_{sm} \mathbf{L}(S) \wedge \bigoplus \mathcal{P}_s \models_{rule} \mathbf{R}(S) \wedge EO \models_{obs} \mathbf{E}(S)\Big\}$$

7.2.4 Executable Commands

The set of executable commands is obtained as in Chapter 5, as all the definitions involved directly apply. Note that all other results carry over to this extended framework, namely the algorithm presented to determine the executable set of commands for statements without command conditions, and the transformation of Definition 96 to determine such sets for the general case.

7.2.5 Successor State

With a coherent set of commands, we are now ready to determine the successor state of the KB, according to the definition:

$$\langle \mathcal{P}_s, SU_s, \mathcal{H}_s, \mathcal{M}_s \rangle \overset{\langle EU_{s+1}, EO_{s+1} \rangle}{\longrightarrow} \langle \mathcal{P}_{s+1}, SU_{s+1}, \mathcal{H}_{s+1}, \mathcal{M}_{s+1} \rangle$$

Definition 118 (Knowledge Base at the Successor State) *Consider a KB at state s, $\langle \mathcal{P}_s, SU_s, \mathcal{H}_s, \mathcal{M}_s \rangle$, where $\mathcal{P}_s = (\mathcal{P}_{D_s}, D_s)$ and where $D_s = (V_s, E_s)$ is a* DAG *and $\mathcal{P}_{D_s} = \{P_v : v \in V_s\}$ and let Δ_{s+1} be a set of executable commands. Let $\Delta_{s+1}^{R@\alpha} \subseteq \Delta_{s+1}$ be the set of all rule commands c in Δ_{s+1} such that $Dest(c) = \alpha$. Let $\Lambda_{s+1} = EU_{s+1} \cup SU_s$. Then the KB at state $s+1$ is $\langle \mathcal{P}_{s+1}, SU_{s+1}, \mathcal{H}_{s+1}, \mathcal{M}_{s+1} \rangle$, where:*

Hierarchy at state $s+1$ $\mathcal{H}_{s+1} = (\mathcal{A}, HE_{s+1}) = (\mathcal{A}, HE_s) = \mathcal{H}_s$. *As we have mentioned before, in the core version of* KABUL^m *the hierarchy relating all the agents is fixed. In a subsequent section we explore the evolution of this DAG.*

Evolution Mode at state $s+1$ $\mathcal{M}_{s+1} = \mathcal{M}_s$. *As we have mentioned before, evolution modes are not used in this core version of* KABUL^m. *Again, evolution modes other than the one giving rise to the equal role representation will be explored below.*

Object Knowledge Base at state $s+1$ $\mathcal{P}_{s+1} = (\mathcal{P}_{D_{s+1}}, D_{s+1})$ *and where* $D_{s+1} = (V_{s+1}, E_{s+1})$ *is a* DAG *and* $\mathcal{P}_{D_{s+1}} = \mathcal{P}_{D_s} \cup \{P_v : v \in (V_{s+1} - V_s)\}$, *such that:*

$$V_{s+1} = V_s \cup \{\alpha_{s+1} : \alpha \in \mathcal{A}\}$$
$$E_{s+1} = E_s \cup \{(\alpha_s, \alpha_{s+1}) : \alpha \in \mathcal{A}\} \cup \{(\alpha^j_{s+1}, \alpha^k_{s+1}) : (\alpha^j, \alpha^k, \_) \in HE_{s+1}\}$$
$$P_{\alpha_{s+1}} = \Gamma_R\left(\Delta_{s+1}^{R@\alpha}, s+1\right)$$

The construction of the next state of the object level knowledge base is quite simple. For each agent we add a node to the MDLP DAG, indexed by the new state $s+1$. The new agents are connected among themselves according to the overall hierarchy. Then each new node is connected from the corresponding agent's node of the previous state. The programs associated with each new node are constructed, as before, from the commands in the set of rule commands that correspond to the node's agent. If D_{s+1} is not a DAG, then $\langle \mathcal{P}_{s+1}, SU_{s+1}, \mathcal{H}_{s+1}, \mathcal{M}_{s+1} \rangle$ is not defined.

Self Update at state $s+1$ *The self update of the next state is* $SU_{s+1} = \Gamma_S(\Delta_{s+1}, \Lambda_{s+1})$. *The construction of the self update at the next state is performed as before.*

Definition 119 (*KABUL*^{m} Semantics) *Let* $\langle \mathcal{P}_s, SU_s, \mathcal{H}_s, \mathcal{M}_s \rangle$ *be a KB at state* s. *A query (where* $q \leq s$*)*

$$\mathbf{holds}\left(\begin{array}{c} L_1@\Theta^1, \ldots, L_k@\Theta^k, \mathbf{in}(R_1@\Theta^1), ..., \mathbf{in}(R_m@\Theta^m), \\ \mathbf{out}(R_{m+1}@\Theta^{m+1}), ..., \mathbf{out}(R_n@\Theta^n) \end{array}\right) \mathbf{at}\ q\ ?$$

is true iff

$$\begin{array}{c} \bigoplus_{\{\alpha_q^j : \alpha^j \in \Theta^1\}} \mathcal{P}_s \models_{sm} L_1 \wedge ... \wedge \bigoplus_{\{\alpha_q^j : \alpha^j \in \Theta^k\}} \mathcal{P}_s \models_{sm} L_k \wedge \\ \wedge \bigoplus_{\{\alpha_q^j : \alpha^j \in \Theta^l\}} \mathcal{P}_s \models_{sm} N(R_1) \wedge ... \wedge \bigoplus_{\{\alpha_q^j : \alpha^j \in \Theta^m\}} \mathcal{P}_s \models_{sm} N(R_1) \wedge \\ \wedge \bigoplus_{\{\alpha_q^j : \alpha^j \in \Theta^{m+1}\}} \mathcal{P}_s \models_{sm} not\, N(R_{m+1}) \wedge ... \wedge \bigoplus_{\{\alpha_q^j : \alpha^j \in \Theta^n\}} \mathcal{P}_s \models_{sm} not\, N(R_n) \end{array}$$

The semantics of *KABUL* coincides with a fragment of *KABUL*^{m}. This fragment is obtained by restricting the set of agents $\mathcal{A}$ to contain just one agent.

Theorem 98 (Embedding of KABUL) *Let* $EU_1, EU_2, ..., EU_s$ *be update programs in* KABUL. *Let* $EO_1, EO_2, ..., EO_s$ *be external observations. Let* $EU'_n, (n \leq s)$ *be update programs in* KABUL^m *with* $\mathcal{A} = \{\alpha\}$, *obtained from* EU_n *by adding* $@\alpha$ *to every rule and literal of every statement. Let* $\langle \mathcal{P}'_s, SU'_s, \mathcal{H}_s, \mathcal{M}_s \rangle$ *be the* KABUL^m *knowledge state produced by* $\langle \mathcal{P}_0, SU_0, \mathcal{H}_0, \mathcal{M}_0 \rangle \otimes \langle EU'_1, EO_1 \rangle \otimes \langle EU'_2, EO_2 \rangle \otimes ... \otimes \langle EU'_s, EO_s \rangle$ *where* $\mathcal{H}_0 = \mathcal{H}_0 = (\mathcal{A}, \{\})$. *Let* $\langle \mathcal{P}_s, SU_s \rangle$ *be the* KABUL *knowledge state produced by* $\langle \mathcal{P}_0, SU_0 \rangle \otimes \langle EU_1, EO_1 \rangle \otimes \langle EU_2, EO_2 \rangle \otimes ... \otimes \langle EU_s, EO_s \rangle$ *(assuming the same* $\models, <$ *and* $Sel(.)$*). Then:*

1. $\langle \mathcal{P}'_s, SU'_s, \mathcal{H}_s, \mathcal{M}_s \rangle$ *is semantically equivalent to* $\langle \mathcal{P}_s, SU_s \rangle$, *i.e. a query*

$$\mathbf{holds}(L_1, ..., L_k, \mathbf{in}(R_1), ..., \mathbf{in}(R_m), \mathbf{out}(R_{m+1}), ..., \mathbf{out}(R_n))\ \mathbf{at}\ q\ ?$$

is true in $\langle \mathcal{P}_s, SU_s \rangle$ *iff the query*

$$\mathbf{holds}\left(\begin{array}{c} L_1@\alpha, \ldots, L_k@\alpha, \mathbf{in}(R_1@\alpha), ..., \mathbf{in}(R_m@\alpha), \\ \mathbf{out}(R_{m+1}@\alpha), ..., \mathbf{out}(R_n@\alpha) \end{array}\right) \mathbf{at}\ q\ ?$$

is true in $\langle \mathcal{P}'_s, SU'_s, \mathcal{H}_s, \mathcal{M}_s \rangle$.

2. SU_s *can be obtained from* SU'_s *by removing every occurrence of* $@\alpha$.

Proof. **1** - Immediately follows from Theorem 91 together with the construction of the DLP $\mathcal{P}_s$, the MDLP $\mathcal{P}'_s$. **2** - Immediately follows from the construction of SU_s and SU'_s. ■

This result immediately implies that *KABUL*^{m} embeds *DLP*, interpretation updates [157] and logic programs under the stable model semantics.

Next we establish the relationship between *KABUL*^{m} and $\mathcal{MDLP}$:

Theorem 99 (Embedding of MDLP) *Let $\mathcal{P} = (\mathcal{P}_D, D)$ be a* Multi-dimensional Dynamic Logic Program, *where $\mathcal{P}_D = \{P_v : v \in V\}$ and $D = (V, E)$. Let S be a set of states such that $S \subseteq V$. Let $\mathcal{A} = V$, $\mathcal{H}_0 = D$ and*

$$EU_1 = \{\textbf{assert}\,(r@v) \Leftarrow : r \in P_v, v \in V\}$$

Let $\phi = L_1, ..., L_k$ be a conjunction of literals of the underlying object language of $\mathcal{P}_D$. Then, $\bigoplus_S \mathcal{P} \models_{sm} \phi$ iff **holds** $L_1@S, ..., L_k@S$ **at** 1? *is true in $\langle \mathcal{P}_1, SU_1, \mathcal{H}_1, \mathcal{M}_1 \rangle = \langle \mathcal{P}_0, SU_0, \mathcal{H}_0, \mathcal{M}_0 \rangle \otimes \langle EU_1, \{\} \rangle$. Furthermore, $SM(\mathcal{P}_1) = SM(\mathcal{P})$ when restricted to the underlying object language of $\mathcal{P}$.*

Proof. *Let $\mathcal{P}$ and $\langle EU_1, \{\} \rangle$ be as defined above. Then, $\langle \mathcal{P}_1, SU_1, \mathcal{H}_1, \mathcal{M}_1 \rangle = \langle \mathcal{P}_0, SU_0, \mathcal{H}_0, \mathcal{M}_0 \rangle \otimes \langle EU_1, \{\} \rangle$ is such that:*

$$\begin{aligned}
\mathcal{P}_1 &= (\mathcal{P}_{D_1}, D_1) \\
\mathcal{P}_{D_1} &= \{P_{v_0} : v_0 \in V_0\} \\
D_1 &= (V_1, E_1) \\
V_1 &= \{v_0, v_1 : v \in V\} \\
E_1 &= \{(v_0^j, v_0^k), (v_1^j, v_1^k) : (v^j, v^k) \in E\} \cup \{(v_0, v_1) : v \in V\} \\
P_{v_0} &= \{\} \\
P_{v_1} &= \{N(r) \leftarrow; H(r) \leftarrow B(r), N(r) : r \in P_v\} \cup \{not\, Ev(R, t-1) \leftarrow; Ev(R, t) \leftarrow\}
\end{aligned}$$

since the atoms $not\, Ev(R, t-1)$ and $Ev(R, t)$ cannot belong to ϕ, nor those of the form $N(R)$, and there are no rules for $not\, N(R)$, and since the nodes v_0 in D_1 and the corresponding programs P_{v_0} can simply be eliminated for being empty (the removed edges do not affect the semantics because the transitive closure of the remaining graph is retained), $SM(\mathcal{P}_1) = SM(\mathcal{P}')$ where $\mathcal{P}' = (\mathcal{P}'_D, D)$ and $\mathcal{P}'_D = \{P'_v : v \in V\}$ is such that:

$$P'_v = \{H(r) \leftarrow B(r) : r \in P_v\}$$

Note that $P'_v = P_v$. It follows that $\bigoplus_S \mathcal{P}_1 \models_{sm} \phi$ iff $\bigoplus_S \mathcal{P}' \models_{sm} \phi$ iff $\bigoplus_S \mathcal{P} \models_{sm} \phi$. i.e. **holds** $L_1@S, ..., L_k@S$ **at** 1? *is true in $\langle \mathcal{P}_1, SU_1, \mathcal{H}_1, \mathcal{M}_1 \rangle$ iff $\bigoplus_S \mathcal{P} \models_{sm} \phi$.* ■

7.3 Introducing DAG Commands

The *KABUL^m* framework presented in the previous section only allows for the evolution of an *MDLP* whose structure, encoded by the *MDLP DAG*, is quite strict in the sense that the hierarchy relating the different agents is fixed, and that there are no edges directly relating different agents at different time states. In this section we propose two general extensions to the core *KABUL^m* that allow a more flexible evolution of the *MDLP DAG*, in particular allowing us to remove these two limitations.

7.3.1 Hierarchy Commands

We start with an extension that allows the hierarchy *DAG* to evolve, instead of the fixed hierarchy *DAG* $\mathcal{H}$ of the previous section. We thus need some way to specify the addition and removal of edges between pairs of agents. To this purpose, to the core *KABUL^m* commands we add commands for the manipulation of the hierarchy *DAG* $\mathcal{H}$ (with $\alpha^j, \alpha^k \in \mathcal{A}$):

$$\textbf{add\_hierarchy\_edge}(\alpha^j \to \alpha^k) \tag{7.9}$$

$$\textbf{remove\_hierarchy\_edge}(\alpha^j \to \alpha^k) \tag{7.10}$$

The intuitive reading of these commands is straightforward: command (7.9) indicates that to the hierarchy *DAG* we must add an edge from α^j to α^k and command (7.10) indicates that from the hierarchy *DAG* we must remove any existing edge from α^j to α^k. We dub these commands *hierarchy commands*. These commands are to be added to the list of commands of $KABUL^m$, and should be treated as basic commands, i.e. can be inhibited, giving rise to the inhibition commands:

$$not\,\mathbf{add\_hierarchy\_edge}(\alpha^j \rightarrow \alpha^k)$$
$$not\,\mathbf{remove\_hierarchy\_edge}(\alpha^j \rightarrow \alpha^k)$$

and can be used to form statements both in their heads as well as in their conditions. Furthermore, these commands can be made persistent or semi-persistent, giving rise to the following four commands:

$$\mathbf{always\_add\_hierarchy\_edge}(\alpha^j \rightarrow \alpha^k)$$
$$\mathbf{once\_add\_hierarchy\_edge}(\alpha^j \rightarrow \alpha^k)$$
$$\mathbf{always\_remove\_hierarchy\_edge}(\alpha^j \rightarrow \alpha^k)$$
$$\mathbf{once\_remove\_hierarchy\_edge}(\alpha^j \rightarrow \alpha^k)$$

There follows examples of such statements:

Example 67 *Consider a scenario where there are two hierarchically unrelated agents α and β. The following statement specifies, in* KABUL^m*, that agent α should always become prevalent over agent β if α has made greater profit than β:*

$$\mathbf{always\_add\_hierarchy\_edge}(\beta \rightarrow \alpha) \Leftarrow profit\,(\alpha, P_\alpha)\,, profit\,(\beta, P_\beta)\,, P_\alpha > P_\beta$$

Example 68 *In a financial advisory company, whenever the market's trend becomes bear, we want the advice of agent adv2 to prevail over that of agent adv1. Also, whenever such an hierarchy edge is added, we want any opposite one to be removed. This is accomplished by the following two statements:*

$$\mathbf{always\_add\_hierarchy\_edge}\,(adv1 \rightarrow adv2) \Leftarrow not\,trend\,(bear, \_)\,, \mathbf{E} : trend\,(bear)$$
$$\mathbf{always\_remove\_hierarchy\_edge}\,\left(\alpha^j \rightarrow \alpha^k\right) \Leftarrow \mathbf{add\_hierarchy\_edge}\,\left(\alpha^k \rightarrow \alpha^j\right)$$

With these commands, we no longer need an initial fixed hierarchy *DAG*. We therefore modify Definition 116 in what concerns the hierarchy relating the set of agents, which ceases to be a global setting and is now empty:

Definition 120 (Initial Knowledge State) *The* initial knowledge state *is the knowledge state at state* 0, $\langle \mathcal{P}_0, SU_0, \mathcal{H}_0, \mathcal{M}_0 \rangle$ *where:*

$$\begin{array}{ll} \mathcal{P}_0 = (\mathcal{P}_{D_0}, D_0) & \mathcal{P}_{D_0} = \{P_{\alpha_0} : \alpha_0 \in V_0\} \\ SU_0 = \{\} & D_0 = (V_0, E_0) \\ \mathcal{H}_0 = (\mathcal{A}, HE_0) & V_0 = \{\alpha_0 : \alpha \in \mathcal{A}\} \\ HE_0 = \{\} & E_0 = \{\} \\ \mathcal{M}_0 = \{\} & P_{\alpha_0} = \{\} \end{array}$$

Note that since there are no edges connecting the agents $\mathcal{A}$ in $\mathcal{H}_0$, the MDLP DAG at the initial state does not contain any edges i.e., $E_0 = \{\}$.

In what concerns the semantics of these commands we have first to determine the sets of executable commands. This is attained as before, with the following minor extensions to some definitions. We start by defining the hierarchy arguments:

Definition 121 (Hierarchy Arguments with respect to U^r) *Let U^r be a set of reduced statements. By the* set of hierarchy arguments of U^r, *denoted by $Args_H(U^r)$, we mean:*

$$Args_R(U^r) = \{Arg(H(S)) \mid Arg(H(S)) = \alpha^j \to \alpha^k[@X], S \in U^r\} \cup \\ \cup \{Arg(C) \mid Arg(C) = \alpha^j \to \alpha^k[@X], C \in B(S), S \in U^r\}$$

As before, we have included the optional construct $@X$, which has not been introduced yet. Its purpose is to allow these definitions to be reused, later on, when such a construct is introduced.

We now define the notion of basic hierarchy commands:

Definition 122 (Basic Hierarchy Commands with respect to U^r) *Let U^r be a set of reduced statements. By the* set of basic hierarchy commands, *given U^r, we mean the set $BasicComm_H(U^r)$ defined as follows:*

$$BasicComm_H(U^r) = \left\{ \begin{array}{c} \textbf{add\_hierarchy\_edge}(\rho), \\ \textbf{remove\_hierarchy\_edge}(\rho) : \rho \in Args_H(U^r) \end{array} \right\}$$

We now modify Definition 83, and define the set of basic commands as follows:

Definition 123 (Basic Commands with respect to U^r) *By the* set of basic commands, *given U^r, we mean the set $BasicComm(U^r)$ defined as follows:*

$$BasicComm(U^r) = BasicComm_R(U^r) \cup BasicComm_S(U^r) \cup BasicComm_H(U^r)$$

All other definitions follow, using this new notion of $BasicComm(U^r)$.

With these modified definitions we can determine a set of executable commands, as before, and define the next state of the knowledge base. This next state is defined as before, except in what concerns the hierarchy DAG, which is now defined as follows:

Definition 124 (Hierarchy DAG at state $s+1$) *Let $\langle \mathcal{P}_s, SU_s, \mathcal{H}_s, \mathcal{M}_s \rangle$ be a KB at state s, where $\mathcal{H}_s = (\mathcal{A}, HE_s)$. Let Δ_{s+1} be a set of executable commands. Let $\Delta^H_{s+1} \subseteq \Delta_{s+1}$ be the set of all hierarchy commands in Δ_{s+1}. The hierarchy DAG at state $s+1$ is $\mathcal{H}_{s+1} = \Gamma_H(\mathcal{H}_s, \Delta^H_{s+1}, s+1) = (\mathcal{A}, HE_{s+1})$ where HE_{s+1} is defined as follows:*

$$HE_{s+1} = HE_s \cup \{(\alpha^j, \alpha^k, s+1) : \textbf{add\_hierarchy\_edge}(\alpha^j \to \alpha^k[@X]) \in \Delta^H_{s+1}\} - \\ - \{(\alpha^j, \alpha^k, t) : t \leq s, \textbf{remove\_hierarchy\_edge}(\alpha^j \to \alpha^k[@X]) \in \Delta^H_{s+1}\}$$

If $(\mathcal{A}, HE_{s+1})$ is not a DAG, then $\mathcal{H}_{s+1}$ is not defined.

The evolution of the hierarchy DAG amounts to the addition and deletion of the specified edges. The label of each edge corresponds to the time state at which such edge was created, which will be needed in the next Section. Again, in this definition, we have introduced the symbol $[@X]$ that was not mentioned before. It is irrelevant at this point, but its inclusion serves the purpose of allowing this definition to be used again below, when we introduce another extension to the framework. One other such occurrence will appear in a definition below, before such extension is set forth, and should be ignored. Note that the definition of the MDLP DAG of state $s+1$ is based on the hierarchy at state $s+1$, i.e. the changes in the hierarchy immediately affect the evolution of the MDLP DAG.

Mark that according to the previous Definition, the addition of a hierarchy edge $\alpha^j \to \alpha^k$ does not imply the automatic retraction of any existing opposite edge $\alpha^k \to \alpha^j$. If such an edge exists, and is not explicitly removed, a cycle will occur and we no longer have a DAG. This particular cause for cycles can be easily dealt with, if we have always the generic statement:

$$\textbf{always\_remove\_hierarchy\_edge}\left(\alpha^k \to \alpha^j\right) \Leftarrow \textbf{add\_hierarchy\_edge}\left(\alpha^j \to \alpha^k\right)$$

But the reader should be aware that non direct cycles can occur in the hierarchy, and this statement only prevents the appearance of direct cycles.

7.3.2 Prevalence Mode Commands

In the previous sections we have proposed $KABUL^m$ to construct *MDLPs* that evolve according to the "*equal role representation*". This evolution mode does not allow relations between a higher ranked older program and a lower ranked newer one. In this section we introduce another extension to $KABUL^m$, by means of a set of commands to allow a flexible evolution of the *MDLP DAG*. In this more general setting, in what concerns the MDLP DAG, we shall allow the specification of arbitrary edges by means of user specified functions.

Such functions specify the evolution of the *MDLP DAG*, by defining which edges should be created or deleted at each time state transition. This allows the construction of more general *MDLP DAGs*, among which those representing the "*hierarchy prevalence representation*" and "*time prevalence representation*" modes as defined in Chapter 6. According to *hierarchy prevalence*, any rule indexed by a higher ranked agent overrides any lower ranked agent's rule, independently of the time state it is indexed by. According to *time prevalence*, any rule indexed by a more recent time state overrides any older rule, independently of to which agents these rules belong.

To this purpose, we consider a set of functions $\mathcal{F}$ such that every function $f \in \mathcal{F}$ has the signature $f : \mathcal{A}^2 \times \{<, \|\} \times \mathcal{T}^3 \longrightarrow 2^{\{+,-\}\times(\mathcal{A}\times\mathcal{T})^2}$. Each function $f \in \mathcal{F}$, defines a set of edges of the forms $+(\alpha^j_{t_1}, \alpha^k_{t_2})$ and $-(\alpha^j_{t_1}, \alpha^k_{t_2})$ where $\alpha^j, \alpha^k \in \mathcal{A}, t_1, t_2 \in \mathcal{T}$, given a pair of agents, their relation, the current time state, and two other time states indicating when the prevalence mode represented by f and the agents relation were set. Below we will show some examples of such functions. The new commands are (with $\alpha^j, \alpha^k \in \mathcal{A}$, and $f \in \mathcal{F}$):

$$\textbf{add\_prevail\_mode}\left(\alpha^j \stackrel{f}{\longleftrightarrow} \alpha^k\right) \tag{7.11}$$

$$\textbf{remove\_prevail\_mode}\left(\alpha^j \stackrel{f}{\longleftrightarrow} \alpha^k\right) \tag{7.12}$$

Since the prevalence modes should persist until removed, we need to keep info about the prevalence mode at each time state. As will become clear when we look closer at some interesting cases of such functions, we also need to keep track of when such prevalence modes were set. Each currently existing prevalence mode is represented by a triplet $\left(\left\{\alpha^j, \alpha^k\right\}, f, n\right)$ where f is the function, set at time state n, specifying the prevalence mode between agents α^j and α^k. We will refer to the set of all such triplets at each time state s as the *Evolution Mode at time state* s, which has the form $\left\{\left(\left\{\alpha^j, \alpha^k\right\}, f, n\right) : \alpha^j, \alpha^k \in \mathcal{A}, f \in \mathcal{F}, n \in \mathcal{T}\right\}$ which is represented by $\mathcal{M}_s$. The way it is obtained will be set forth below.

As before, these new commands are to be added to the list of commands of $KABUL^m$, and should be treated as basic commands, i.e. can be inhibited, giving rise to the inhibition commands:

$$not\ \mathbf{add\_prevail\_mode}\left(\alpha^j \overset{f}{\longleftrightarrow} \alpha^k\right)$$
$$not\ \mathbf{remove\_prevail\_mode}\left(\alpha^j \overset{f}{\longleftrightarrow} \alpha^k\right)$$

and can be used to form statements both in their heads as well as in their conditions. Furthermore, these commands can be made persistent or semi-persistent giving rise to the following four commands:

$$\mathbf{always\_add\_prevail\_mode}\left(\alpha^j \overset{f}{\longleftrightarrow} \alpha^k\right)$$
$$\mathbf{once\_add\_prevail\_mode}\left(\alpha^j \overset{f}{\longleftrightarrow} \alpha^k\right)$$
$$\mathbf{always\_remove\_prevail\_mode}\left(\alpha^j \overset{f}{\longleftrightarrow} \alpha^k\right)$$
$$\mathbf{once\_remove\_prevail\_mode}\left(\alpha^j \overset{f}{\longleftrightarrow} \alpha^k\right)$$

Before we define the semantics for these newly added commands, we modify all the definitions that allow us to determine the sets of executable commands. Since such modifications are quite similar to the ones set forth in the previous Section, we refrain from giving their motivation, unless needed.

In what concerns the semantics of these commands we have first to determine the sets of executable commands. This is accomplished as before, with the following modifications. We start by defining the prevalence mode arguments:

Definition 125 (Prevalence Mode Arguments with respect to U^r) *Let U^r be a set of reduced statements. By the* set of prevalence mode arguments of U^r, *denoted by $Args_M(U^r)$, we mean:*

$$Args_M(U^*) = \left\{Arg(H(S)) \mid Arg(H(S)) = \alpha^j \overset{f}{\longleftrightarrow} \alpha^k [@X], S \in U^r\right\} \cup$$
$$\cup \left\{Arg(C) \mid Arg(C) = \alpha^j \overset{f}{\longleftrightarrow} \alpha^k [@X], C \in B(S), S \in U^r\right\}$$

Again, in this definition, we have introduced the symbol $[@X]$, not defined before, whose inclusion serves the purpose of allowing this definition to be used below, when we introduce another extension to the framework.

We now define the notion of basic prevalence mode commands:

Definition 126 (Basic Prevalence Mode Commands with respect to U^r) *Let U^r be a set of reduced statements. By the set of basic prevalence mode commands, given U^r, we mean the set $BasicComm_M(U^r)$ defined as:*

$$BasicComm_M(U^r) = \left\{ \begin{array}{c} \mathbf{add\_prevail\_mode}(\rho), \mathbf{remove\_prevail\_mode}(\rho) : \\ : \rho \in Args_M(U^r) \end{array} \right\}$$

And we modify the set of basic commands as follows:

Definition 127 (Basic Commands with respect to U^r) *By the set of basic commands, given U^r, we mean the set $BasicComm(U^r)$ defined as:*

$$BasicComm(U^r) = BasicComm_R(U^r) \cup BasicComm_S(U^r) \cup \\ \cup BasicComm_H(U^r) \cup BasicComm_M(U^r)$$

All other definitions follow, using this new notion of $BasicComm(U^r)$.

In these prevalence mode commands, an argument of the form $\alpha^j \overset{f}{\longleftrightarrow} \alpha^k$ should be considered equal to an argument of the form $\alpha^k \overset{f}{\longleftrightarrow} \alpha^j$, i.e. such arguments should be considered as the pair $(\{\alpha^k, \alpha^j\}, f)$. This is important when determining the set of executable commands, in what concerns command conditions. Consider the two reduced statements:

$$\textbf{assert}(r@\alpha) \Leftarrow \textbf{add\_prevail\_mode}\left(\alpha^j \overset{f}{\longleftrightarrow} \alpha^k\right)$$
$$\textbf{add\_prevail\_mode}\left(\alpha^k \overset{f}{\longleftrightarrow} \alpha^j\right) \Leftarrow$$

We wish rule r to be asserted. This has to be taken into account, syntactically, when determining the set of executable commands. We have two options: either we assume that every argument of this form, between two agents, is always written in the same order, or we add generic statements such as:

$$\textbf{add\_prevail\_mode}\left(\alpha^k \overset{f}{\longleftrightarrow} \alpha^j\right) \Leftarrow \textbf{add\_prevail\_mode}\left(\alpha^j \overset{f}{\longleftrightarrow} \alpha^k\right)$$

for all prevalence mode commands. Throughout, we assume that this issue is dealt with without further ado.

With these definitions in hand we can determine the executable commands and are now ready to define the semantics of this extended language. To determine the semantics we need to define the Evolution Mode at the subsequent state, $\mathcal{M}_{s+1}$. Finally, we also need to determine the *MDLP* DAG according to the specified prevalence modes.

The Evolution Mode is defined as follows:

Definition 128 (Evolution Mode at state $s+1$) *Let $\langle \mathcal{P}_s, SU_s, \mathcal{H}_s, \mathcal{M}_s \rangle$ be a KB at state s. Let Δ_{s+1} be a set of executable commands. Let $\Delta^M_{s+1} \subseteq \Delta_{s+1}$ be the set of all prevalence mode commands in Δ_{s+1}. The Evolution Mode at state $s+1$ is $\mathcal{M}_{s+1} = \Gamma_M(\mathcal{M}_s, \Delta^M_{s+1}, s+1)$, defined as follows:*

$$\Gamma_M\left(\mathcal{M}_s, \Delta^M_{s+1}, s+1\right) = \mathcal{M}_s \cup \left\{ \begin{array}{c} (\{\alpha^j, \alpha^k\}, f, s+1) : \\ : \textbf{add\_prevail\_mode}\left(\alpha^j \overset{f}{\longleftrightarrow} \alpha^k [@X]\right) \in \Delta^M_{s+1} \end{array} \right\} - \\ - \left\{ \begin{array}{c} (\{\alpha^j, \alpha^k\}, f, t) : \\ : \textbf{remove\_prevail\_mode}\left(\alpha^j \overset{f}{\longleftrightarrow} \alpha^k [@X]\right) \in \Delta^M_{s+1}, t \leq s \end{array} \right\}$$

This simply amounts to adding and removing the references to the specified prevalence modes indexed by the states at which they were set.

After establishing the current evolution mode, we can determine which edges, other than the basic ones representing the equal role prevalence mode, should be added or removed from the MDLP DAG. These edges will be obtained by means of the functions defining each of the evolution modes between pairs of agents.

Definition 129 (Added and Removed Prevalence Edges at state $s+1$) *Let $\mathcal{M}_{s+1}$ be the Evolution Mode at state $s+1$, and $\mathcal{H}_{s+1} = (\mathcal{A}, HE_{s+1})$ the hierarchy at state $s+1$. The set of added (resp. removed) prevalence edges at state $s+1$ is $\Gamma^{+}_{PE}(\mathcal{H}_{s+1}, \mathcal{M}_{s+1})$ (resp. $\Gamma^{-}_{PE}(\mathcal{H}_{s+1}, \mathcal{M}_{s+1})$), is defined as follows:*

$$\Gamma^{+}_{PE}(\mathcal{H}_{s+1}, \mathcal{M}_{s+1}) = \left\{(\alpha^j_{t_1}, \alpha^k_{t_2}) : +(\alpha^j_{t_1}, \alpha^k_{t_2}) \in \Gamma_{PE}(\mathcal{H}_{s+1}, \mathcal{M}_{s+1})\right\}$$
$$\Gamma^{-}_{PE}(\mathcal{H}_{s+1}, \mathcal{M}_{s+1}) = \left\{(\alpha^j_{t_1}, \alpha^k_{t_2}) : -(\alpha^j_{t_1}, \alpha^k_{t_2}) \in \Gamma_{PE}(\mathcal{H}_{s+1}, \mathcal{M}_{s+1})\right\}$$

where $\Gamma_{PE}(\mathcal{H}_{s+1}, \mathcal{M}_{s+1}) = PE^{<}_{s+1} \cup PE^{\|}_{s+1}$ and

$$PE^{<}_{s+1} = \bigcup f\left(\alpha^j, \alpha^k, <, s+1, n, m\right)$$

for all $f, \alpha^j, \alpha^k, n, m$ such that $\left(\left\{\alpha^j, \alpha^k\right\}, f, n\right) \in \mathcal{M}_{s+1}$, and $\left(\alpha^j, \alpha^k, m\right) \in HE_{s+1}$.

$$PE^{\|}_{s+1} = \bigcup f\left(\alpha^j, \alpha^k, \|, s+1, n, 0\right)$$

for all $f, \alpha^j, \alpha^k, n, m$ such that $\left(\left\{\alpha^j, \alpha^k\right\}, f, n\right) \in \mathcal{M}_{s+1}$, and $\left(\alpha^j, \alpha^k, \_\right), \left(\alpha^k, \alpha^j, \_\right) \notin HE_{s+1}$.

Since some of the functions that specify which edges are to be added or removed are sensitive to the existence (or not) of a hierarchical relation between the pair of involved agents, a test is first performed ($\left(\alpha^j, \alpha^k, m\right) \in HE_{s+1}$ or $\left(\alpha^j, \alpha^k, \_\right), \left(\alpha^k, \alpha^j, \_\right) \notin HE_{s+1}$) resulting in the parameter $<$ or $\|$ being passed to the function. Then $\Gamma_{PE}(\mathcal{H}_{s+1}, \mathcal{M}_{s+1})$ will contain all edges (added and removed) defined by all current prevalence modes, defined by the functions f, for each pair of agents. Such edges are then separated into two sets, $\Gamma^{+}_{PE}(\mathcal{H}_{s+1}, \mathcal{M}_{s+1})$ and $\Gamma^{-}_{PE}(\mathcal{H}_{s+1}, \mathcal{M}_{s+1})$, containing the edges to be added and those to be removed, respectively.

The *MDLP DAG* at state $s+1$ is now defined as:

Definition 130 (MDLP DAG at state $s+1$) *Let $\langle \mathcal{P}_s, SU_s, \mathcal{H}_s, \mathcal{M}_s \rangle$ be a KB at state s. Let Δ_{s+1} be a set of executable commands. Let $\Delta^{M}_{s+1} \subseteq \Delta_{s+1}$ be the set of all prevalence mode commands in Δ_{s+1}. The* MDLP DAG *at state $s+1$ is $D_{s+1} = (V_{s+1}, E_{s+1})$, where V_{s+1} is as defined before and E_{s+1} is defined as follows:*

$$\begin{aligned} E_{s+1} = E_s \cup \left\{\left(\alpha^k_s, \alpha^k_{s+1}\right) : \alpha^k \in \mathcal{A}\right\} \cup \left\{(\alpha^j_{s+1}, \alpha^k_{s+1}) : \left(\alpha^j, \alpha^k, \_\right) \in HE_{s+1}\right\} \cup \\ \cup\, \Gamma^{+}_{PE}(\mathcal{H}_{s+1}, \mathcal{M}_{s+1}) - \Gamma^{-}_{PE}(\mathcal{H}_{s+1}, \mathcal{M}_{s+1}) \end{aligned}$$

if D_{s+1} is a DAG. Otherwise, it is undefined and there is no KB at state $s+1$.

A pair of agents can have more than one prevalence mode at each time. By allowing a general class of functions to be used, and more than one function adding and removing edges among the nodes of the MDLP DAG, we open the door for possible conflicts where one such edge is specified to be both added and deleted. As per the previous definition, in all such cases, those edges will not belong to the MDLP DAG i.e., they will be deleted. Even though some scenarios could take advantage of such situation, we will not present any such example, and advise towards the avoidance of such function(s). Note that we could have made some restrictions on the individual functions allowed, as well as on the sets of functions to be used for each pair of agents, but those restrictions would cost us unnecessary overheads which we believe can do without at this stage.

It is important to remark that since we are allowing arbitrary functions (as long as they have the correct signature) to be used in order as to establish the prevalence modes, we cannot guarantee that D_{s+1} is in fact a DAG. The result of applying those functions can produce a graph that is cyclic which would render the knowledge state useless because the semantics of *MDLP* has not been defined for cyclic graphs. How to deal with such situations? The first option would be, of course, to avoid it. If the cycles indeed occur, several solutions could be set forth which we now briefly mention, but which will not be explored in this work:

- Detect that D_{s+1} is going to be cyclic and discard this state transition altogether;
- Detect that D_{s+1} is going to be cyclic and use only the basic version, to which we do not add PE^{+}_{s+1};
- Perform some form of belief revision, minimally removing edges until no cycles occur. This option is computationally expensive;
- Enter some exception mode where the knowledge state is preserved until an external update containing prevalence mode commands, without conditions that require querying the *MDLP*, sets the evolution mode so that the cycles are removed;
- Extend the semantics of *MDLP* to deal with cycles, although the epistemic meaning of cycles in this framework is still not a clear issue to us.

Since the study of cycles in graphs falls outside the scope of this work, we have opted to simply undefine the knowledge state as per the above definition.

In the next Chapter we present an example to partially illustrate the use of this extended language.

Prevalence Mode Functions

We follow up with some (possibly) interesting examples of functions. Each function f has signature $f : \mathcal{A}^2 \times \{<, \|\} \times \mathcal{T}^3 \longrightarrow 2^{\{+,-\}\times(\mathcal{A}\times\mathcal{T})^2}$ and its parameters $f\left(\alpha^j, \alpha^k, h, s, n, m\right)$ have the following meaning: α^j and α^k are the two agents involved; $h \in \{<, \|\}$ contains the hierarchy relation between α^j and α^k: $h =$ " $<$ " means that $\alpha^j < \alpha^k$, and $h =$ " $\|$ " means that α^j and α^k are not directly hierarchically related; s is the current time state; n is the time state when the prevalence mode f was set; m is the time state when the current hierarchical relation between α^j and α^k was set. Not all parameters will be used by all functions.

Time Prevalence: According to this prevalence mode, previously explained in Chapter 6, any rule indexed by a more recent time state overrides any older rule, independently of to which of the two agents these rules belong. The function specifying this mode is defined as:

$$f_{tp}\left(\alpha^j, \alpha^k, \_, s, \_, \_\right) = \left\{+(\alpha^j_{s-1}, \alpha^k_s), +(\alpha^k_{s-1}, \alpha^j_s)\right\}$$

Example 69 *Consider the following program:*

$$EU_1 = \left\{\textbf{add\_prevail\_mode}\left(\alpha^j \overset{f_{tp}}{\longleftrightarrow} \alpha^k\right) \Leftarrow\right\}$$

The transition from time states $i-1$ to i is represented in Figure 7.1[4].

[4]In these examples we consider a sufficiently large i. For example, $i = 20$.

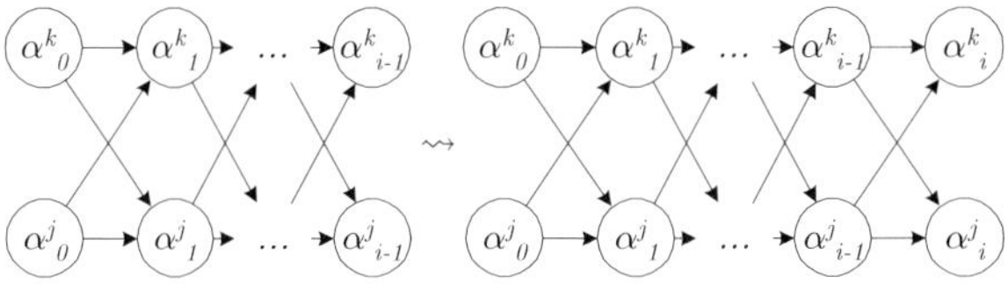

Figure 7.1: Time Prevalence Mode

The previous function only makes time prevail after being issued. We may want a function that also sets the past to the same time prevalence mode. Such function would be:

$$f_{atp}\left(\alpha^j, \alpha^k, \_, s, \_, \_\right) = \left\{+\left(\alpha^j_{p-1}, \alpha^k_p\right), +\left(\alpha^k_{p-1}, \alpha^j_p\right) : 1 < p \leq s\right\}$$

Example 70 *Consider the following program:*

$$EU_i = \left\{\textbf{add\_prevail\_mode}\left(\alpha^j \overset{f_{atp}}{\longleftrightarrow} \alpha^k\right) \Leftarrow\right\}$$

The transition from time states $i-1$ to i is represented in Figure 7.2.

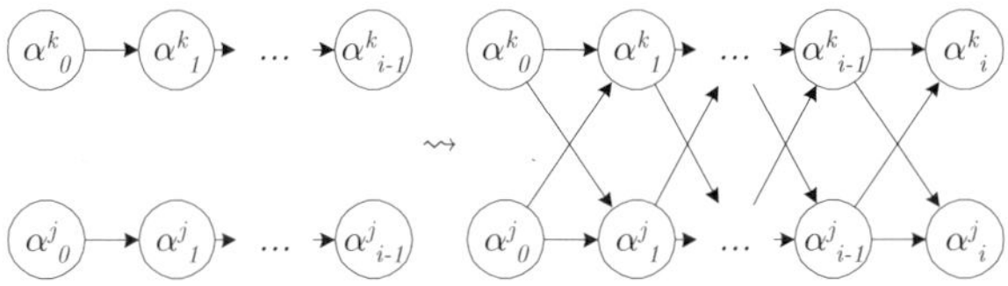

Figure 7.2: Set the Past to Time Prevalence Mode

Hierarchy Prevalence: According to this prevalence mode, any rule indexed by a higher ranked agent overrides any lower ranked agent's rule, starting when both the prevalence mode and the hierarchy between the two agents are set. Motivation for this prevalence mode can be found in Chapter 6.

$$\begin{aligned} f_{hp}\left(\alpha^j, \alpha^k, <, s, n, m\right) &= \left\{+\left(\alpha^j_s, \alpha^k_p\right) : p = max\left(n, m\right), 0 < p < s\right\} \cup \\ &\cup \left\{-\left(\alpha^j_{s-1}, \alpha^k_p\right) : p = max\left(n, m\right), 0 < p < s-1\right\} \\ f_{hp}\left(\_, \_, \|, \_, \_, \_\right) &= \{\} \end{aligned}$$

Note that if there is no hierarchical relation between the two agents, no edges are added nor removed.

Example 71 *Suppose the following program:*

$$EU_1 = \left\{\begin{array}{c} \textbf{add\_prevail\_mode}\left(\alpha^j \overset{f_{hp}}{\longleftrightarrow} \alpha^k\right) \Leftarrow \\ \textbf{add\_hierarchy\_edge}\left(\alpha^j \rightarrow \alpha^k\right) \Leftarrow \end{array}\right\}$$

The transition from state $i-1$ to state i is represented in Figure 7.3.

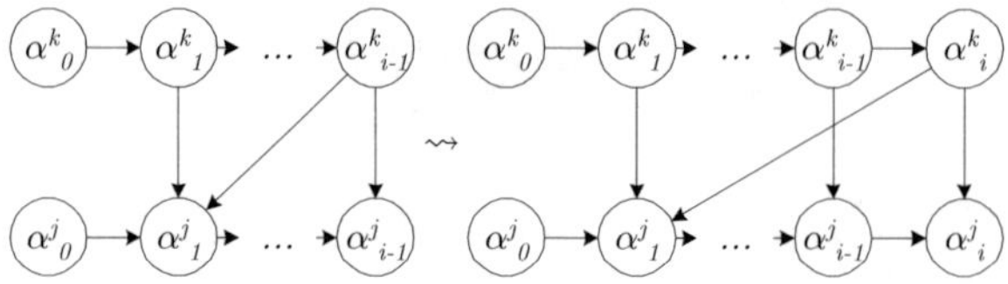

Figure 7.3: Hierarchy Prevalence Mode

Example 72 *Consider the following programs:*

$$EU_1 = \left\{ \begin{array}{c} \textbf{add\_prevail\_mode}\left(\alpha^j \stackrel{f_{hp}}{\longleftrightarrow} \alpha^k\right) \Leftarrow \\ \textbf{add\_hierarchy\_edge}\left(\alpha^j \rightarrow \alpha^k\right) \Leftarrow \end{array} \right\}$$

$$EU_{i-2} = \left\{ \begin{array}{c} \textbf{remove\_hierarchy\_edge}\left(\alpha^j \rightarrow \alpha^k\right) \Leftarrow \\ \textbf{add\_hierarchy\_edge}\left(\alpha^k \rightarrow \alpha^j\right) \Leftarrow \end{array} \right\}$$

The transition from time states $i-1$ to i is represented in Figure 7.4.

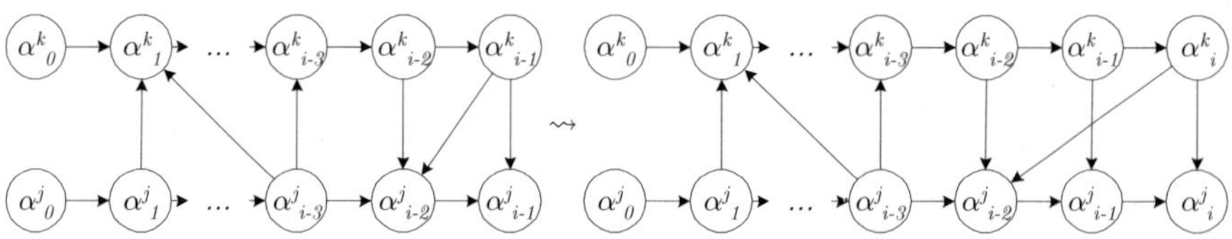

Figure 7.4: Hierarchy Change under Hierarchy Prevalence Mode

Clear: This function removes all edges set by any previous prevalence modes except those defined by the basic $KABUL^m$ semantics that encode the equal role representation.

$$f_{clear}\left(\alpha^j, \alpha^k, \_, s, \_, \_\right) = \left\{-\left(\alpha^j_p, \alpha^k_q\right), -\left(\alpha^k_p, \alpha^j_q\right) : p, q \in \mathcal{T}, p, q < s, p \neq q\right\}$$

Example 73 *Consider the following program:*

$$EU_1 = \left\{ \begin{array}{c} \textbf{add\_prevail\_mode}\left(\alpha^j \stackrel{f_{tp}}{\longleftrightarrow} \alpha^k\right) \Leftarrow \\ \textbf{add\_hierarchy\_edge}\left(\alpha^j \rightarrow \alpha^k\right) \Leftarrow \end{array} \right\}$$

$$EU_{i-3} = \left\{ \begin{array}{c} \textbf{add\_hierarchy\_edge}\left(\alpha^k \rightarrow \alpha^j\right) \Leftarrow \\ \textbf{remove\_hierarchy\_edge}\left(\alpha^j \rightarrow \alpha^k\right) \Leftarrow \\ \textbf{add\_prevail\_mode}\left(\alpha^j \stackrel{f_{hp}}{\longleftrightarrow} \alpha^k\right) \Leftarrow \\ \textbf{remove\_prevail\_mode}\left(\alpha^j \stackrel{f_{tp}}{\longleftrightarrow} \alpha^k\right) \Leftarrow \end{array} \right\}$$

$$EU_i = \left\{ \textbf{add\_prevail\_mode}\left(\alpha^j \stackrel{f_{clear}}{\longleftrightarrow} \alpha^k\right) \Leftarrow \right\}$$

The transition from time states $i-1$ to i is represented in Figure 7.5. Note that f_{clear} only removes those edges linking two nodes indexed by previous time states, not affecting the new edge $(\alpha^k_i, \alpha^j_{i-3})$ added by the hierarchy prevalence mode.

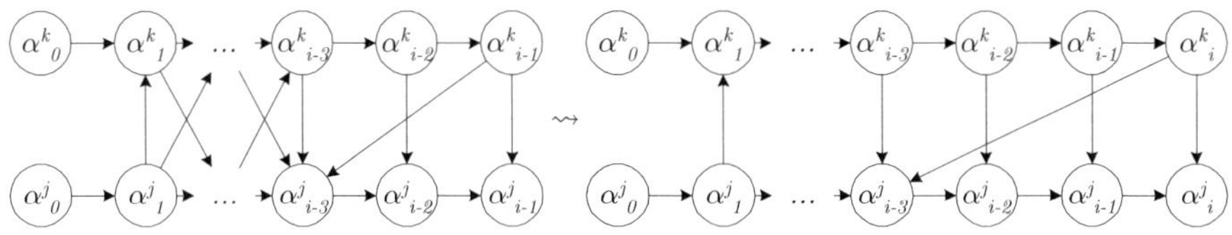

Figure 7.5: Clear all Past Prevalence Modes

Recent Time Prevail (δ) According to this prevalence mode, in the most recent δ states, there are edges encoding the time prevalence mode. In states older that δ, time does not prevail, prevalence being set by any other existing mode.

$$f_{rtp}(\delta) : N \longrightarrow \mathcal{A}^2 \times \{<,=\} \times \mathcal{T}^3 \longrightarrow 2^{\{+,-\}\times(\mathcal{A}\times\mathcal{T})^2}$$

$$f_{rtp}(\delta)\left(\alpha^j, \alpha^k, \_, s, n, \_\right) = \left\{+\left(\alpha^j_{s-1}, \alpha^k_s\right), +\left(\alpha^k_{s-1}, \alpha^j_s\right)\right\} \cup \\ \cup \left\{-\left(\alpha^j_{s-1-\delta}, \alpha^k_{s-\delta}\right), -\left(\alpha^k_{s-1-\delta}, \alpha^j_{s-\delta}\right) : s - n \geq \delta\right\}$$

Example 74 *Suppose the following program:*

$$EU_1 = \left\{ \textbf{add\_prevail\_mode}\left(\alpha^j \overset{f_{rtp}(2)}{\longleftrightarrow} \alpha^k\right) \Leftarrow \right\}$$

The transition from state $i-1$ to state i is represented in Figure 7.6.

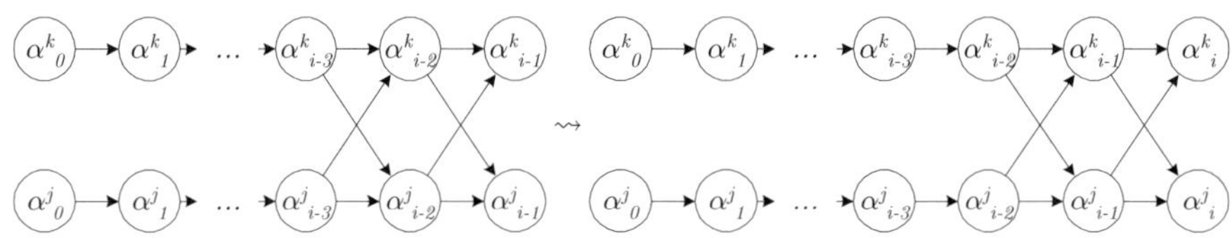

Figure 7.6: Recent Time Prevalence with $\delta = 2$

7.3.3 Agent Commands

In the previous Sections we have extended *KABUL* with several features, namely with the ability to:

- construct MDLPs instead of just sequences of programs, introducing $KABUL^m$;
- change the otherwise fixed hierarchy that relates the agents in the system, introducing the *hierarchy commands*;
- allow a flexible evolution of the MDLP DAG, introducing the *prevalence mode commands.*

It would be fair to ask why do we still have to rely on a fixed set of agents $\mathcal{A}$ and not allow it to be dynamic. If this framework is to be used to represent an agent system situated in a dynamic environment where different sources of information (agents) exist, it seems reasonable to expect that new agents would be brought about and others would cease to exist. This would suggest that instead of a fixed set of agents $\mathcal{A}$ we should have a set of agents for each state, $\mathcal{A}_s$, that would be allowed to be updated by yet another new set of commands. Such commands could look like:

$$\textbf{add\_agent}\ (\alpha)$$
$$\textbf{remove\_agent}\ (\alpha)$$

and their semantics would update the set $\mathcal{A}_s$ and start another "line" of nodes in the MDLP DAG for this new agent.

Even though it would not be a difficult task to do, we will not introduce these commands simply because they are irrelevant if only we assume to have an initial set of agents $\mathcal{A}$ containing enough elements, one for each agent that will eventually appear in the system. This is so because of some properties of MDLP among which the one that states that an empty program does not affect the semantics at any other state and can be removed as long as the relations between all other nodes are preserved (Proposition 84). Furthermore, since those "yet to exist" agents will not be related to any other agent, they will fall outside of the relevancy graph when determining the semantics at any other agent and thus, do not have to be considered, and can be eliminated. Therefore, we can simply assume that every agent has always been in the system, although all its programs are empty.

As for the elimination of agents, the way it is emulated depends on what we want such elimination to represent. Two alternatives:

1. If, when eliminating an agent, we want to preserve all its past contributions to the system, then we simply cease to issue commands to that agent and, if needed, adapt the hierarchy according to the new situation. Note that the old programs indexed by the nodes of this agent will still contribute to the semantics of the overall system because they may still be linked to other nodes.

2. If, when eliminating an agent, we want it to completely disappear, then we simply disconnect all the nodes of this agent from all other agents, and clear all its links in the hierarchy. Disconnecting the nodes can be achieved by a suitable function to be used as a prevalence mode.

7.4 Multiple Update Programs

In the previous Section we have extended KABUL to deal with the flexible construction of MDLPs. This was accomplished by first extending the language with the capabilities of updating individual nodes in the MDLP and subsequently by the introduction of new commands to flexibly manipulate the way such MDLP grows. According to this extended framework, we have a set of agents $\mathcal{A}$ that represents different sources of information. However, these agents can also be made to represent different kinds of knowledge. For example, we can have a subset of $\mathcal{A}$ representing the goals of the system, where such goals are dynamically changed by means of updates. Other subsets of $\mathcal{A}$ can represent other modalities such as intentions, beliefs, etc. Recall that having just one set of agents $\mathcal{A}$ and one hierarchy $\mathcal{H}$ relating them does not mean that all such nodes must be connected. In fact, the MDLP DAG can encode several DAGs, and thus several MDLPs. Suppose a very simple framework with $\mathcal{A} = \{goals, knowledge\}$ such that $\mathcal{H}$ does not contain any edges. Suppose further that we execute the two commands:

$$\textbf{assert}\,(rich \leftarrow win\_lottery@knowledge)$$
$$\textbf{assert}\,(rich@goals)$$

At the subsequent state we observe that $rich@goals$ is true and that $rich@knowledge$ is false, indicating that we are not rich but we have a goal to be so. This reading of $\mathcal{A}$ as representing not only agents (or sources of information) but also as different modalities is at the heart of the applicability of this framework within the context of multi-agent systems. We are not concerned with the meaning assigned to those MDLPs, but rather with it being possible in principle. More on this in the next Chapter. But before that, we need to introduce the last extension to the framework, related with the desire to have a modular design of agents, where one such agent is composed of several sub-agents with different functionalities/capabilities. We have already briefly mentioned this view of agents when, in Chapter 6, we explained how MDLP can be used to represent inter- and intra-agent relationships. Accordingly, we need to allow the construction and evolution of the KB to be jointly specified by more than one sub-agent. Since we've adopted the stance that an agent's behaviour is to be encoded by a KABUL program, then so should the agent's sub-agents. For this we need to have concurrent extended *KABUL* programs manipulating the same MDLP. We will be referring to this new extension of the framework as $KABUL^+$.

7.4.1 Framework and Syntax

In this new extension, besides the initial set of agents $\mathcal{A}$, we introduce a set of sub-agents $\mathcal{SA}$. Associated with each of those sub-agents there is one $KABUL^+$ program. Each of these programs will be jointly manipulating an MDLP DAG. Furthermore, for each agent in $\mathcal{A}$ there corresponds a hierarchy relating the sub-agents in $\mathcal{SA}$. The rationale behind this is that each new node in the MDLP DAG will now consist of a set of nodes, one corresponding to each sub-agent, linked according to the sub-agent hierarchy for that particular agent. Suppose for example that one of the agents represents the goals of the system and another agent represents some outside agent. Further suppose that we have two sub-agents, one of them specialized in communication and the other in goal management. We want to differentiate the hierarchical status of each of those sub-agents when updating to each of the two agents' nodes. We want to be able to give higher priority to the goal manager when updating to the goals nodes and higher priority to the communication expert when updating to the node corresponding to the outside agent. Accordingly, associated with each knowledge state there will be a set of sub-agent hierarchies, one for each agent. We will denote such set of DAGs at state s by $\mathcal{SH}_s$. It has the generic form:

$$\mathcal{SH}_s = \{SD_{\alpha_s} : \alpha \in \mathcal{A}\}$$

where $SD_{\alpha_s} = (\mathcal{SA}, SE_{\alpha_s})$ is a DAG.

We will also introduce an extension to the language to allow for sub-agents to communicate. This will be achieved by means of inter-sub-agent updates. We do so with minor changes to both the syntax and semantics, by extending the statement assertion commands with a reference to which sub-agent such statement is to be asserted. Accordingly, such statement assertion commands have now the form:

$$[\mathbf{always\_} \mid \mathbf{once\_}]\,\mathbf{assert}\,(S@\beta) \tag{7.13}$$

where $\beta \in \mathcal{SA}$. If $@\beta$ is omitted from a statement command, we assume that it refers to the sub-agent represented by the program to which the statement belongs, i.e. it will be treated as before and so statement S will be asserted to the sub-agent's own self update at the next state. We also introduce the corresponding inhibition command:

$$not\,\mathbf{assert}\,(S@\beta)$$

Finally, to allow for sub-agents having private capabilities, we extend the framework so as to concede a private knowledge base associated with each sub-agent, and extend statement bodies to permit conditions on this private knowledge base. For simplicity, we define such notions as we have done for external observations, except that they are evaluated over what can be considered a set of private observations. Our goal here is to open the door for sub-agents to access private procedure calls so as to perform their own private capabilities. The formal definitions for using such private procedure calls can be established with notions similar to the notion of code calls found in [219] which could be imported, *mutandis mutatis*, into our framework. Here, we consider a capabilities language which is common to every sub-agent, and the actual capabilities each possesses is determined by the set of atoms it observes in its private capabilities set. We extend statements to allow for conditions on this new language, appended to the body of statements, with the form:

$$\mathbf{P} : \mathbf{in}\,(E_1)\,, ..., \mathbf{in}\,(E_p)\,, \mathbf{out}\,(E_{p+1})\,, ..., \mathbf{out}\,(E_q)$$

Then each sub-agent will have, at each state, a private set of capabilities which is just a subset of the capabilities language. The condition is evaluated just as is the one on external observations, except that it is over this private set.

Overall, there will be a set of agents and a set of sub-agents. To each sub-agent, at each state, there corresponds a set of nodes, one for each agent. Rule commands are executed at those nodes, according to the agent specified in the commands. Each set of sub-agents will observe the same set of external observations used, as before, to partially evaluate its statements. The external update will now be a set of external update programs, one for each agent. Of course one could assign to a single sub-agent the task of dealing with all external updates and forward them to the proper sub-agents. Sub-agents will now be able to communicate at a level other than by means of asserting rules in the object knowledge base. They can update other sub-agents with statements. This is particularly important for coordination tasks where asserting a statement can mean delegating a task to some agent which has the proper capabilities to perform it. Such inter-sub-agent updates will require another entry in our notion of knowledge state. Accordingly, for each sub-agent and at each state, there is a set of update programs each of them originating in one of the other sub-agents. As the reader may have noticed, each sub-agent, at each state, must now deal with several update programs, namely its own self update, the external update, and one internal update from every other sub-agent. To deal with such families of update programs, the notion of executable set of commands (Definition 95) can be directly adapted, using the same notion of rejected statements, if only the relation $<$ used to establish precedence criteria between the self and external updates is extended to deal with all the new programs, in a similar manner to the extension of the semantics of DLP to that of MDLP.

Each knowledge state will have the form $\langle \mathcal{P}_s, \mathcal{SA}_s, \mathcal{H}_s, \mathcal{SH}_s, \mathcal{M}_s, \mathcal{SM}_s, \mathcal{IU}_s \rangle$ where:

- $\mathcal{P}_s$ is an MDLP representing the object level knowledge base.
- $\mathcal{SA}_s$ is a set of tuples of the form $\left\{\left(SU_s^\beta, <_\beta, C_s^\beta\right) : \beta \in \mathcal{SA}\right\}$, where SU_s^β is the (self) update program of sub-agent β at state s, $<_\beta$ is a partial order, of sub-agent β, relating the positive and inhibition statements of the self, external and all updates incoming from other sub-agents and C_s^β is the set containing the private capabilities of sub-agent β at state s. For simplicity, we will assume that $<_\beta$ and C_s^β are initially given and fixed throughout. Therefore, we leave $<_\beta$ and C_s^β implicit and reduce $\mathcal{SA}_s$ to be a set of programs $\left\{SU_s^\beta : \beta \in \mathcal{SA}\right\}$, one for each sub-agent. We dub these programs *sub-agent programs*.
- $\mathcal{H}_s$ is a DAG of the form $(\mathcal{A}, HE_s)$ representing the hierarchy between agents.
- $\mathcal{SH}_s$ is a Set of DAGs of the form $\{SD_{\alpha_s} : \alpha \in \mathcal{A}\}$ each representing the hierarchy between the sub-agents, for each agent. Each DAG SD_{α_s} has the form $(\mathcal{SA}, SAE_{\alpha_s})$ where SAE_{α_s} is the set of edges relating the sub-agents within agent α, at state s.
- $\mathcal{M}_s$ is a set of triplets of the form $\left\{\left(\left\{\alpha^j, \alpha^k\right\}, f, n\right) : \alpha^j, \alpha^k \in \mathcal{A}, f \in \mathcal{F}, n \in \mathcal{T}\right\}$, defined as before, representing the evolution mode of agents.
- $\mathcal{SM}_s$ is a set of sets of the form $\{\mathcal{SM}_s^\alpha : \alpha \in \mathcal{A}\}$ where each $\mathcal{SM}_s^\alpha$ represents the evolution mode of the sub-agents within agent α and, as for the case of agent's evolution modes, is a set of triplets of the form $\left\{\left(\left\{\beta^j, \beta^k\right\}, f, n\right) : \beta^j, \beta^k \in \mathcal{SA}, f \in \mathcal{SF}, n \in \mathcal{T}\right\}$.
- $\mathcal{IU}_s$ is a set of sets of update programs, $\left\{\mathcal{IU}_s^\beta : \beta \in \mathcal{SA}\right\}$, where each $\mathcal{IU}_s^\beta$ represents the internal updates to sub-agent β, from every other sub-agent i.e. $\mathcal{IU}_s^\beta$ is of the form $\left\{IU_s^{\beta',\beta} : \beta', \beta \in \mathcal{SA}, \beta \neq \beta'\right\}$ where $IU_s^{\beta',\beta}$ is the update from β' to β at state s.

At each state transition, the system receives, besides the set of external observations which will be visible to all sub-agents, a set of external update programs, one for each sub-agent, as follows:

$$\mathcal{EU}_{s+1} = \left\{EU_{s+1}^\beta : \beta \in \mathcal{SA}\right\}$$

As before, state transitions are of the form:

$$\langle \mathcal{P}_s, \mathcal{SA}_s, \mathcal{H}_s, \mathcal{SH}_s, \mathcal{M}_s, \mathcal{SM}_s, \mathcal{IU}_s \rangle \overset{\langle \mathcal{EU}_{s+1}, EO_{s+1} \rangle}{\longrightarrow}$$
$$\langle \mathcal{P}_{s+1}, \mathcal{SA}_{s+1}, \mathcal{H}_{s+1}, \mathcal{SH}_{s+1}, \mathcal{M}_{s+1}, \mathcal{SM}_{s+1}, \mathcal{IU}_{s+1} \rangle$$

At each state transition, each of the sub-agents independently partially evaluates all its corresponding update programs, namely its own self update program, its external update program, and all the internal updates incoming from other sub-agents. Then, based on these partially evaluated statements and its relation $<_\beta$, it determines a set of executable updates. This set of executable updates will contain:

- self-update statement commands that will be used to totally determine its own self update at the next state, SU^{β}_{s+1};
- statement commands to other sub-agents that will be used to partly determine the internal updates at the next state $\mathcal{IU}_{s+1}$;
- hierarchy commands that will be used to partly determine $\mathcal{H}_{s+1}$ and $\mathcal{SH}_{s+1}$;
- prevalence mode commands that will be used to partly determine the evolution modes $\mathcal{M}_{s+1}$ and $\mathcal{SM}_{s+1}$;
- rule commands that will be used to partly determine the object level knowledge base $\mathcal{P}_{s+1}$.

Note that when we mention that some set of commands will be used to partially determine some component of the next state, we mean that the executable commands of other sub-agents will also be needed in order to totally determine such next state component.

Besides the extension in the statement assertion commands, to refer to the proper sub-agent, we also need to extend the commands to manipulate the hierarchies to be able to deal with the new sub-agent hierarchies. Note that rule commands need not be extended because they are always executed at the corresponding sub-agent node in the specified agent. As for the hierarchy commands, besides the existing:

$$[\textbf{always\_} \mid \textbf{once\_}]\textbf{add\_hierarchy\_edge}(\alpha^j \rightarrow \alpha^k) \tag{7.14}$$

$$[\textbf{always\_} \mid \textbf{once\_}]\textbf{remove\_hierarchy\_edge}(\alpha^j \rightarrow \alpha^k) \tag{7.15}$$

where $\alpha^j, \alpha^k \in \mathcal{A}$, which we now dub *agent hierarchy commands*, we introduce the commands:

$$[\textbf{always\_} \mid \textbf{once\_}]\textbf{add\_hierarchy\_edge}(\beta^j \rightarrow \beta^k@\alpha) \tag{7.16}$$

$$[\textbf{always\_} \mid \textbf{once\_}]\textbf{remove\_hierarchy\_edge}(\beta^j \rightarrow \beta^k@\alpha) \tag{7.17}$$

where $\beta^j, \beta^k \in \mathcal{SA}$ and $\alpha \in \mathcal{A}$. Their intuitive reading is the same as the previous two, except that they are executed on the DAG $SD_{\alpha_s} \in \mathcal{SH}_s$. We dub these two newly introduced commands *sub-agent hierarchy commands.*

As for the prevalence mode commands, besides the existing

$$[\textbf{always\_} \mid \textbf{once\_}]\ \textbf{add\_prevail\_mode}\left(\alpha^j \overset{f}{\longleftrightarrow} \alpha^k\right) \tag{7.18}$$

$$[\textbf{always\_} \mid \textbf{once\_}]\ \textbf{remove\_prevail\_mode}\left(\alpha^j \overset{f}{\longleftrightarrow} \alpha^k\right) \tag{7.19}$$

where $\alpha^j, \alpha^k \in \mathcal{A}$ and $f \in \mathcal{F}$, which we now dub *agent prevalence mode commands*, we introduce the commands:

$$[\textbf{always\_} \mid \textbf{once\_}]\ \textbf{add\_prevail\_mode}\left(\beta^j \overset{f}{\longleftrightarrow} \beta^k@\alpha\right) \tag{7.20}$$

$$[\textbf{always\_} \mid \textbf{once\_}]\ \textbf{remove\_prevail\_mode}\left(\beta^j \overset{f}{\longleftrightarrow} \beta^k@\alpha\right) \tag{7.21}$$

where $\beta^j, \beta^k \in \mathcal{SA}$, $\alpha \in \mathcal{A}$ and f is a function with signature

$$f : \mathcal{SA}^2 \times \{<, \|\} \times \mathcal{T}^3 \longrightarrow 2^{\{+,-\}\times(\mathcal{SA}\times\mathcal{T})^2}$$

i.e. f is a function similar to the one previously used, except that agents are replaced with sub-agents. We call the set of all such functions $\mathcal{SF}$. We dub these two newly introduced commands *sub-agent prevalence mode commands*. The intuitive reading of these commands is the same as the previous two, except that they are executed on the set $\mathcal{SM}_s^\alpha$.

There follows a table summarizing the syntax of this general language, in BNF:

⟨*statement*⟩	::=	⟨*command*⟩ [⇐ ⟨*conditions*⟩] ;
⟨*base_comm*⟩	::=	**assert** [**_event**] (⟨*rule*⟩ @ ⟨*agent*⟩) |
		| **retract** [**_event**] (⟨*rule*⟩ @ ⟨*agent*⟩) |
		| **assert** (⟨*statement*⟩ [@ ⟨*sub_agent*⟩]) |
		| **retract** (⟨*statement*⟩) |
		| **add_hierarchy_edge**(⟨*h_arg*⟩) |
		| **remove_hierarchy_edge**(⟨*h_arg*⟩) |
		| **add_prevail_mode** (⟨*m_arg*⟩) |
		| **remove_prevail_mode** (⟨*m_arg*⟩) ;
⟨*per_comm*⟩	::=	**always_** ⟨*base_comm*⟩ | **once_** ⟨*base_comm*⟩ ;
⟨*inhib_comm*⟩	::=	*not* ⟨*base_comm*⟩ ;
⟨*command*⟩	::=	⟨*base_comm*⟩ | ⟨*per_comm*⟩ | ⟨*inhib_comm*⟩ ;
⟨*h_arg*⟩	::=	⟨*agent*⟩ → ⟨*agent*⟩ |
		| ⟨*sub_agent*⟩ → ⟨*sub_agent*⟩ @ ⟨*agent*⟩ ;
⟨*m_arg*⟩	::=	⟨*agent*⟩ $\overset{\langle function \rangle}{\longleftrightarrow}$ ⟨*agent*⟩ |
		| ⟨*sub_agent*⟩ $\overset{\langle function \rangle}{\longleftrightarrow}$ ⟨*sub_agent*⟩ @ ⟨*agent*⟩ ;
⟨*conditions*⟩	::=	[⟨*comm_conds*⟩ ,] [⟨*lit_conds*⟩ ,] [**R** : ⟨*rule_conds*⟩ ,] [**E** : ⟨*env_conds*⟩ ,] [**P** : ⟨*prv_conds*⟩] ;
⟨*comm_conds*⟩	::=	⟨*base_comm*⟩ [, ⟨*comm_conds*⟩] |
		| ⟨*inhib_comm*⟩ [, ⟨*comm_conds*⟩] ;
⟨*lit_conds*⟩	::=	⟨*literal*⟩ @ ⟨*agents*⟩ [, ⟨*lit_conds*⟩] ;
⟨*rule_conds*⟩	::=	**in** (⟨*rule*⟩ @ ⟨*agents*⟩) [, ⟨*rule_conds*⟩] |
		| **out** (⟨*rule*⟩ @ ⟨*agents*⟩) [, ⟨*rule_conds*⟩] ;
⟨*env_conds*⟩	::=	**in** (⟨*observ*⟩) [, ⟨*env_conds*⟩] |
		| **out** (⟨*observ*⟩) [, ⟨*env_conds*⟩] ;
⟨*prv_conds*⟩	::=	**in** (⟨*capability*⟩) [, ⟨*prv_conds*⟩] |
		| **out** (⟨*capability*⟩) [, ⟨*prv_conds*⟩] ;
⟨*agents*⟩	::=	{⟨*agent*⟩ [, ⟨*agents*⟩]}

7.4.2 Semantics

We now provide the semantics for *KABUL*$^+$. For this purpose, we start with the definition of the initial state:

Definition 131 (*KABUL*$^+$ Initial Knowledge State) *Let A be a set of agents and SA a set of sub-agents. The initial knowledge state is the knowledge state at state* 0,

$\langle \mathcal{P}_0, \mathcal{SA}_0, \mathcal{H}_0, \mathcal{SH}_0, \mathcal{M}_0, \mathcal{SM}_0, \mathcal{IU}_0 \rangle$ *where:*

$$
\begin{array}{ll}
\mathcal{P}_0 = (\mathcal{P}_{D_0}, D_0) & D_0 = (V_0, E_0) \\
\mathcal{SA}_0 = \left\{ SU_0^\beta : \beta \in \mathcal{SA} \right\} & V_0 = \left\{ \alpha_0^+, \alpha_0^-, \beta_0^\alpha : \beta \in \mathcal{SA}, \alpha \in \mathcal{A} \right\} \\
SU_0^\beta = \{\} & E_0 = \left\{ \left(\beta_0^\alpha, \alpha_0^+\right), \left(\alpha_0^-, \beta_0^\alpha\right) : \beta \in \mathcal{SA}, \alpha \in \mathcal{A} \right\} \\
\mathcal{H}_0 = (\mathcal{A}, HE_0) & \mathcal{P}_{D_0} = \left\{ P_{\beta_0^\alpha} : \beta \in \mathcal{SA}, \alpha \in \mathcal{A}, \beta_0^\alpha \in V_0 \right\} \\
HE_0 = \{\} & P_{\beta_0^\alpha} = \{\} \\
\mathcal{SH}_0 = \{ SD_{\alpha_0} : \alpha \in \mathcal{A} \} & \mathcal{IU}_0 = \left\{ \mathcal{IU}_0^\beta : \beta \in \mathcal{SA} \right\} \\
SD_{\alpha_0} = (\mathcal{SA}, SAE_{\alpha_0}) & \mathcal{IU}_0^\beta = \left\{ IU_0^{\beta^j,\beta} : \beta^j, \beta \in \mathcal{SA}, \beta^j \neq \beta \right\} \\
SAE_{\alpha_0} = \{\} & IU_0^{\beta^j,\beta^k} = \{\} \\
\mathcal{SM}_0 = \{ \mathcal{SM}_0^\alpha : \alpha \in \mathcal{A} \} & \mathcal{M}_0 = \{\} \\
\mathcal{SM}_0^\alpha = \{\} &
\end{array}
$$

At this point it is worth explaining how the MDLP DAG is constructed, and how it evolves. With each agent's node being composed of a set of nodes corresponding each to one of the sub-agents, there is no longer the notion of one single program associated with each agent, at each time state. Nevertheless, the notion of agent is still necessary inasmuch as queries to the KB are posed with respect to agents, i.e. a literal $L@\alpha$ is still to be evaluated at agent α, and agents are still to be related according to the agent hierarchy and prevalence modes. To this purpose, to each agent α at each time state s there corresponds a pair of nodes in the MDLP DAG, namely α_s^+ and α_s^-. These nodes enable queries to agent α at state s to be performed at α_s^+. Note however that since there is no program associated with this node, these queries are equivalent to queries to the set of states $\{\beta_s^\alpha\}$. Furthermore, all edges linking agents, namely those specified by the agent hierarchy, prevalence modes, etc, are defined in terms of these nodes. All incoming edges link to α_s^- and all outgoing edges link from α_s^+. We dub α_s^- the source of agent α at state s, and α_s^+ the sink of agent α at state s.

The partial evaluation of the statements in all update programs is performed as before, having in mind that literal and rule conditions are now evaluated at the agent's sink of the corresponding state, i.e. α_s^+. Consequently, at each state s each sub-agent β partially evaluates update programs SU_s^β, those in $\mathcal{IU}_s^\beta$, and the external update EU_{s+1}^β, with respect to $\mathcal{P}_s$ and EO_{s+1}, thus obtaining its reduced forms. The corresponding logic programs are also obtained as before.

The notion of executable commands, for each sub-agent β, is given by Definition 95, where

$$W = W_\beta = \left\{ EU_{s+1}^\beta, SU_s^\beta \right\} \cup \left\{ IU_s^{\beta^j,\beta} : IU_s^{\beta^j,\beta} \in \mathcal{IU}_s^\beta \right\}$$

and the order relation is $<_\beta$. Accordingly, a coherent set of commands Δ_{s+1}^β is a set of *executable commands* for sub-agent β, iff

$$I_{\Delta_{s+1}^\beta} = least\left(\mathcal{W}_\beta^* - Rejected\left(W_\beta, <_\beta, \Delta_{s+1}^\beta \right) \cup Common\left(\mathcal{W}_\beta^*, \Delta_{s+1}^\beta \right) \right)$$

$$\mathcal{W}_\beta^* = \bigcup_{U^* \in W_\beta} U^*$$

$$Common\left(\mathcal{W}_\beta^*, \Delta_{s+1}^\beta \right) = \Omega\left(\mathcal{W}_\beta^* \right) \cup Coh\left(\mathcal{W}_\beta^* \right) \cup Default\left(\mathcal{W}_\beta^*, \Delta_{s+1}^\beta \right)$$

In line with the above definitions, at each state transition we obtain one set of executable commands Δ_{s+1}^β for each sub-agent β in $\mathcal{SA}$. It is important to mention that the conditions on the concurrent execution of commands only refer to the commands that are self executed. Although this may seem like an inconvenience inasmuch some sub-agents will not execute some commands because they are conditional on the concurrent execution of other commands that will in fact be executed by other sub-agents, this only matters for a restricted class of commands, namely those concerning the hierarchy and prevalence mode commands. The advantage of this approach is that it caters for a completely autonomous determination of executable commands by each sub-agent, thus enabling its direct and efficient distribution. Nevertheless, at the cost of efficiency, some coordination policies could be established to determine the executability of such statements. These could be accomplished, for example, by incorporating the framework of [46].

With these sets of executable commands we can determine the next state of the knowledge base.

Definition 132 (Knowledge Base at state $s+1$) *Consider a knowledge base at state s, $\langle \mathcal{P}_s, \mathcal{SA}_s, \mathcal{H}_s, \mathcal{SH}_s, \mathcal{M}_s, \mathcal{SM}_s, \mathcal{IU}_s \rangle$, and let $\left\{\Delta^{\beta}_{s+1} : \beta \in \mathcal{SA}\right\}$ be the set of executable commands, one for each sub-agent, determined as per the definitions above. Let:*

- $\Delta^{\beta R@\alpha}_{s+1}$ *be the set of rule commands C in Δ^{β}_{s+1} such that $Dest\,(C) = \alpha$;*
- $\Delta^{\beta S@\beta'}_{s+1}$ *be the set of statement commands C in Δ^{β}_{s+1} such that $Arg\,(C) = S@\beta'$;*
- $\Delta^{\beta H}_{s+1}$ *be the set of agent hierarchy commands in Δ^{β}_{s+1};*
- $\Delta^{\beta H@\alpha}_{s+1}$ *be the set of sub-agent hierarchy commands C in Δ^{β}_{s+1} such that $Arg\,(C) = \beta^j \rightarrow \beta^k@\alpha$;*
- $\Delta^{\beta M}_{s+1}$ *be the set of agent prevalence mode commands in Δ^{β}_{s+1};*
- $\Delta^{\beta M@\alpha}_{s+1}$ *be the set of sub-agent prevalence mode commands C in Δ^{β}_{s+1} such that $Arg\,(C) = \beta^j \overset{f}{\longleftrightarrow} \beta^k@\alpha$.*

The knowledge base at state $s+1$ is

$$\langle \mathcal{P}_{s+1}, \mathcal{SA}_{s+1}, \mathcal{H}_{s+1}, \mathcal{SH}_{s+1}, \mathcal{M}_{s+1}, \mathcal{SM}_{s+1}, \mathcal{IU}_{s+1} \rangle$$

where[5]*:*

Agent Hierarchy at state $s+1$:

$$\mathcal{H}_{s+1} = \Gamma_H \left(\mathcal{H}_s, \bigcup_{\beta \in \mathcal{SA}} \Delta^{\beta H}_{s+1}, s+1 \right)$$

The agent hierarchy at the next state is obtained, as before, starting from the previous agent hierarchy to which we add and remove the specified edges.

[5]As before, the knowledge state is only defined if every graph involved is a DAG.

Sub-Agent Hierarchy at state $s+1$: $\mathcal{SH}_{s+1} = \left\{SD_{\alpha_{s+1}} : \alpha \in \mathcal{A}\right\}$ *where*

$$SD_{\alpha_{s+1}} = \Gamma_H \left(SD_{\alpha_s}, \bigcup_{\beta \in \mathcal{SA}} \Delta_{s+1}^{\beta H@\alpha}, s+1 \right)$$

The sub-agent hierarchy at the next state is the set of all individual hierarchies, one for each agent, each obtained as for the case of the general agent hierarchy.

Agent Evolution Mode at state $s+1$:

$$\mathcal{M}_{s+1} = \Gamma_M \left(\mathcal{M}_s, \bigcup_{\beta \in \mathcal{SA}} \Delta_{s+1}^{\beta M}, s+1 \right)$$

The agent evolution mode at the next state is obtained, as before, starting from the previous agent evolution mode to which we add and remove the newly specified prevalence modes.

Sub-Agent Evolution Mode at state $s+1$: $\mathcal{SM}_{s+1} = \left\{\mathcal{SM}_{s+1}^{\alpha} : \alpha \in \mathcal{A}\right\}$ *where*

$$\mathcal{SM}_{s+1}^{\alpha} = \Gamma_M \left(\mathcal{SM}_s^{\alpha}, \bigcup_{\beta \in \mathcal{SA}} \Delta_{s+1}^{\beta M@\alpha}, s+1 \right)$$

As for the sub-agent hierarchy, the sub-agent evolution mode is the set of all individual evolution modes, one for each agent, each obtained as for the case of the general agent evolution mode.

Sub-Agent Programs at $s+1$: $\mathcal{SA}_{s+1} = \left\{SU_{s+1}^{\beta} : \beta \in \mathcal{SA}\right\}$ *where*

$$SU_{s+1}^{\beta} = \Gamma_S \left(\Delta_{s+1}^{\beta}, \Lambda_{s+1}^{\beta} \right)$$

and where $\Lambda_{s+1}^{\beta} = SU_s^{\beta} \cup EU_{s+1}^{\beta} \cup \left(\bigcup_{\beta' \in \mathcal{SA}, \beta' \neq \beta} \mathcal{IU}_s^{\beta} \right)$. *The sub-agent programs, one for each sub-agent, which correspond to the self updates of the previous sections, are obtained in a similar manner as before.*

Internal Updates at state $s+1$: $\mathcal{IU}_{s+1} = \left\{\mathcal{IU}_{s+1}^{\beta} : \beta \in \mathcal{SA}\right\}$ *where*

$$\mathcal{IU}_{s+1}^{\beta} = \left\{ IU_{s+1}^{\beta',\beta} : \beta', \beta \in \mathcal{SA}, \beta' \neq \beta \right\}$$

and where $IU_s^{\beta',\beta}$ *is defined as:*

$$IU_s^{\beta',\beta} = \left\{ S : \textbf{assert}\,(S@\beta) \in \Delta_{s+1}^{\beta' S@\beta} \right\}$$

The internal updates from sub-agent β' *to sub-agent* β *are simply the set of all statements* S *such that sub-agent* β' *executed a command of the form* **assert** $(S@\beta)$.

Object Knowledge Base at state $s+1$: $\mathcal{P}_{s+1} = \left(\mathcal{P}_{D_{s+1}}, D_{s+1}\right)$ *where* $D_{s+1} = (V_{s+1}, E_{s+1})$ *is a* DAG *and* $\mathcal{P}_{D_{s+1}} = \mathcal{P}_{D_s} \cup \left\{ P_{\beta_{s+1}^{\alpha}} : \beta \in \mathcal{SA}, \alpha \in \mathcal{A} \right\}$, *such that:*

$$V_{s+1} = V_s \cup \left\{ \alpha_{s+1}^{+}, \alpha_{s+1}^{-}, \beta_{s+1}^{\alpha} : \beta \in \mathcal{SA}, \alpha \in \mathcal{A} \right\}$$

The set of nodes of the previous state MDLP DAG is augmented with two nodes for each agent, α^+_{s+1} and α^-_{s+1}, corresponding to the sink and the source of each agent, and with a set of nodes β^α_{s+1} for each sub-agent β and each agent α.

$$\begin{aligned}E_{s+1} = E_s &\cup \left\{\left(\beta^\alpha_s, \beta^\alpha_{s+1}\right) : \beta \in \mathcal{SA}, \alpha \in \mathcal{A}\right\} \cup \left\{\left(\alpha^{j+}_{s+1}, \alpha^{k-}_{s+1}\right) : \left(\alpha^j, \alpha^k, \_\right) \in HE_{s+1}\right\} \cup \\ &\cup \left\{\left(\beta^{j\alpha}_{s+1}, \beta^{k\alpha}_{s+1}\right) : \left(\beta^j, \beta^k, \_\right) \in SAE_{\alpha_{s+1}}\right\} \cup \\ &\cup \Gamma^+_{PE}\left(\mathcal{H}_{s+1}, \mathcal{M}_{s+1}\right) \cup \left(\bigcup_{\alpha\in\mathcal{A}} \Gamma^+_{PE}\left(SD_{\alpha_{s+1}}, \mathcal{SM}^\alpha_{s+1}\right)\right) - \\ &- \Gamma^-_{PE}\left(\mathcal{H}_{s+1}, \mathcal{M}_{s+1}\right) - \left(\bigcup_{\alpha\in\mathcal{A}} \Gamma^-_{PE}\left(SD_{\alpha_{s+1}}, \mathcal{SM}^\alpha_{s+1}\right)\right)\end{aligned}$$

where $\Gamma^+_{PE}\left(\mathcal{H}_{s+1}, \mathcal{M}_{s+1}\right)$ and $\Gamma^-_{PE}\left(\mathcal{H}_{s+1}, \mathcal{M}_{s+1}\right)$ are as defined above, except that every edge $\left(\alpha^j_{s+1}, \alpha^k_{s+1}\right)$ is replaced by an edge $\left(\alpha^{j+}_{s+1}, \alpha^{k-}_{s+1}\right)$. The set of edges of the previous MDLP DAG is augmented with: edges of the form $\left(\beta^\alpha_s, \beta^\alpha_{s+1}\right)$ stating that sub-agents at state $s+1$, inside any agent, override themselves at state s; edges of the form $\left(\alpha^{j+}_{s+1}, \alpha^{k-}_{s+1}\right)$ encoding the agent hierarchy; edges of the form $\left(\beta^{j\alpha}_{s+1}, \beta^{k\alpha}_{s+1}\right)$ encoding the sub-agent hierarchies; the set of edges $\Gamma^+_{PE}\left(\mathcal{H}_{s+1}, \mathcal{M}_{s+1}\right)$ corresponding to the current agent evolution mode; and all the edges, for each agent, included $\Gamma^+_{PE}\left(SD_{\alpha_{s+1}}, \mathcal{SM}^\alpha_{s+1}\right)$ corresponding to the evolution modes of sub-agents inside each agent. Furthermore, the edges $\Gamma^-_{PE}\left(\mathcal{H}_{s+1}, \mathcal{M}_{s+1}\right)$ and all the edges, for each agent, included $\Gamma^+_{PE}\left(SD_{\alpha_{s+1}}, \mathcal{SM}^\alpha_{s+1}\right)$ corresponding to the evolution modes of agents and sub-agents inside each agent, respectively, are removed. Also,

$$P_{\beta^\alpha_{s+1}} = \Gamma_R\left(\Delta^{\beta R@\alpha}_{s+1}, s+1\right)$$

The programs associated with each sub-agent inside each agent are obtained in a similar manner as before.

As the reader may have noticed, a sub-agent may issue agent hierarchy commands that are mutually conflicting with those executed by another sub-agent. Consider a situation where sub-agent β executes the command **add_hierarchy_edge**($\alpha^j \to \alpha^k$), while at the same state transition sub-agent β' executes command **remove_hierarchy_edge**($\alpha^j \to \alpha^k$). Since the agent hierarchy is determined using the union of the executable hierarchy commands of all sub-agents, i.e.

$$\mathcal{H}_{s+1} = \Gamma_H\left(\mathcal{H}_s, \bigcup_{\beta\in\mathcal{SA}} \Delta^{\beta H}_{s+1}, s+1\right)$$

these two commands constitute a potential conflict. When we defined the operator Γ_H, we gave preference to the removal of hierarchy edges. This means that if two such commands are executed, the edge $\alpha^j \to \alpha^k$ will not belong to the agent hierarchy. Other options could have been endorsed here. The most obvious one would be to define yet two more hierarchies, between sub-agents, establishing their power in what concerns both agent hierarchy commands and prevalence mode commands. Then, based on such hierarchies, those conflicts could be resolved.

As before, the semantics of a $KABUL^+$ query is based on a direct semantics evaluation at the object level MDLP, as follows:

Definition 133 (*KABUL*$^+$ Semantics) *Let $\langle \mathcal{P}_s, \mathcal{SA}_s, \mathcal{H}_s, \mathcal{SH}_s, \mathcal{M}_s, \mathcal{SM}_s, \mathcal{IU}_s \rangle$ be a KB at state s. A query (where $q \leq s$)*

$$\mathbf{holds}\left(\begin{array}{c} L_1@\Theta^1, \ldots, L_k@\Theta^k, \mathbf{in}(R_1@\Theta^1), ..., \mathbf{in}(R_m@\Theta^m), \\ \mathbf{out}(R_{m+1}@\Theta^{m+1}), ..., \mathbf{out}(R_n@\Theta^n) \end{array}\right) \mathbf{at}\ q\ ?$$

is true iff

$$\begin{array}{c} \bigoplus_{\{\alpha_q^{j+}:\alpha^j\in\Theta^1\}} \mathcal{P}_s \models_{sm} L_1 \wedge ... \wedge \bigoplus_{\{\alpha_q^{j+}:\alpha^j\in\Theta^k\}} \mathcal{P}_s \models_{sm} L_k \wedge \\ \wedge \bigoplus_{\{\alpha_q^{j+}:\alpha^j\in\Theta^l\}} \mathcal{P}_s \models_{sm} N(R_1) \wedge ... \wedge \bigoplus_{\{\alpha_q^{j+}:\alpha^j\in\Theta^m\}} \mathcal{P}_s \models_{sm} N(R_1) \wedge \\ \wedge \bigoplus_{\{\alpha_q^{j+}:\alpha^j\in\Theta^{m+1}\}} \mathcal{P}_s \models_{sm} not\, N(R_{m+1}) \wedge ... \wedge \bigoplus_{\{\alpha_q^{j+}:\alpha^j\in\Theta^n\}} \mathcal{P}_s \models_{sm} not\, N(R_n) \end{array}$$

The *KABUL*$^+$ framework embeds all previously presented ones. It directly embeds *KABUL*^{m} if we consider only one sub-agent in *KABUL*$^+$, whose program is the self-update in *KABUL*^{m}. All other results follow. We have:

Theorem 100 KABUL$^+$ *embeds* KABUL^m, KABUL, DLP, MDLP, *interpretation updates [157] and logic programs under the stable model semantics.*

7.5 Summary and Open Issues

In this Chapter we have presented *KABUL*$^+$. This last piece of the puzzle, which embeds all previously introduced ones, allows the specification, with a precise semantical characterization, of rather elaborate *Evolving Knowledge Bases* including features like the abilities to:

- combine knowledge from different sources;
- specify external updates to the knowledge of each individual source;
- relate the sources of knowledge according to elaborate precedence relations;
- update such precedence relations;
- specify and update the evolution of such precedence relations;
- specify and update the internal behaviour of the knowledge base;
- access and reason about external observations;
- specify multiple entities (sub-agents), within an evolving knowledge base, each independently carrying out part of the internal behaviour;
- specify and update precedence relations among such sub-agents;

In the next Chapter we proffer two illustrative examples. The first explores the applicability of the language to model a dynamic financial advisory system. The second explores the applicability of *KABUL*$^+$ in the context of agent systems. We will leave any further comments and open issues to the final Chapter, right after the illustrative examples.

Chapter 8

Illustrative Examples

In this Chapter, we present two applications of the framework presented, rather more elaborate than the examples presented throughout. The first concerns the modelling of a financial advisory knowledge base which combines the advice with provenance from different advisors, together with stock market data, to produce stock recommendations. The second concerns the use of KABUL *as the basis for representing agents' epistemic states. Parts of this Chapter appeared in [135, 138].*

8.1 A Dynamic Knowledge Base for Stock Ratings

8.1.1 Scenario Overview

Let us consider a financial advisory company. One of the primary goals of one such financial advisory companies is to rate shares in the stock market in what concerns their potential for investment. Such ratings are usually given as an advice, for each stock, to either buy, hold or sell.

To perform the evaluation of stock potential, several models of the market exist, leading to several evaluation methods, such as for example the *technical analysis* and the *fundamental analysis*, among many others. Such methods differ from one another mainly due to the underlying model employed, leading thus to prediction rules that are based on different characteristics of shares and market.

The *fundamental analysis* typically focuses on key statistics in a company's financial statements. From these statements a number of useful ratios can be calculated. The ratios fall under five main categories: profitability (e.g. Net Profit Margin), price (e.g. Book Value Per Share and Price/Earnings Ratio), liquidity (e.g. Current Ratio), leverage (e.g. Debt Ratio), and efficiency (e.g. Inventory Turnover). After determining the condition and outlook of the company, together with some factors rating the economy and the industry sector, the fundamental analyst is prepared to determine if the company's stock is overvalued, undervalued, or correctly valued. To learn more about the fundamental analysis we recommend the book [53].

Technical analysis is the process of analyzing a security's historical prices in an effort to determine probable future prices. This is done by comparing current price action (i.e., current expectations) with comparable historical price action to predict a reasonable outcome. Technical analysis is based almost entirely on the analysis of price (e.g. open, high, low, close, etc.) and volume. These simple fields are used to create literally hundreds of indicators that study price relationships, trends, patterns, etc. (e.g. Moving Average, Moving Average Convergence Divergence, Commodity Channel Index, Accumulation/Distribution, etc.). By analyzing such indicators, the technical analyst is prepared to determine if the company's stock price will rise, fall, or maintain. To learn more about the technical analysis we recommend the book [74].

It is important to stress that no one such method is guaranteed: each performs better under certain situations. Furthermore, each method is not static and is constantly evolving in the sense that the set of rules that serves as the basis to evaluate the fundamental values and technical factors change as more research is done and the market evolves. Note that since most of these techniques are available to the public, their widespread use affects the market itself, causing its behaviour to change, i.e. we are in the presence of an evolving scenario amenable to description by updates.

Since the primary goal of the company is (should be) to issue correct stock ratings, any available information is useful, such as for example (illegal) insider information.

In this example we show how to use $KABUL^m$ to represent such a financial advisory company, with special emphasis on how to represent and combine knowledge obtained by the different methods of rating stocks. The model adopted is a very simple and naive view of how things actually work, merely for illustrative purposes. All the rules and values utilized do not have any relationship with those that constitute the technical and fundamental analysis. They are pure fiction, so please do not try this at home!

8.1.2 Knowledge Base Specification

In this example, we consider three distinct ways to rate stock: based on the *technical analysis* (*TA*), based on fundamental analysis (*FA*), and based on insider information (*II*). To further simplify this example, we consider that all the values and indicators used by all analysts are determined outside the knowledge base and entered as external observations, just as stock prices, index values, etc. With the simple rules provided by these three entities, together with the data obtained from the stock market (share prices, indexes, etc), the company has to combine all such information to obtain share ratings. Since the rules provided by the several sources may be different for each share, the company must assign preference to the information incoming from each of them. For illustrative purposes, we assume that the company perceives that the technical analysis performs better when the market trend is *bull* (bull is the word used to describe a market with an upward trend), the fundamental analysis performs better when the market is *bear* (bear is the word used to describe a market with a downward trend), and that the insider information should be treated as the information from the technical analysis. We also consider another trend value, *trade*, describing a market which is neither *bull* nor *bear*. The market trend will also be an external observation.

In our example, for illustrative purposes, we consider three basic types of data that is received form the environment:

Volatile By this kind of data we mean all those values that change at every tick of the clock, and whose value we do not want to keep for future use. In this kind of data we include the share prices (note that although past share prices are needed to determine some important values, by assuming that such values are determined outside, we can discard such past share prices). We use atoms of the form $price\,(StockName, Value)$ to represent share prices;

Non-Volatile By this kind of data we mean all those indicators, representing stock and industry characteristics, that should be kept until a new value is determined, which replaces the previous one. Among these are the indicators needed for the technical and fundamental analysis. We use atoms of the form $char\,(CharName, Name, Value)$ to represent the value $Value$ of the characteristic $CharName$, of stock or industry $Name$ (either $Stockname$ or $Industryname$) observed from the environment. Since this information is stored in the knowledge base for an undetermined period of time, we assert atoms that also refer to the time at which they were first determined. To this purpose, we use atoms of the form $char\,(CharName, Name, Value, Time)$. Of non-volatile nature will also be considered the atoms that represent the trend of the market: $trend\,(bull)$, $trend\,(bear)$ and $trend\,(trade)$ as observations and $trend\,(bull, Time)$, $trend\,(bear, Time)$ and $trend\,(trade, Time)$ as the atoms to be asserted.

Historical By this kind of data we mean all those values that we wish to keep to perform some sort of historical analysis. For illustrative purposes, in this example we only consider market indexes, such as the Nasdaq and Dow Jones, as data of this sort. The observed atoms are of the form $index\,(IndexName, Value)$ and the asserted atoms of the form $index\,(IndexName, Value, Time)$.

In this example we consider some names of stocks (e.g. msf, $intl$, son, tel, edp, $epal$...), names of industries (e.g. $comm$, tmt,...) names of indexes (e.g. dow, $nasdaq$, $psi20$, ...), names of characteristics (e.g. ma, $macd$, cci, ...), and integers for the values and time. The stock ratings are represented by atoms of the form: $buy(StockName)$, $sell(StockName)$ and $hold(StockName)$.

There follows examples of atoms in the language, together with their meaning:

- $char\,(ma, son, 23, 7)$: at time 7, the moving average (ma) for Sonae SGPS (son) is 23;
- $price\,(intl, 48)$: the latest price for Intel ($intl$) is 48;
- $index\,(nasdaq, 3465, 8)$: at time 8, the value of the Nasdaq ($nasdaq$) index is 3465;
- $trend\,(bull)$: the market trend is Bull ($bull$);
- $hold(son)$: the advice is to hold Sonae SGPS stock;
- $char\,(ma, tmt, 34, 9)$: at time 9, the moving average (ma) for the TMT (Technology, Media and Telecommunications) industry sector (tmt) is 27;

The knowledge base contains some atoms that will not change, representing the associations between the various stocks and their corresponding industries. Such atoms have the form $type\,(Stockname, IndustryName)$. Examples are $type\,(msn, tmt)$ and $type\,(intl, tmt)$, representing the facts that both Microsoft and Intel belong to the TMT industry sector, and $type\,(edp, comm)$ and $type\,(epal, comm)$, representing the facts that both EDP and EPAL belong to the commodities industry sector.

In what concerns the agents involved in the scenario, we have one agent representing the advisory company (*cmpny*), one agent representing the stock market (*mrkt*), one agent representing the technical analysis (*ta*), one agent representing the fundamental analysis (fa) and one agent representing the insider information (*ii*). To represent these entities we use the set of agents:

$$\mathcal{A} = \{cmpny, mrkt, ta, fa, ii\}$$

The agents *ta*, fa and *ii* contain the information obtained by the corresponding source, and we dub them *rating agents.* The agent *mrkt* contains the information obtained from the Stock Market (including all the values and characteristics determined outside our system, that in real life might not be related to the stock market). The agent *cmpny* contains all remaining information.

Before we specify the hierarchy that relates these agents, we define what and how information can be received from the environment. The knowledge base will be able to perceive raw data from the Stock Market, i.e. share prices and indexes and indirect information referring to stock characteristics and the market trend. Accordingly, we assume that environment observations are simply atoms of the form $index\,(IndexName, Value)$, $price\,(StockName, Value)$, $trend(MarketType)$ and $char\,(CharName, StockName, Value)$.

The first two figures one must keep track of when dealing with the stock market is the price of the shares and the several indexes that reflect the behaviour of the market. The stock market indexes, like the NASDAQ and the DOW JONES, represent the overall price of specific portfolios, providing valuable information as to the overall behaviour of the market, which can be obtained not only from its current values but also from their fluctuations. It is therefore important to keep track of such indexes over time. To this purpose, we store the value of every observed index, referenced by the time at which such value held. If the external observations are atoms of the form $index\,(IndexName, Value)$, we assert atoms of the form $index\,(IndexName, Value, Time)$. For this, we use the following simple persistent assertion statement:

$$\textbf{always\_assert}\,(index\,(N, V, T)\,@mrkt) \Leftarrow time\,(T)\,, \mathbf{E} : index\,(N, V)$$

Of course, one must keep track of prices for individual shares, represented by atoms of the form $price\,(StockName, Value)$. As we have mentioned before, even though from the historical sequence of such prices one can obtain valuable characteristics with respect to the evolution of shares, such as the *rate of valuation*, etc., for illustrative purposes we assume that these and other characteristics of stock are determined from outside our knowledge base and observable. This way, we can deal with stock prices as values that we do not retain i.e. we are only interested in their current value, whose assertion is thus performed by the non-inertial statement:

$$\textbf{always\_assert\_event}\,(price\,(S, V)\,@mrkt) \Leftarrow \mathbf{E} : price\,(S, V)$$

In what concerns the stock characteristics, since we do not know when these will be determined (observed), and every time a new value for some such characteristic is determined we want to remove the previous one, we resort to the following pair of statements, that precisely achieves such a replacement:

$$\textbf{always\_assert}\,(char\,(N, S, V, T)\,@mrkt) \Leftarrow time\,(T)\,, \mathbf{E} : char\,(N, S, V)$$
$$\textbf{always\_retract}\,(char\,(N, S, V', T')\,@mrkt) \Leftarrow \textbf{assert}\,(char\,(N, S, V, T)\,@mrkt)\,, \mathbf{R} : \textbf{in}\,(char\,(N, S, V', T'))\,@mrkt$$

Mark the need for the rule condition $\textbf{in}\,(char\,(N, S, V', T')\,@mrkt)$ in the second statement, to ensure that we retract the correct previously asserted characteristic (for the same name and stock). In what concerns the market trend, since there cannot be two simultaneously trends of the market, at least in our simplified example, the assertion of one trend must imply the removal of the other. This is achieved by the two statements (where again we index the atoms with time).

$$\begin{aligned}\textbf{always\_assert}\,(trend\,(X,T)\,@mrkt) &\Leftarrow not\,trend\,(X,\_)\,, time\,(T)\,, \mathbf{E} : trend\,(X)\\ \textbf{always\_retract}\,(trend\,(X,T)\,@mrkt) &\Leftarrow \textbf{assert}\,(trend\,(Y,\_)\,@mrkt)\,,\\ &\quad\ \mathbf{R} : \textbf{in}\,(trend\,(X,T))\,@mrkt\end{aligned}$$

The atoms of the form $time\,(T)$, used in previous statements, are updated with the following two statements. We use the agent *cmpny* to store these values.

$$\begin{gathered}\textbf{assert\_event}\,(time\,(1)\,@cmpny) \Leftarrow\\ \textbf{always\_assert\_event}\,(time\,(X+1)\,@cmpny) \Leftarrow time\,(X)\end{gathered}$$

Note that the statements used to represent this scenario are just one of many possible ways to encode it. Often we do not presented the simplest encoding, mainly for illustrative purposes, this being the main goal of this example.

We now turn to the hierarchical relations between all these agents. To start with, we have the company prevail over every rating agent. It seems rather natural to allow for the company to have the final saying with respect to any advice, i.e. the advice provided by the rating agents can be overridden by the company itself. In what concerns the relationship between the company and the agent representing the market, they will be unrelated: it doesn't make much sense to override stock prices for example. Of course one may say that the company could have its own view of the stock market trend and that this view should prevail over the externally observed one. If we wish to encode such a situation where the agent *mrkt* contains two kinds of rules, some overridable and some not, we would have to split such an agent in two and establish the relationships accordingly. In this example, to keep things simple, we will consider the market as an unrelated agent. These relationships with the company are set by the following non-persistent statements:

$$\begin{gathered}\textbf{add\_hierarchy\_edge}\,(ta \rightarrow cmpny) \Leftarrow\\ \textbf{add\_hierarchy\_edge}\,(fa \rightarrow cmpny) \Leftarrow\\ \textbf{add\_hierarchy\_edge}\,(ii \rightarrow cmpny) \Leftarrow\end{gathered}$$

In what concerns the hierarchy between the *ta* and *fa* rating agents, as we have mentioned before, it will depend on the market trend. We wish the technical analysis to prevail over the fundamental analysis when the market becomes *bull*, achieved by the following persistent statement:

$$\textbf{always\_add\_hierarchy\_edge}\,(fa \rightarrow ta) \Leftarrow not\,trend\,(bull,\_)\,, \mathbf{E} : trend\,(bull)$$

We want the fundamental analysis to prevail over the technical analysis when the market becomes *bear*, enforced by the statement:

$$\textbf{always\_add\_hierarchy\_edge}\,(ta \rightarrow fa) \Leftarrow not\,trend\,(bear,\_)\,, \mathbf{E} : trend\,(bear)$$

When the market is *trade*, we want fa and ta agents to be considered as equal. This is assured by the statements:

$$\textbf{always\_remove\_hierarchy\_edge}\,(fa \to ta) \Leftarrow trend\,(bull, \_)\,, \mathbf{E} : trend\,(trade)$$
$$\textbf{always\_remove\_hierarchy\_edge}\,(ta \to fa) \Leftarrow trend\,(bear, \_)\,, \mathbf{E} : trend\,(trade)$$

In any kind of market, we wish the insider information to prevail over the other two sources. This is ensured by the non-persistent statements:

$$\textbf{add\_hierarchy\_edge}\,(fa \to ii) \Leftarrow$$
$$\textbf{add\_hierarchy\_edge}\,(ta \to ii) \Leftarrow$$

In the previous statements, besides the conditions on the environment observations there is a condition for the current market trend. Its purpose is to have the statement executed only if the market trend actually changes. In this example, the overall semantics would be the same if such condition was not present, but we would be unnecessarily executing one of such statements every time a market trend was observed, even though no change occurred.

Of course, when we add one such hierarchy edge, we must remove any existing opposite ones. This is guaranteed by the statement:

$$\textbf{always\_remove\_hierarchy\_edge}\left(\alpha^j \to \alpha^k\right) \Leftarrow \textbf{add\_hierarchy\_edge}\left(\alpha^k \to \alpha^j\right)$$

We now have to define the prevalence modes between the different agents. We define two simple prevalence mode functions that combine the time prevalence and hierarchy prevalence modes with a reset to the current mode, i.e. if the relationship between two agents was set to time prevalence mode and is, at some point, changed to hierarchy prevalence mode, we want to change the past as if it had always been set to this mode, and vice versa.

Such modified time prevalence function is defined as follows:

$$\begin{aligned} f_{tp^*}\left(\alpha^j, \alpha^k, \_, s, \_, \_\right) = {} & \left\{+(\alpha^j_{p-1}, \alpha^k_p), +(\alpha^k_{p-1}, \alpha^j_p) : 0 < p \leq s\right\} \cup \\ & \cup \left\{-\left(\alpha^j_n, \alpha^k_m\right), -\left(\alpha^k_n, \alpha^j_m\right), 0 \leq n < s, 0 \leq m < s\right\} - \\ & - \left\{-(\alpha^j_{p-1}, \alpha^k_p), -(\alpha^k_{p-1}, \alpha^j_p) : 0 < p < s\right\} \end{aligned}$$

and the hierarchy prevalence function is defined below (to define this function we are using the result according to which the MDLP semantics is preserved with any transitive closures and reductions of the MDLP DAG, this being the reason why only one edge is set at each state):

$$\begin{aligned} f_{hp^*}\left(\alpha^j, \alpha^k, <, s, \_, \_\right) = {} & \{+\left(\alpha^j_s, \alpha^k_0\right)\} \cup \\ & \cup \left\{-\left(\alpha^j_n, \alpha^k_m\right), -\left(\alpha^k_n, \alpha^j_m\right), 0 \leq n < s, 0 \leq m < s\right\} \\ f_{hp^*}\left(\alpha^j, \alpha^k, \|, s, \_, \_\right) = {} & \{\} \end{aligned}$$

These two prevalence modes are utilized to relate the various agents. In what concerns the relationship between the company and all the rating agents, we set it to the hierarchical prevalence mode to encode the fact that, no matter what, company policy always prevails. This is enacted by the initial prevalence mode statements:

$$\textbf{add\_prevail\_mode}\left(ii \overset{f_{hp^*}}{\longleftrightarrow} cmpny\right) \Leftarrow$$

$$\textbf{add\_prevail\_mode}\left(fa \overset{f_{hp^*}}{\longleftrightarrow} cmpny\right) \Leftarrow$$

$$\textbf{add\_prevail\_mode}\left(ta \overset{f_{hp^*}}{\longleftrightarrow} cmpny\right) \Leftarrow$$

Since the rating agents and the one representing the stock market do not have rules for the same atoms, there is no need to establish neither a hierarchy relation nor a prevalence mode between them. Concerning the prevalence modes between the rating agents, we set it to the hierarchy prevalence mode between the insider information and each of ta and fa, specified by the statements:

$$\textbf{add\_prevail\_mode}\left(ii \overset{f_{hp^*}}{\longleftrightarrow} ta\right) \Leftarrow$$

$$\textbf{add\_prevail\_mode}\left(ii \overset{f_{hp^*}}{\longleftrightarrow} fa\right) \Leftarrow$$

Concerning the prevalence modes between the technical analysis and the fundamental analysis, they depend on the current trend of the market, coinciding with their hierarchical relationship. As a result, initially we set this prevalence mode to the time prevailing mode, induced by the statement:

$$\textbf{add\_prevail\_mode}\left(fa \overset{f_{tp^*}}{\longleftrightarrow} ta\right) \Leftarrow$$

Then we specify the changes in prevalence modes between these two agents to become hierarchy prevailing whenever some hierarchy relation is set between them, and time prevailing when the hierarchy relation is removed. Accordingly, such prevalence settings will be specified by the persistent statements:

$$\textbf{always\_add\_prevail\_mode}\left(fa \overset{f_{hp^*}}{\longleftrightarrow} ta\right) \Leftarrow not\, trend\,(bear, \_)\,, \mathbf{E} : trend\,(bear)$$

$$\textbf{always\_add\_prevail\_mode}\left(fa \overset{f_{hp^*}}{\longleftrightarrow} ta\right) \Leftarrow not\, trend\,(bull, \_)\,, \mathbf{E} : trend\,(bull)$$

$$\textbf{always\_add\_prevail\_mode}\left(fa \overset{f_{tp^*}}{\longleftrightarrow} ta\right) \Leftarrow not\, trend\,(trade, \_)\,, \mathbf{E} : trend\,(trade)$$

$$\textbf{always\_remove\_prevail\_mode}\left(fa \overset{f_{hp^*}}{\longleftrightarrow} ta\right) \Leftarrow \textbf{add\_prevail\_mode}\left(fa \overset{f_{tp^*}}{\longleftrightarrow} ta\right)$$

$$\textbf{always\_remove\_prevail\_mode}\left(fa \overset{f_{tp^*}}{\longleftrightarrow} ta\right) \Leftarrow \textbf{add\_prevail\_mode}\left(fa \overset{f_{hp^*}}{\longleftrightarrow} ta\right)$$

Before we show the assertion of some rules to determine stock ratings, we show how the MDLP DAG looks like according to the market trend. With this purpose, we first consider the external update EU_1 containing a statement $\textbf{assert}\,(S) \Leftarrow$ for each of the above specified statements (S). Then we consider the knowledge state $\langle \mathcal{P}_s, SU_s, \mathcal{H}_s, \mathcal{M}_s\rangle = \langle EU_1, EO_1\rangle \otimes ... \otimes \langle EU_i, EO_i\rangle \otimes ... \otimes \langle EU_s, EO_s\rangle$ $(1 < i \leq s)$, such that $EU_j = \{\}$ for all $1 < j \leq s$. Now, according to the market trend, defined by the

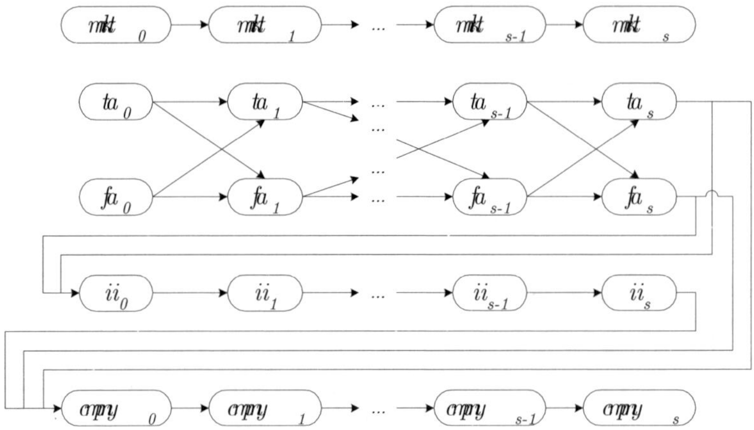

Figure 8.1: Trade Market

external observations, we show the MDLP DAG as well as some other characteristics of the knowledge state $\langle \mathcal{P}_s, SU_s, \mathcal{H}_s, \mathcal{M}_s \rangle$ (where $\mathcal{P}_s = (\mathcal{P}_{D_s}, D_s)$, $\mathcal{H}_s = (\mathcal{A}, HE_s)$, $D_s = (V_s, E_s)$):

Trade market: This situation occurs after $trend\,(trade)$ is observed, and before any other $trend\,(bull)$ or $trend\,(bear)$ is observed, i.e. $EO_i = \{trend\,(trade)\}$ and $EO_j = \{\}$ for all $1 < j \leq s, j \neq i$. There follow some characteristics of this knowledge state (whose MDLP DAG D_s is depicted in Figure 8.1):

$$\textbf{holds}\,(not\,trend\,(bear, \_)\,, not\,trend\,(bull, \_)\,, trend\,(trade, i))\ \textbf{at}\ s\ ?\ \text{is true}$$

$$HE_s = \{(ii, cmpny, 1)\,, (fa, cmpny, 1)\,, (ta, cmpny, 1)\,, (ta, ii, 1)\,, (fa, ii, 1)\}$$

$$\mathcal{M}_s = \left\{ \begin{array}{c} (\{ii, cmpny\}\,, f_{hp^*}, 1)\,, (\{fa, cmpny\}\,, f_{hp^*}, 1)\,, (\{ta, cmpny\}\,, f_{hp^*}, 1)\,, \\ (\{ii, fa\}\,, f_{hp^*}, 1)\,, (\{ii, ta\}\,, f_{hp^*}, 1)\,, (\{ta, fa\}\,, f_{tp^*}, i) \end{array} \right\}$$

$$V_s = \{\alpha_i : 0 \leq i \leq s, \alpha \in \mathcal{A}\}$$

$$\begin{aligned} E_s = {} & \{(\alpha_i, \alpha_{i+1}) : 0 \leq i < s, \alpha \in \mathcal{A}\} \cup \\ & \cup \{+(fa_j, ta_{j+1}), +(ta_j, fa_{j+1}) : 0 \leq j < s\} \cup \\ & \cup \{(ii_s, cmpny_0)\,, (fa_s, cmpny_0)\,, (ta_s, cmpny_0)\,, (fa_s, ii_0)\,, (ta_s, ii_0)\} \end{aligned}$$

Bull market: This situation occurs after $trend\,(bull)$ is observed, and before the observation of any other $trend\,(trade)$ or $trend\,(bear)$, i.e. $EO_i = \{trend\,(bull)\}$ and $EO_j = \{\}$ for all $1 < j \leq s, j \neq i$. There follow some characteristics of this knowledge state (whose MDLP DAG D_s is depicted in Figure 8.2):

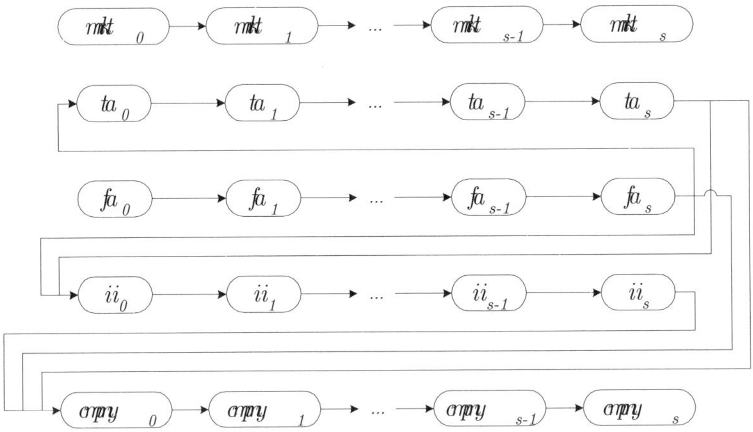

Figure 8.2: Bull Market

holds $(not\, trend\,(bear, \_)\,, trend\,(bull, i)\,, not\, trend\,(trade, \_))$ **at** s ? is true

$$HE_s = \left\{ \begin{array}{c} (ii, cmpny, 1)\,, (fa, cmpny, 1)\,, (ta, cmpny, 1)\,, \\ (ta, ii, 1)\,, (fa, ii, 1)\,, (fa, ta, i) \end{array} \right\}$$

$$\mathcal{M}_s = \left\{ \begin{array}{c} (\{ii, cmpny\}\,, f_{hp^*}, 1)\,, (\{fa, cmpny\}\,, f_{hp^*}, 1)\,, (\{ta, cmpny\}\,, f_{hp^*}, 1)\,, \\ (\{ii, ta\}\,, f_{hp^*}, 1)\,, (\{ii, fa\}\,, f_{hp^*}, 1)\,, (\{ta, fa\}\,, f_{hp^*}, i) \end{array} \right\}$$

$$V_s = \{\alpha_i : 0 \leq i \leq s, \alpha \in \mathcal{A}\}$$

$$E_s = \{(\alpha_i, \alpha_{i+1}) : 0 \leq i < s, \alpha \in \mathcal{A}\} \cup$$

$$\cup \left\{ \begin{array}{c} (ii_s, cmpny_0)\,, (fa_s, cmpny_0)\,, (ta_s, cmpny_0)\,, \\ (fa_s, ii_0)\,, (ta_s, ii_0)\,, (fa_s, ta_0) \end{array} \right\}$$

Bear market: This situation occurs after $trend\,(bear)$ is observed, and before the observation of any other $trend\,(trade)$ or $trend\,(bull)$, i.e. $EO_i = \{trend\,(bear)\}$ and $EO_j = \{\}$ for all $1 < j \leq s, j \neq i$. There follow some characteristics of this knowledge state (whose MDLP DAG D_s is depicted in Figure 8.3):

holds $(trend\,(bear, i)\,, not\, trend\,(bull, \_)\,, not\, trend\,(trade, \_))$ **at** s ? is true

$$HE_s = \left\{ \begin{array}{c} (ii, cmpny, 1)\,, (fa, cmpny, 1)\,, (ta, cmpny, 1)\,, \\ (ta, ii, 1)\,, (fa, ii, 1)\,, (ta, fa, i) \end{array} \right\}$$

$$\mathcal{M}_s = \left\{ \begin{array}{c} (\{ii, cmpny\}\,, f_{hp^*}, 1)\,, (\{fa, cmpny\}\,, f_{hp^*}, 1)\,, (\{ta, cmpny\}\,, f_{hp^*}, 1)\,, \\ (\{ii, ta\}\,, f_{hp^*}, 1)\,, (\{ii, fa\}\,, f_{hp^*}, 1)\,, (\{ta, fa\}\,, f_{hp^*}, i) \end{array} \right\}$$

$$V_s = \{\alpha_i : 0 \leq i \leq s, \alpha \in \mathcal{A}\}$$

$$E_s = \{(\alpha_i, \alpha_{i+1}) : 0 \leq i < s, \alpha \in \mathcal{A}\} \cup$$

$$\cup \left\{ \begin{array}{c} (ii_s, cmpny_0)\,, (fa_s, cmpny_0)\,, (ta_s, cmpny_0)\,, \\ (fa_s, ii_0)\,, (ta_s, ii_0)\,, (ta_s, fa_0) \end{array} \right\}$$

No market type: This situation occurs at the beginning, before the first observation regarding the market trend, i.e. $EO_j = \{\}$ for all $1 \leq j \leq s$. This knowledge state is in all respects similar to the flat market situation (depicted in Figure 8.1)

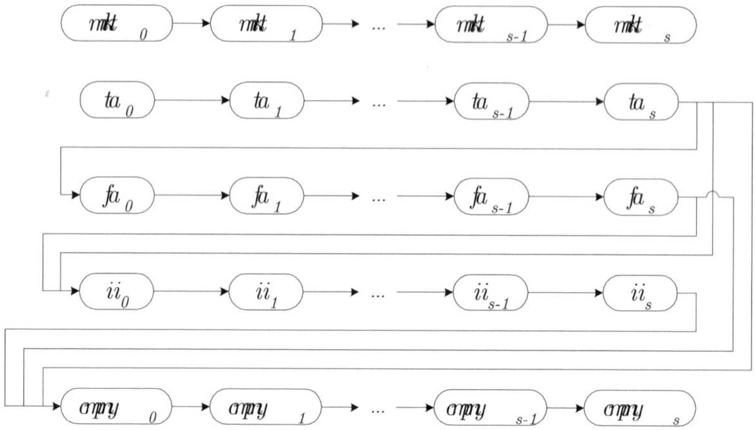

Figure 8.3: Bear Market

except that:

$$\textbf{holds}\left(not\,trend\left(bear,\_\right), not\,trend\left(bull,\_\right), trend\left(trade,i\right)\right) \textbf{ at } s \text{ ? is false}$$
$$\textbf{holds}\left(not\,trend\left(bear,\_\right), not\,trend\left(bull,\_\right), not\,trend\left(trade,\_\right)\right) \textbf{ at } s \text{ ? is true}$$

8.1.3 Knowledge Base Evolution

We now illustrate the evolution of the system, with some sequences of external observations and external updates representing the rating rules issued by the market researchers.

$t = 1$ The knowledge base starts with the initial state $\langle \mathcal{P}_0, SU_0, \mathcal{H}_0, \mathcal{M}_0 \rangle$ and we first consider the external update EU_1 containing a statement $\textbf{assert}\,(S) \Leftarrow$ for each of the above specified statements (S). Furthermore, included in this first external update we also have other statements which we now describe.

First of all, in order to properly perform the kinds of reasoning in the fundamental analysis, we need to establish the relationships between the several stock and the corresponding industry sectors. These will be one time assertions that remain constant throughout, unless of course the companies represented by the stock change their line of business, something that will not happen in this example but would nevertheless be trivial to accomplish in $KABUL^m$. Accordingly, we include in EU_1 the statements:

$$\textbf{assert}\left(type\left(msn, tmt\right)@mrkt\right) \Leftarrow$$
$$\textbf{assert}\left(type\left(intl, tmt\right)@mrkt\right) \Leftarrow$$
$$\textbf{assert}\left(type\left(son, tmt\right)@mrkt\right) \Leftarrow$$
$$\textbf{assert}\left(type\left(sonc, tmt\right)@mrkt\right) \Leftarrow$$
$$\textbf{assert}\left(type\left(telc, tmt\right)@mrkt\right) \Leftarrow$$
$$\textbf{assert}\left(type\left(edp, comm\right)@mrkt\right) \Leftarrow$$
$$\textbf{assert}\left(type\left(epal, comm\right)@mrkt\right) \Leftarrow$$

to the effect that stocks $msn, intl, son, sonc$ and $telc$ all belong to the TMT industry sector, and that stocks edp and $epal$ are commodities.

Also at this first state transition, the knowledge base is updated with the first rating rules of the technical analysis. These rules are:

$$\begin{aligned}buy(S) \leftarrow\ & char(ma, S, V_{ma}, \_), char(macd, S, V_{macd}, \_), not\, trend(trade, \_), \\ & price(S, V), V_{ma} > V, V_{macd} > 0\end{aligned}$$

$$\begin{aligned}hold(S) \leftarrow\ & char(ma, S, V_{ma}, \_), char(macd, S, V_{macd}, \_), not\, trend(trade, \_), \\ & price(S, V), V_{ma} < V, V_{macd} > -1\end{aligned}$$

$$sell(S) \leftarrow char(macd, S, V_{macd}, \_), not\, trend(trade, \_), V_{macd} < -1$$

$$\begin{aligned}sell(S) \leftarrow\ & char(cci, S, V_{cci}, \_), char(sgr, S, V_{sgr}, \_), trend(trade, \_), \\ & V_{cci} * V_{sgr} < -2, V_{cci} < 0\end{aligned}$$

$$\begin{aligned}buy(S) \leftarrow\ & char(cci, S, V_{cci}, \_), char(sgr, S, V_{sgr}, \_), trend(trade, \_), \\ & V_{cci} * V_{sgr} < -2, V_{sgr} < 0\end{aligned}$$

For example, the first rule says that some stock should be rated *buy* if the trend of the market is not *trade*, and the stock's Moving Average (ma) is higher than its current price and the Moving Average Convergence Divergence ($macd$) is greater than 0. The other rules have similar readings. Before we continue, we must add that each stock, at each state, should only have one rating (it makes no sense to recommend to both buy and sell the same stock). This indicates that each of these rules should in fact specify a set of conditions under which the corresponding rating should follow, but such conditions should also imply the negation of any other rating. If for example the TA rates some share as *buy*, and the FA rates this share as *sell*, and the market is *bull* (TA prevails over FA), then *sell* should not follow, i.e. under these circumstances the rule for *sell* of FA should be rejected. This is similar to what happens when we use strong negation where an atom $-a$ should override an atom a. For the case of extended logic programs, we used the notion of expanded program to deal with this issue. Here, we will use a similar notion according to which every time we specify some rule for a positive atom (*sell*, *buy* or *hold*), we add two rules with the same body but whose heads are the default negation of the other two atoms. In this example, we dub these extra rules *companion rules*. For example, when we assert the first rule above, we should also assert the two rules:

$$\begin{aligned}not\, sell(S) \leftarrow\ & char(ma, S, V_{ma}, \_), char(macd, S, V_{macd}, \_), not\, trend(trade, \_), \\ & price(S, V), V_{ma} > V, V_{macd} > 0\end{aligned}$$

$$\begin{aligned}not\, hold(S) \leftarrow\ & char(ma, S, V_{ma}, \_), char(macd, S, V_{macd}, \_), not\, trend(trade, \_), \\ & price(S, V), V_{ma} > V, V_{macd} > 0\end{aligned}$$

Accordingly, for each rule as above and its companion rules (r), we include in EU_1 the statement:

$$\textbf{assert}\,(r@ta) \Leftarrow$$

We also have an update with the first rating rules of the fundamental analysis. These rules are:

$$\begin{aligned} buy(S) \leftarrow & char(bvps, S, V_{bvps}, T_{bvps}), char(npm, S, V_{npm}, T_{npm}), \\ & char(per, S, V_{per}, T_{per}), char(npm, I, V_{inpm}, T_{inpm}), char(per, I, V_{iper}, T_{iper}), \\ & price(S, V), type(S, I), V_{bvps} > V, V_{npm} > V_{inpm}, V_{per} < V_{iper}, time(T), \\ & T_{bvps} > T-8, T_{npm} > T-8, T_{per} > T-8, T_{inpm} > T-8, T_{iper} > T-8 \end{aligned}$$

$$\begin{aligned} hold(S) \leftarrow & char(bvps, S, V_{bvps}, T_{bvps}), char(npm, S, V_{npm}, T_{npm}), \\ & char(per, S, V_{per}, T_{per}), char(npm, I, V_{inpm}, T_{inpm}), char(per, I, V_{iper}, T_{iper}), \\ & price(S, V), type(S, I), V_{bvps} > V, V_{npm} < V_{inpm}, V_{per} = V_{iper}, time(T), \\ & T_{bvps} > T-8, T_{npm} > T-8, T_{per} > T-8, T_{inpm} > T-8, T_{iper} > T-8 \end{aligned}$$

$$\begin{aligned} sell(S) \leftarrow & char(bvps, S, V_{bvps}, T_{bvps}), char(npm, S, V_{npm}, T_{npm}), \\ & char(per, S, V_{per}, T_{per}), char(npm, I, V_{inpm}, T_{inpm}), char(per, I, V_{iper}, T_{iper}), \\ & price(S, V), type(S, I), V_{bvps} < V, V_{npm} < V_{inpm}, V_{per} > V_{iper}, time(T), \\ & T_{bvps} > T-8, T_{npm} > T-8, T_{per} > T-8, T_{inpm} > T-8, T_{iper} > T-8 \end{aligned}$$

For example, the first rule states that some stock should be rated *buy* whenever the Book value Per Share is higher that the current stock price, and the Net Profit Margin of the stock is higher than the Net Profit Margin of the industry sector, and the Price/Earnings Ratio is lower than the Price/Earnings Ration of the industry sector, and all such used characteristics are recent (in our example more recent than 8 states). Consequently, for each rule as above and its companion rules (r), we include in EU_1 the following statement:

$$\textbf{assert}\,(r@fa) \Leftarrow$$

At this state transition there is no insider information.

We view this first state transition as a specification of the knowledge base, thus still not connected to the stock market. As a result, the external observation set is empty. We are now ready to start receiving data from the stock market, and of course any other updates to any of the agents involved.

$t = 2$ At this state transition we do not have any external updates i.e. $EU_2 = \{\}$. As for the external observations EO_2, they are summarized in the next table. It is important to stress that not every characteristic is observed at every state transition, and in this short running of the example not every characteristic is actually used by the rating rules.

$t=2$	*stock*					*market indexes*			*industry idx*	
bull	*msf*	*son*	*sonc*	*edp*	*epal*	*nasdaq*	*dow*	*psi20*	*tmt*	*comm*
ma	110	28	19	12	10	–	–	–	–	–
macd	1	−2	1	0	0	–	–	–	–	–
cci	1	−2	1	1	0	–	–	–	–	–
sgr	−1	3	−1	−1	0	–	–	–	–	–
price	100	27	18	13	10	3000	8000	7000	1000	1570
bvps	140	–	–	14	–	–	–	–	–	–
npm	22	–	–	18	–	–	–	–	20	17
per	2	–	–	1	–	–	–	–	3	2
yvar	–	–	–	–	2	–	–	–	–	–

To each entry in the table (different from $-$) there corresponds one atom in EO_2. For example the cell that contains the number 110 would correspond to an atom $char(ma, msf, 110)$ in EO_2. The entry 8000 would correspond to the atom $index(dow, 8000)$ in EO_2. Furthermore, the table also contains information about the trend of the market which, in this case, would correspond to an atom $trend(bull)$ in EO_2. For this first external observation input, unlike for subsequent ones where we only provide the table, we show the entire set of external observations:

$$\begin{aligned} EO_2 = \{ & char(macd, msf, 1), char(cci, msf, 1), char(per, msf, 2), price(msf, 100), \\ & char(ma, msf, 110), char(bvps, msf, 140), char(npm, msf, 22), \\ & char(sgr, msf, -1), char(ma, son, 28), char(macd, son, -2), \\ & char(cci, son, -2), char(sgr, son, 3), price(son, 27), char(ma, sonc, 19), \\ & char(macd, sonc, 1), char(cci, sonc, 1), char(sgr, sonc, -1), price(sonc, 18), \\ & char(ma, edp, 12), char(macd, edp, 0), char(cci, edp, 1), char(sgr, edp, -1), \\ & char(bvps, edp, 14), price(edp, 13), char(npm, edp, 18), char(per, edp, 1), \\ & char(ma, epal, 10), char(macd, epal, 0), price(epal, 10), char(cci, epal, 0), \\ & char(sgr, epal, 0), char(ivar, epal, 2), char(npm, tmt, 20), char(per, tmt, 3), \\ & char(npm, comm, 17), char(per, comm, 2), index(dow, 8000), \\ & index(psi20, 7000), index(tmt, 1000), index(comm, 1570), \\ & index(nasdaq, 3000), trend(bull)\} \end{aligned}$$

With this EU_2 and EO_2 we obtain the knowledge state $\langle \mathcal{P}_2, SU_2, \mathcal{H}_2, \mathcal{M}_2 \rangle$, and with it the stock ratings:

	msf	*son*	*sonc*	*edp*	*epal*
stock ratings	**buy**	**sell**	**buy**	**hold**	–

These stock ratings are obtained by determining the stable model semantics of $\mathcal{P}_2$. In particular, $\mathcal{P}_2$ has a single stable model M_2 and:

$$\begin{aligned} \{buy(msf), sell(son), buy(sonc), hold(edp)\} &\subset M_2 \\ sell(epal) &\notin M_2 \\ hold(epal) &\notin M_2 \\ buy(epal) &\notin M_2 \end{aligned}$$

Instead of presenting all the details of the knowledge state, we provide rather a brief informal explanation of the reason why these ratings were obtained. Since the market trend is *bull*, the MDLP DAG is the one depicted in Fig. 8.2 where *ta* hierarchically prevails over *fa*. In what concerns the rating for *son*, we have that it rates *sell* if we were to use the rules of *ta* and *fa* individually. Therefore such result also carries over to the overall semantics, i.e. no rules are rejected. In what concerns the rating of *epal*, there are no rules whose body is true so this stock is not rated. With respect to *sonc* stocks, the *ta* rates them as a *buy* and they are unrated by the *fa*, so no conflict arises. Same with respect to the *son* stocks which are rated *sell* by the *ta* and unrated by the *fa*. About *edp* stocks, they are rated *hold* by the *ta* and *buy* by the *fa*. But since there is a rule for $hold(edp)$ in *ta* with a true body, then there is also a (companion) rule for $not\,buy(edp)$ with the same true body. Since *ta* hierarchically prevails over *fa* in this *bull* market, the rule for $buy(edp)$ in *ta* is rejected by its companion rule, and thus the *hold* rating.

$t = 3$ At the subsequent state transition, the external update EU_3 is empty again, and we receive external observations summarized in the next table (with respect to the previous table, we have removed some characteristics for which there were no observed values):

$t = 3$			*stock*				*market indexes*			*industry indexes*
bull	*msf*	*son*	*sonc*	*edp*	*epal*	*nasdaq*	*dow*	*psi20*	*tmt*	*comm*
ma	120	27	18	12	11	–	–	–	–	–
macd	1.2	−2	0	0	0	–	–	–	–	–
cci	1	−3	1	1	0	–	–	–	–	–
sgr	−1	3	−1	−1	0	–	–	–	–	–
price	120	26	19	13	11	3200	8070	7100	1200	1560

With this EU_3 and EO_3 we obtain the knowledge state $\langle \mathcal{P}_3, SU_3, \mathcal{H}_3, \mathcal{M}_3 \rangle$ and with it the stock ratings:

	msf	*son*	*sonc*	*edp*	*epal*
stock ratings	**buy**	**sell**	**hold**	**hold**	–

From now on, we shall only explain the relevant changes with respect to the previous ratings. In this new state, the only major difference is the drop in *ma* and increase in price for *sonc*, causing its rating to drop from *buy* to *hold*. All other ratings remain the same, for the same reasons as before.

$t = 4$ At state 4, the technical analyst decided to update the way to rate stock, to be somehow more aggressive. Three new rules were issued, two for service in *bull* markets and one in *bear* markets. They are more aggressive because, for example, to rate stock *buy*, in a *bull* market, all that is required, according to this new rule, is that the Moving Average of some stock be higher than its stock price. The rules are:

$$\begin{aligned} sell\,(S) &\leftarrow char\,(macd, S, V_{macd}, \_)\,, trend\,(bear, \_)\,, V_{macd} < 0 \\ buy\,(S) &\leftarrow char\,(ma, S, V_{ma}, \_)\,, trend\,(bull, \_)\,, price\,(S, V)\,, V_{ma} > V \\ not\ sell\,(S) &\leftarrow char\,(macd, S, V_{macd}, \_)\,, trend\,(bull, \_)\,, V_{macd} > -2 \end{aligned}$$

Like before, for each rule and its companion rule (r), we include in EU_4 the statement:

$$\textbf{assert}\,(r@ta) \Leftarrow$$

We receive external observations summarized in the table:

$t = 4$			*stock*				*market indexes*			*industry indexes*
bull	*msf*	*son*	*sonc*	*edp*	*epal*	*nasdaq*	*dow*	*psi20*	*tmt*	*comm*
ma	130	26	19	11	11	–	–	–	–	–
macd	1.2	−2	−1	0	0	–	–	–	–	–
cci	1	−3	1	1	0	–	–	–	–	–
sgr	−1	2	−1	−1	0	–	–	–	–	–
price	120	26	20	12	10	3400	8160	7200	1600	1580

With this EU_4 and EO_4 we obtain the knowledge state $\langle \mathcal{P}_4, SU_4, \mathcal{H}_4, \mathcal{M}_4 \rangle$ and with it the stock ratings:

	msf	*son*	*sonc*	*edp*	*epal*
stock ratings	**buy**	**sell**	–	**hold**	**buy**

The new rules already asserted caused the *epal* rating to be upgraded to *buy*: note that the Moving Average of *epal* is above its share price. Stock *sonc* is now unrated because no rules apply. All other results are preserved.

$t = 5$ At the subsequent state transition, the external update EU_5 is empty again, and we receive external observations summarized in the table:

$t = 5$	*stock*					*market indexes*			*industry indexes*	
bull	*msf*	*son*	*sonc*	*edp*	*epal*	*nasdaq*	*dow*	*psi20*	*tmt*	*comm*
ma	140	25	21	12	10	–	–	–	–	–
macd	1.1	−2	−2	0	0	–	–	–	–	–
cci	1	−3	1	1	0	–	–	–	–	–
sgr	−1	2	−1	−1	0	–	–	–	–	–
price	130	25	22	13	10	4000	8270	7300	2000	1540

With this EU_5 and EO_5 we obtain the knowledge state $\langle \mathcal{P}_5, SU_5, \mathcal{H}_5, \mathcal{M}_5 \rangle$, and with it the stock ratings:

	msf	*son*	*sonc*	*edp*	*epal*
stock ratings	**buy**	**sell**	**sell**	**hold**	–

Stock *epal* is unrated once again because its Moving Average is again equal to its share price. The stock *sonc* has been rated a *sell* because of its low *macd*.

$t = 6$ At this state transition several events occurred. New reports about the state of the economy were released, including new *bvps*, *npm* and *per* for several key companies and key sectors. This caused the stock market to enter a *bear* trend. All this is summarized by the table:

$t = 6$	*stock*					*market indexes*			*industry indexes*	
bear	*msf*	*son*	*sonc*	*edp*	*epal*	*nasdaq*	*dow*	*psi20*	*tmt*	*comm*
ma	100	25	21	12	10	–	–	–	–	–
macd	−1.7	−2	−2	1	0	–	–	–	–	–
cci	1	−4	1	1	0	–	–	–	–	–
sgr	−1	2	−1	−1	0	–	–	–	–	–
price	110	24	21	13	9	3800	8200	7200	1300	1550
bvps	80	–	–	15	–	–	–	–	–	–
npm	9	–	–	17	–	–	–	–	10	15
per	–	–	–	1	–	–	–	–	1	2

But not all was bad news. The company has just received valuable insider information according to which there was going to be a major takeover and the share price for *sonc* would rise above 28 to then drop back again. The order would then be to buy until that value and, once the price rises above 28, sell it all. This can be encoded by the four statements which constitute EU_6:

$$\begin{aligned} \textbf{assert}\,(buy\,(sonc)\,@ii) &\Leftarrow \\ \textbf{once\_retract}\,(buy\,(sonc)\,@ii) &\Leftarrow price\,(sonc, V)\,, V > 28 \\ \textbf{once\_assert}\,(sell\,(sonc)\,@ii) &\Leftarrow price\,(sonc, V)\,, V > 28 \end{aligned}$$

$$\textbf{once\_assert}\,(\textbf{once\_retract}\,(sell\,(sonc)\,@ii) \Leftarrow price\,(sonc, V)\,, V < 24) \Leftarrow price\,(sonc, V)\,, V > 28$$

The first one immediately asserts a *buy* rating for *sonc*. The second retracts such recommendation once the price reaches 28, at which point a *sell* recommendation is issued by the third one. Then, when the price drops below 24, the *sell* rating is removed. Note that the last statement, the one that effectively retracts the *sell* recommendation, is only asserted after the price rises, or otherwise it would be executed immediately because the current price is 21.

With this EU_6 and EO_6 we obtain the knowledge state $\langle \mathcal{P}_6, SU_6, \mathcal{H}_6, \mathcal{M}_6 \rangle$, and with it the stock ratings:

	msf	*son*	*sonc*	*edp*	*epal*
stock ratings	**sell**	**sell**	**buy**	**buy**	–

There are two major changes that need to be noticed in these ratings. The first concerns the rating of *sonc* which, even though all technical data points to a *sell* recommendation, receives a *buy* recommendation because the insider information prevails over the technical analysis one. The other change concerns the *edp* recommendation, which has changed from *hold* to *buy*. The major reason for this is the change in the market trend which is now a *bear* one. Accordingly, the ratings obtained according to the more conservative fundamental analysis, which rate it as a *buy*, now prevail over the technical analysis which rates it as a *hold*. The other change concerns the *msf* stock which is now rated *sell* by both technical and fundamental analyses.

$t = 7$ At this state transition the previous *bear* market trend is declared over and a period of a more flattish market starts. Also, new reports about the economy, always important for the fundamental analysis are presented. The external update is empty for this state transition. This table summarizes the received data:

$t = 7$	*stock*					*market indexes*			*industry indexes*	
trade	*msf*	*son*	*sonc*	*edp*	*epal*	*nasdaq*	*dow*	*psi20*	*tmt*	*comm*
ma	82	23	24	13	10	–	–	–	–	–
macd	−1	−1	−4	1	0	–	–	–	–	–
cci	1	−4	1	1	0	–	–	–	–	–
sgr	−1	1	−1	−1	0	–	–	–	–	–
price	91	22	27	14	10	3090	7970	7060	1100	1550
bvps	100	–	–	15	15	–	–	–	–	–
npm	11	–	–	18	17	–	–	–	15	16
per	–	–	–	1	1	–	–	–	2	2
yvar	–	–	–	–	2	–	–	–	–	–

With this EU_7 and EO_7 we obtain the knowledge state $\langle \mathcal{P}_7, SU_7, \mathcal{H}_7, \mathcal{M}_7 \rangle$, and with it the stock ratings:

	msf	*son*	*sonc*	*edp*	*epal*
stock ratings	**hold**	**sell**	**buy**	**buy**	**buy**

To be noted in this new state is the change from a *bear* to a *trade* market, characterized by the non-existing hierarchical relation between the technical and fundamental analysis. In relation to stock ratings, we observe that *msf* now rates *hold*. This rating is obtained by means of rules from the fundamental analysis, given the new economical data since this analysis rated this stock as *sell* in the previous state. Regarding the rating by the technical analysis for this stock, there are no applicable rules. About *epal*, it is now rated *buy* because of its high *bvps* when compared to its current price, and its good *npm* and *per* values when compared to those of the corresponding industry sector. The rating of *sonc* stock is *buy*, still due to the insider information - note that its share price has not reached 28 yet. The rating for *edp* is kept, as for now the technical analysis does not rate it.

$t = 8$ At this state transition we receive the data summarized in the table.

$t = 8$	*stock*					*market indexes*			*industry indexes*	
trade	*msf*	*son*	*sonc*	*edp*	*epal*	*nasdaq*	*dow*	*psi20*	*tmt*	*comm*
ma	81	22	24	13	10	–	–	–	–	–
macd	0	0	−3	0	0	–	–	–	–	–
cci	1	−3	1	1	0	–	–	–	–	–
sgr	−1	1	−1	−1	0	–	–	–	–	–
price	90	22	29	14	10	3150	8030	7040	1150	1540

The most relevant fact observed is that the share price for *sonc* is over the insider information threshold of 28. This means the executable set of commands for this state transition includes the commands:

$$\textbf{once\_retract}\,(buy\,(sonc)\,@ii)$$
$$\textbf{once\_assert}\,(sell\,(sonc)\,@ii)$$
$$\textbf{once\_assert}\,(\textbf{once\_retract}\,(sell\,(sonc)\,@ii) \Leftarrow price\,(sonc, V)\,, V < 24)$$

Accordingly, we obtain the knowledge state $\langle \mathcal{P}_8, SU_8, \mathcal{H}_8, \mathcal{M}_8 \rangle$, in which the statement

$$\textbf{once\_retract}\,(sell\,(sonc)\,@ii) \Leftarrow price\,(sonc, V)\,, V < 24$$

belongs to SU_8, and the ratings obtained are:

	msf	*son*	*sonc*	*edp*	*epal*
stock ratings	**hold**	**sell**	**sell**	**buy**	**buy**

The most relevant fact is that *sonc* stock now rates *sell*, by means of the rule asserted due to the insider information.

$t = 9$ At this state transition, the fundamental analyst noticed that some of his ratings were obtaining not so good results, such as for example the case of *epal* stock which was rated *sell* in the previous two states because of its very good fundamental indicators, but nevertheless its price remaining the same. He recognized that some companies with good fundamental indicators still do not do well in the market and, to overcome this problem, an update to the rating policies was issued so as not to rate *buy* any stock whose Year Variation was very low. This is expressed by the rule r:

$$not\,buy\,(S) \leftarrow char\,(yvar, S, V_{yvar}, T_{yvar})\,, V_{yvar} < 3, T_{yvar} > T - 8$$

and the corresponding statement in EU_9:

$$\mathbf{assert}\,(r@fa) \Leftarrow$$

The external observations are summarized in the table:

$t = 9$	*stock*					*market indexes*			*industry indexes*	
trade	*msf*	*son*	*sonc*	*edp*	*epal*	*nasdaq*	*dow*	*psi20*	*tmt*	*comm*
ma	81	22	24	13	10	–	–	–	–	–
macd	0	0	−2	0	0	–	–	–	–	–
cci	1	1	1	1	0	–	–	–	–	–
sgr	−1	−3	−1	−1	0	–	–	–	–	–
price	88	21	27	14	10	3100	8000	7055	1160	1560

With this EU_8 and EO_8 we obtain the knowledge state $\langle \mathcal{P}_8, SU_8, \mathcal{H}_8, \mathcal{M}_8 \rangle$, and with it the stock ratings:

	msf	*son*	*sonc*	*edp*	*epal*
stock ratings	**hold**	**buy**	**sell**	**buy**	–

Note that with respect to the rating for *epal*, even though there is a rule issued by the *ta* at state 1 according to which this stock should be rated *buy*, the rule just asserted, together with the low *yvar* for *epal*, causes the rejection of the earlier rule. Since no other rules provide for rating this stock, it becomes unrated. Noticeable is the change in rating for the *son* stock since it represents the first rating of any share by the *ta* during a *trade* market.

$t = 10$ At this state transition we receive the data summarized in the table.

$t = 10$	*stock*					*market indexes*			*industry indexes*	
trade	*msf*	*son*	*sonc*	*edp*	*epal*	*nasdaq*	*dow*	*psi20*	*tmt*	*comm*
ma	80	23	22	14	10	–	–	–	–	–
macd	0	1	0	1	0	–	–	–	–	–
cci	1	2	1	1	0	–	–	–	–	–
sgr	−1	−3	−1	−1	0	–	–	–	–	–
price	87	23	22	15	10	3150	8010	7045	1140	1550

The most relevant fact observed is that the share price for *sonc* is below the insider information threshold of 24. This means that the executable set of commands for this state transition includes the command:

$$\mathbf{once\_retract}\,(sell\,(sonc)\,@ii)$$

Forthwith, we obtain the knowledge state $\langle \mathcal{P}_{10}, SU_{10}, \mathcal{H}_{10}, \mathcal{M}_{10} \rangle$, and with it the stock ratings:

	msf	son	$sonc$	edp	$epal$
stock ratings	–	**buy**	–	**buy**	–

Two relevant occurrences in this state transition should be noticed. First, the *sell* recommendation for *sonc* no longer holds because it has been explicitly retracted by the command resulting from the previous update due to the insider information, and there are no other rules to rate this stock with its current market values. Second, the msf rating no longer holds because one of the fundamental values previously used to rate it *hold* (*per*) is now too old (it was last updated at $t = 2$), and the body of the rating rule that was used before is now false, no other rules for this stock being applicable.

8.1.4 Further Elaborations

Several features of KABUL have not been made the most in this example to keep it in manageable size. In particular, the employment of sub-agents as introduced before was left out of this example completely. Nevertheless, such a notion of sub-agents could play an important role in further elaborations of the example, as in the scenario that we now informally describe.

Consider the same financial company which now employs several researchers whose job description is to use various ways to come up with stock ratings. For simplicity we consider, like before, that there are three distinct ways to do so: fundamental analysis, technical analysis and insider information. Each of the hired market researchers, even though a specialist in one (or more) of such methods, from time to time will also establish some ratings based on methods for which he is not a specialist by far. The company has to set up the knowledge base so as to keep the hierarchical relationships between the various methods which depend on the market trend, and at the same time to establish the relationships among the various researchers, which may vary from method to method. This could be easily encoded in $KABUL^{+}$, where each of the rating methods is, as before, an agent in the system, and each of the researchers is a sub-agent. Consider three researchers Joe Fundamental, Mike Technical, and Nick Insider. Joe is a specialist in the Fundamental Analysis. He also knows quite a lot about the Technical Analysis, but not as much as Mike. Nick is the best at obtaining insider information, but does not have a clue about analysis. This scenario, for example, could be partially encoded by the sub-agent hierarchy (where $\mathcal{SA} = \{joe, mike, nick\}$):

$$\begin{aligned} \mathcal{SH}_s &\subset \{SD_{ta_s}, SD_{fa_s}, SD_{ii_s}\} \\ SD_{ta_s} &= (\mathcal{SA}, \{(joe, mike), (nick, joe), (nick, mike)\}) \\ SD_{fa_s} &= (\mathcal{SA}, \{(mike, joe), (nick, joe), (nick, mike)\}) \\ SD_{ii_s} &= (\mathcal{SA}, \{(joe, nick), (mike, nick)\}) \end{aligned}$$

In it each sub-agent would have a sub-agent program to encode its behaviour. The internal updates between sub-agents could be used to perform some form of cooperative work. For example, imagine a situation where Nick Insider, before issuing a buy recommendation on any company, wants to check with Joe Fundamental if the company's overall situation is good. In this scenario, Nick's tips are private capabilities and so are Joe's overall evaluations. To encode such a situation, we could have the statement in Nick's sub-agent program:

$$\mathbf{always\_assert}\,(\mathbf{assert}\,(\mathbf{assert}\,((buy\,(S)\,@ii) \Leftarrow)\,@nick) \Leftarrow \mathbf{P} : good\,(S)\,@joe) \Leftarrow \mathbf{P} : tip\,(S)$$

According to it, whenever Nick has a tip on stock s, he sends the statement

$$\mathbf{assert}\,(\mathbf{assert}\,((buy\,(s)\,@ii) \Leftarrow)\,@nick) \Leftarrow \mathbf{P} : good\,(s)$$

to Joe. Then, if Joe can determine according to his private capabilities that s is a good company, he sends the statement

$$\mathbf{assert}\,(buy\,(s)\,@ii) \Leftarrow$$

back to Nick, who then executes it and asserts $buy\,(s)$ in his corresponding node of the Insider Information agent.

8.2 An Agent Architecture

8.2.1 Introduction

Over recent years, the notion of agency has claimed a major role in defining the trends of modern research. Influencing a broad spectrum of disciplines such as Sociology, Psychology, among others, the agent paradigm virtually invaded every sub-field of Computer Science [57, 114, 123, 160, 211]. Although commonly implemented by means of imperative languages, mainly for reasons of efficiency, the agent concept has recently increased its influence in the research and development of computational logic based systems. Since efficiency is not always the crucial issue, but clear specification and correctness is, *Logic Programming* and *Non-monotonic Reasoning* have been revived back into the spotlight.

The *Logic Programming* paradigm provides a well-defined, general, integrative, encompassing, and rigorous framework for systematically studying computation, be it syntax, semantics, procedures, or attending implementations, environments, tools, and standards. *LP* approaches problems, and provides solutions, at a sufficient level of abstraction so that they generalize from problem domain to problem domain. This is afforded by the nature of its very foundation in logic, both in substance and method, and constitutes one of its major assets. To this accrues the recent significant improvements in the efficiency of *Logic Programming* implementations for *Non-monotonic Reasoning* [69, 176, 216, 231]. Besides allowing for a unified declarative and procedural semantics, eliminating the traditional wide gap between theory and practice, the use of several and quite powerful results in the field of non-monotonic extensions to *Logic Programming (LP)*, such as belief revision, inductive learning, argumentation, preferences, abduction, etc. [211] can represent an important composite added value to the design of rational agents. These results, together with the improvement in efficiency, allow the referred mustering of *Logic Programming* and *Non-monotonic Reasoning* to accomplish a felicitous degree of combination between reactive and rational behaviours of agents, the *Holy Grail* of modern *Artificial Intelligence*, whilst preserving clear and precise specification enjoyed by declarative languages.

If we are to move Logic Programming to a more open and dynamic environment, typical of the agency paradigm, we need to consider ways of representing and integrating knowledge from different sources which may evolve in time. Moreover, an agent not only comprises knowledge about each states, but also some form of knowledge about the transitions between states. This knowledge about state transitions can represent the agent's knowledge about the environment's evolution, as well as its own behaviour and evolution. Recent developments, among which those described in this work, open *Logic Programming* to these otherwise unreachable dynamic worlds.

Based on the strengths of $\mathcal{MDLP}$ as a framework capable of simultaneously represent several aspects of a system in a dynamic fashion, and of *KABUL*[1] as a powerful language to specify the evolution of such representations, by means of transitions, we have launched ourselves in the design of an agent architecture, $\mathcal{MINERVA}$. Named after the Goddess of Wisdom, the $\mathcal{MINERVA}$ agent architecture is being designed with the intention of providing, on a sound theoretical basis, a common agent framework based on the strengths of Logic Programming, to allow the combination of several non-monotonic knowledge representation and reasoning mechanisms developed in recent years. Rational agents, in our opinion, will require an admixture of any number of those reasoning mechanisms to carrying out their tasks.

The work on the design of such architecture has just started and there are many issues that have not been addressed yet. Accordingly, this Section should be viewed as a rather speculative description of the possible role *KABUL* may play within agent systems.

Our view of an agent situated in a multi-agent system is that of an essentially epistemic entity, where from its mental state its actions follow.

Mental states are about knowledge about the external environment, but also about what is often referred to as modalities such as goals, intentions. But a mental state is also about the behaviour that characterizes its evolution. We adopt the stance of such behaviour being carried out by a composition of specialized function related subagents, that execute their various specialized tasks. Examples of such subagents are those implementing the reactive, planning, scheduling, belief revision, goal management, learning, dialogue management, information gathering, preference evaluation, strategy, and diagnosis functionalities. To this end, a $\mathcal{MINERVA}$ agent will be based on a modular design where a *Common Knowledge Base*, containing object knowledge about the world, as well as the mentioned modalities is concurrently manipulated by specialized sub-agents (schematically depicted in Fig. 8.4). Based on this view, and assuming the possibility of a uniform logic programming rule based knowledge representation, we adopt the definition of an agent state as being a *KABUL* knowledge state that evolves according to the common observe-think-act cycle.

We now provide a description of the main components of such an agent, and how they are defined.

8.2.2 Overall Architecture

An agent will consist of several specialized, possibly concurrent, sub-agents performing various tasks while reading and manipulating a common knowledge base. We now establish the correspondence between the agent components and *KABUL* knowledge states. To distinguish a $\mathcal{MINERVA}$ agent from the agents which constitute the *KABUL* set $\mathcal{A}$, we will refer to those elements of $\mathcal{A}$ as k-agents.

By default, we will assume that the agent we are describing is named α. Agent α is situated in a community where other agents exist. Let the set of such multi-agent system agents, excluding agent α, be $\mathcal{A}_{mas} = \{\beta, \gamma, \mu, \nu, ...\}$. Each element of $\mathcal{A}_{mas}$, together with α, will be a k-agent in *KABUL*. But, as we mentioned before, k-agents can also be used to represent other aspects of a system such as what we have called the *modalities*. We then need to define which of these *modalities* will exist for agent α. Examples of such are *intentions*, *goals*, *reactions*, or any other distinct

[1]We will refer to *KABUL*, although we will be using, when required, its most general form, *KABUL*$^+$.

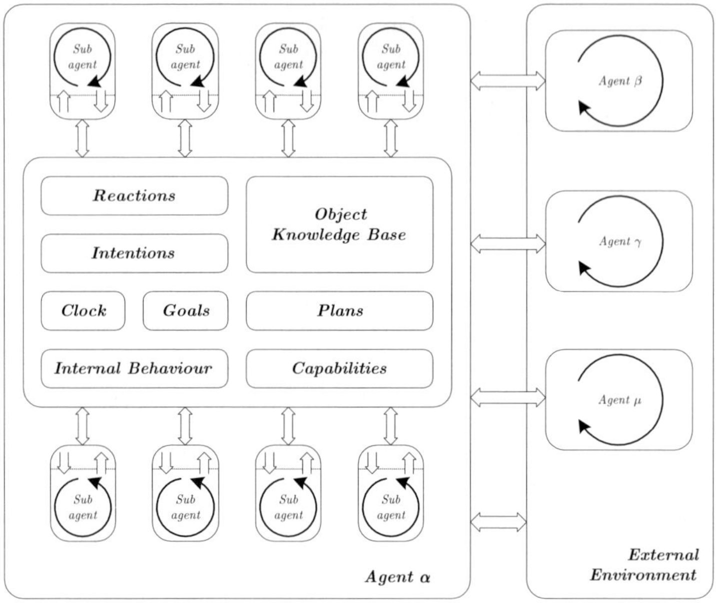

Figure 8.4: The $\mathcal{MINERVA}$ agent architecture

form of knowledge. Let $\mathcal{A}_{mod} = \{intentions, goals, reactions, ...\}$ be such set. We have mentioned that those actions that an agent is to execute follow from its mental state. To simplify the extraction of such actions from the mental state, we will require any agent specified according to this architecture to have a reserved k-agent node representing such actions to be executed. We will call such k-agent *exec*. According to some agency theories, such commitments are referred to as the intentions of the agent. Opting for a special reserved k-agent, in this case named *exec*, does not exclude such view for one can always make it reflect the content of any other k-agent in the MDLP DAG, either by connecting them with DAG edges or by asserting (resp. retracting) there, everything that is also asserted (resp. retracted) on such other k-agent. Then, the KABUL set of k-agents is $\mathcal{A}$, defined as:

$$\mathcal{A} = \mathcal{A}_{mas} \cup \mathcal{A}_{mod} \cup \{\alpha\} \cup \{exec\}$$

Then we need to define the set of sub-agents which constitute agent α. To each of these sub-agents corresponds a set of specialized tasks that can be independently carried out. Each of these sub-agents' behaviour is to be specified by a set of statements, and each can access its own private set of capabilities. As before, we assume that such capabilities are given in the form of a set of atoms that are only accessible to each sub-agent, and serve to evaluate the private conditions in its statements. Examples of such sub-agents would be the dialoguer, scheduler, reactor, learner, goal manager, hierarchy manager, etc., and more than one sub-agent can co-exist for each task: we can for example specify an agent with more than one learning sub-agent, each learning according to a different method. Let the set of KABUL sub-agents be equal to such sub-agents, i.e.

$$\mathcal{SA} = \{\alpha_a, \alpha_b, \alpha_d, \alpha_e, ...\}$$

For each of these sub-agents we need to define its set of private capabilities and the hierarchy relating itself with other sub-agents in what concerns the way to combine update statements according to their provenance.

Finally, we need to define the set of functions, encoding the prevalence modes, $\mathcal{F}$, that will be used by the agent. These are all the required elements, together with the underlying object language defined by $\mathcal{K}$, to launch the agent, its initial knowledge state being $\langle \mathcal{P}_0, \mathcal{SA}_0, \mathcal{H}_0, \mathcal{SH}_0, \mathcal{M}_0, \mathcal{SM}_0, \mathcal{IU}_0 \rangle$, as defined in the previous chapter.

At each state, the agent evolves according to the observe-think-act cycle:

---

cycle $(s, \langle \mathcal{P}_s, \mathcal{SA}_s, \mathcal{H}_s, \mathcal{SH}_s, \mathcal{M}_s, \mathcal{SM}_s, \mathcal{IU}_s \rangle)$
observe (determine $\langle \mathcal{EU}_{s+1}, EO_{s+1} \rangle$)
think (determine $\langle \mathcal{P}_{s+1}, \mathcal{SA}_{s+1}, \mathcal{H}_{s+1}, \mathcal{SH}_{s+1}, \mathcal{M}_{s+1}, \mathcal{SM}_{s+1}, \mathcal{IU}_{s+1} \rangle$)
act (determine and execute actions)
cycle $(s+1, \langle \mathcal{P}_{s+1}, \mathcal{SA}_{s+1}, \mathcal{H}_{s+1}, \mathcal{SH}_{s+1}, \mathcal{M}_{s+1}, \mathcal{SM}_{s+1}, \mathcal{IU}_{s+1} \rangle)$

We shall not be concerned with the steps *observe* and *act*. We only assume that actions are selected by consulting the object level MDLP $\mathcal{P}_{s+1}$ at the current state of *exec* i.e., the agent executes those actions ω such that

$$\textbf{holds}\,(\omega@exec)\ \textbf{at}\ s+1\ ?$$

and that the names of those actions that are successfully executed will be included in the subsequent state's external observations. For example, if the agent, after consulting $\mathcal{P}_{s+1}$, successfully executes actions ω_1 and ω_2, then the set of external observations at the subsequent cycle, EO_{s+2}, will be such that $\{\omega_1, \omega_2\} \subseteq EO_{s+2}$. For this we must assume that the set of actions $\mathcal{K}_\omega \subseteq \mathcal{K}$ is known.

Now that we have launched the agent, the first cycle should be used to program it. We now describe such programming stage, which basically consists of specifying the initial hierarchies, sub-agent programs, and prevalence modes. Note however that there is complete freedom in what concerns the use of KABUL statements for this purpose. We will just describe some possibilities and common options.

Agent Hierarchies and Prevalence Modes

In what concern k-agent hierarchies, typically there will be edges linking those k-agents in $\mathcal{A}_{mas}$ amongst themselves and with k-agent α, according to α's trust. There is no need for k-agent α to be the most trusted and therefore the prevalent one. Establishing the hierarchy is performed as in the previous example, where statements of the form

$$\textbf{add\_hierarchy\_edge}\,(\gamma \rightarrow \mu) \Leftarrow$$

belong to the external update of the sub-agent responsible for carrying out the task represented by such statement, and where $\gamma, \mu \in \mathcal{A}_{mas} \cup \{\alpha\}$. Typically there will be one (or more) sub-agent(s) in charge of managing the agent hierarchies. Such sub-agent(s) should also be programmed (updated) with those statements describing the hierarchies' evolutions. The same applies to agent prevalence modes. Either the same sub-agent, or a different one if those tasks are independent, should be updated with a set of statements establishing such prevalence mode related behaviour.

Not all k-agents will be linked and, at each state, $\mathcal{P}_s$ will encode a set of DAGs. For example, if one of the k-agents represents the goals, it makes no sense to have a link between this node and the ones representing outside agents' knowledge. We refer to the scenario previously mentioned where a very simple framework exists, with $\mathcal{A} = \{goals, knowledge\}$ such that $\mathcal{H}$ does not contain any edges. Further suppose that we execute the two commands:

$$\textbf{assert}\,(rich \leftarrow win\_lottery@knowledge)$$
$$\textbf{assert}\,(rich@goals)$$

At the subsequent state, we observe that $rich@goals$ is true and $rich@knowledge$ false, indicating that we are not rich but we have a goal to be so. If there were an edge linking $knowledge$ and $goals$, we would not be able to obtain the truth valuation we want when the goal is evaluated at the prevailing node.

Then, within each k-agent, one must specify the hierarchies relating the different sub-agents in what concerns their position with respect to such k-agent. For example, it is only natural that, if there is a sub-agent acting as a scheduler, such sub-agent be higher in the *exec* k-agent hierarchy than for example a learner sub-agent. Or, another example, a dialoguer sub-agent should be hierarchically superior than a reactor sub-agent within the k-agent node corresponding to some outside agent γ. Or we may want Joe Fundamental to be hierarchically superior than Mike Technical when it comes to asserting rules in the fundamental analysis node, and the opposite situation when dealing with the technical analysis one. Again, one sub-agent could be specified to deal with such sub-agent hierarchies.

Sub-agent Programs

The sub-agents manipulate the common knowledge base. Each is specified by a KABUL program which encodes its behaviour. There is total flexibility in what concerns the division of tasks among sub-agents. We now draw some considerations on how some specific behaviours, within the context of agent systems, can be encoded. We assume that, as in the previous example, there is a k-agent in $\mathcal{A}_{mod}$, representing a clock, specified by the statements:

$$\textbf{assert\_event}\,(time\,(1)\,@clock) \Leftarrow$$
$$\textbf{always\_assert\_event}\,(time\,(X+1)\,@clock) \Leftarrow time\,(X)$$

The first issue we consider is that of recording observations. Suppose for example that agent α has some sensor that observes its current position as an atom of the form $at\,(X,Y)$. Every time there is a new observation for its position, the previous position must be retracted and the current one asserted, say at α's node. This could be accomplished by:

$$\textbf{always\_assert}\,(at\,(X,Y,T)\,@\alpha) \Leftarrow time\,(T)\,@clock, \mathbf{E} : \textbf{in}\,(at\,(X,Y))$$
$$\textbf{always\_retract}\,(at\,(X,Y,T)\,@\alpha) \Leftarrow \mathbf{R} : \textbf{in}\,(at\,(X,Y,T)\,@\alpha)\,, \mathbf{E} : \textbf{in}\,(at\,(X,Y))$$

A behaviour characteristic of a Dialoguer sub-agent is similar to a sensor in what concerns receiving input from the environment. It is different in the sense that it processes messages incoming from the other agents in the multi-agent system $(\beta, \gamma, \mu, \nu, ...)$ and the *KABUL* commands are executed by asserting the information into the corresponding k-agent's node. Also it is this sub-agent's responsibility, according to the message, to generate new goals, issue replies, etc. Examples of *KABUL* statements typical of this sub-agent would be (we assume that elements of $\mathcal{A}$ are also terms of the observation language):

$$\textbf{always\_assert}\,(R@Agent) \Leftarrow \mathbf{R}:\textbf{out}(R@Agent), \mathbf{E}:\textbf{in}\,(message\,(Agent, R))$$

representing that every rule R sent by agent $Agent$ should be asserted in the corresponding $Agent$'s node if such rule was not present at $Agent$'s node;

$$\begin{aligned}\textbf{always\_assert}\,(goal(G, Agent)@goals) \Leftarrow & cooperative(Agent)@\alpha,\\ & \mathbf{E}:\textbf{in}\,(request\,(Agent, G))\end{aligned}$$

representing that any request to solve a goal, received by a cooperative agent, should be adopted as its own goal. Here the choice of goal representation is just for illustrative purposes;

$$\begin{aligned}\textbf{always\_assert}\,(msgTo(Agent, plan\,(G, Plan))@exec) \Leftarrow & \; goal\,(G, Agent)\,@goals,\\ & Agent \neq \alpha, plan(G, Plan)@plans\end{aligned}$$

representing that a message with a plan (here represented by $plan\,(G, Plan)$) should be sent to an agent every time agent α has a goal G requested by that agent and it has a plan for such a goal. Here we are assuming that this message represents an action to be executed immediately. These are asserted at k-agent $exec$. We have mentioned before that every action that is executed will appear in the subsequent set of external observations. The purpose of this is to allow for the update of the knowledge state with the effects of actions. In the previous case, such an action could have the effect of removing the goal, specified as follows:

$$\textbf{always\_retract}\,(goal(G, Agent)@goals) \Leftarrow \mathbf{E}:\textbf{in}\,(msgTo(Agent, plan\,(G, Plan)))$$

Every action in $exec$, after being executed, should be either retracted or falsified. There are several ways in which this can be achieved, depending on the design of the agent. One way would be to have the following statement being executed by some sub-agent:

$$\textbf{always\_retract}\,(\Omega@exec) \Leftarrow \mathbf{E}:\textbf{in}\,(\Omega)$$

The previous statements indicate the direct assertion and retraction of all actions in $exec$. It is possible however to differentiate between different kinds of actions such as for example those resulting from reactions from those proposed by more deliberative sub-agents. These could be asserted in different nodes and a sub-agent, with scheduling capabilities, would manage and combine such actions and assert the action into the $exec$ node for execution. Such a scheduler could be specified to give preference to reactions, or even to block them.

These are just a few simple examples of statements that can be mustered. Other possible statements have been shown throughout previous examples.

8.2.3 Related Work

As we have mentioned before, this Section just aims at showing the possible use of *KABUL* in agent systems. The characteristic of $\mathcal{MINERVA}$ that makes it most distinct from other existing agent architectures is that its knowledge is represented by non-monotonic theories, expressed by logic programs, with default negation in both the heads and bodies of clauses, organized according to acyclic digraphs. This permits the use of the richer knowledge representation capabilities afforded by such logic programs, for example to represent the relations amongst the agents themselves in a MAS, as well as for a direct and simple mechanism to represent and reason about dynamic environments where the governing rules change with time. It has been shown that updating non-monotonic theories is quite different from updating theories represented in classical propositional logic, governed by the update postulates in [116], and far different from the mere assertion and deletion of formulas. To the best of our knowledge, $\mathcal{MINERVA}$ is the only agent architecture that proposes to incorporate such update capabilities. Most other agent architectures incorporate some update facilities, but all in line with the model update postulates of [116], or by simple assertion and retraction of formulas. We should also make clear at this point that the assertions and retractions specified by the *KABUL* commands differ substantially from those approaches employing simple assertion and retraction of formulas. The former are dealt with by the semantics of $\mathcal{MDLP}$, which further rejects other existing rules on the grounds of the newly asserted ones, and may as well reinstate other previously rejected rules, while the latter only deal with "physical" assertions and retractions of formulas, the semantics being determined according to the new set of formulas.

Clearly, not all situations require such update features as our's and, in those, other existing agent proposals may perform better. Nevertheless, when the governing rules change dynamically, new rules possibly invalidating existing rules, as for example in legal reasoning scenarios, a semantics like the one provided for by $\mathcal{MDLP}$ will be required. $\mathcal{MDLP}$ additionally caters for a clear framework, with a precise semantics, for representing societies of hierarchically related agents.

The use of computational logic for modelling single and multi-agent systems has been widely investigated (e.g., see [211] for a quite recent roadmap). The agent-based architecture described in [123] aims at reconciling rationality and reactivity. Agents are logic programs which continuously perform an "observe-think-act" cycle, and their behaviour is defined via a proof procedure which exploits iff-definitions and integrity constraints. One difference between such approach and ours is that in [123] the semantics is a proof-theoretic operational one, while our approach provides a declarative, model-theoretic characterization of environment-aware agents. The semantical differences between exploiting iff-definitions and logic programs under the stable models semantics have been extensively studied and are naturally inherited when comparing both systems. But most important, the theory update performed by the observation part of the cycle in [123] amounts to a simple monotonic addition of facts and integrity constraints which, unlike in our proposal, does not allow for the full fledged rule updates supported by LUPS.

Different action languages [95, 101] have been proposed to describe and reason on the effects of actions (c.f. [96] for a survey). Intuitively, while action languages and update languages are both concerned with modelling changes, action languages focus on the notions of causality and fluents, while update languages focusses its features on declarative updates for general knowledge bases . As shown in before, it is possible, in some cases, to establish a correspondence between actions languages such as the languages $\mathcal{A}$ of [95] and $\mathcal{C}$ of [101], and update languages such as KUL and LUPS. Since update languages were specifically designed to allow assertions and retraction of rules to allow for a knowledge base to evolve, action languages by only allowing the effects of actions to be fluents restrict themselves to purely extensional updates. From this purely syntactical point of view update languages are more expressive. Action languages such as $\mathcal{C}$, on the other hand, were designed to express the notion of causality which is semantically different from the underlying notion of inertia found in the DLP semantics. It is thus natural to observe differences in the semantics between action languages and update languages (see [16] for a more detailed discussion of the relation between the two approaches).

In [106], Hindriks et al. they propose the agent programming language *3APL*, together with a transition system based operational semantics. Knowledge is represented as a set of first order formulas (although the authors claim it could be any logical language) in a database, and goals are sequences of imperative and logic constructs. On top of these there are so-called practical reasoning rules to specify changes to the agent state. *3APL*, as claimed by the authors, intends to be a language to serve both as a sound basis for theoretical work on agents and as a vehicle for practical applications. The approach to the design of *3APL* is predicated on the premise that an agent programming language amounts to providing a way to specify the dynamics of the mental state of an agent, be it its knowledge and beliefs or its goals, intentions, and commitments. This intention and premise are shared by $\mathcal{MINERVA}$ in the sense that the first is the ground for the choice of non-monotonic logic programming in general as the basic framework, and the second amounts to the motivation for using multi-dimensional dynamic logic programming, and *KABUL* as knowledge representation and evolution specification language. In some sense, we can compare the *3APL* database to the object knowledge base of a $\mathcal{MINERVA}$ agent, and the *3APL* practical reasoning rules to the *KABUL* commands in $\mathcal{MINERVA}$. The differences being that, in $\mathcal{MINERVA}$, updates to the environment (and to the agent mental state) that can bring about contradictory theories (if formulas are simply regarded as having all the same strength) are automatically dealt with by *KABUL* and $\mathcal{MDLP}$. As noted above, updates are not simple assertions and retractions of formulas. In particular, a newly asserted rule is not equal in "power" to an old rule (in that case it would be a revision and not an update) and does not simply replace it. Katsuno and Mendelzon [116] study updates for theories in classical propositional logic. But updating a belief base depends on the representation language. In particular, updates of non-monotonic knowledge bases, for example represented by logic programs under the stable models semantics, require a substantially different mechanism from those of classical propositional logic based representations, as discussed in Chapter 3. It seems that, unlike its authors claim, the belief base used by *3APL* agents cannot be represented by an arbitrary logic language. In particular, their belief base cannot use the representational capabilities of default negation. $\mathcal{MINERVA}$ has been specifically designed to use logic programs with default negation both in the heads and in the bodies of rules as the basic representation mechanism. Programs written in this language are arranged according to several acyclic digraphs whose semantics is precisely characterized by $\mathcal{MDLP}$. The use of *KABUL*, which has an imperative reading, provides for the mental state transitions by means of the necessary update operations. In *3APL* there is no notion of sub-agents concurrently changing the mental state of the agent, possibly with contradictory information. In $\mathcal{MINERVA}$, these contradictions are resolved by the semantics of $\mathcal{MDLP}$ according to a specified hierarchy between sub-agents. Like in *3APL*, action specifications in *KABUL* are static inasmuch as *KABUL* commands cannot be updated. We are currently extending *KABUL* programs with self-update capabilities to overcome this drawback, and to enrich the behaviour specification power of *KABUL*.

AgentSpeak(L) [201] is a logical language for programming Belief-Desire-Intention (BDI) agents, originally designed by abstracting the main features of the PRS and dMARS systems [58]. Our approach shares with AgentSpeak(L) the objective of using a simple logical specification language to model the execution of an agent, rather than employing modal operators. On the other hand, while AgentSpeak(L) programs are described by means of a proof-theoretic operational semantics, our approach provides a declarative, model-theoretic characterization of environment-aware agents. The relation of our approach with the agent language 3APL (which has been shown to embed AgentSpeak(L) in [107]) is similar, inasmuch as 3APL is provided only with an operational characterization.

MetateM (and *Concurrent MetateM*), introduced by Fisher et al. [31, 84], is a programming language based on the notion of direct execution of temporal formulae, primarily used to specify reactive behaviours of agents. It shares similarities with the *KABUL* language inasmuch as both employ rules to represent a relationship between past and future, i.e. each rule in *MetateM* or in *KABUL* consists of conditions about the past (or present) and a conclusion about the future. While the use of temporal logics in MetateM allows for the specification of rather elaborate temporal conditions, something for which *KABUL* was not designed for, the underlying $\mathcal{MDLP}$ semantics of *KABUL* allows for the specification of agents capable of being deployed in dynamic environments where the governing laws change over time. If we move to the more general class of logic programs with non-monotonic default negation both in the premises and conclusions of rules, *KABUL* and $\mathcal{MDLP}$ directly provide an update semantics needed to resolve contradictions naturally arising from conflicting rules acquired at different time instants, something apparently not possible in *MetateM*. This partially amounts to the distinction between updating theories represented in classical logic and those represented by non-monotonic logic programs (cf. Chapter 3).

The *IMPACT* agent architecture, introduced by Subrahmanian et al. [219], provides a framework to build agents on top of heterogeneous sources of knowledge. To "agentize" such sources, the authors introduce the notion of agent program written over a language of so-called code-calls, which can be seen as encapsulations of whatever the source represents, and the actions the agent can execute. Such agent programs and their semantics resemble logic programs extended with deontic modalities. In *IMPACT*, at every state transition, the agent determines a set of actions to be executed, abiding by some notion of deontic consistency, which simultaneously corresponds to a basic change in the agent's mental state. *IMPACT* agents do not incorporate the rule based update mechanisms of $\mathcal{MINERVA}$ although, in principle, it appears to be possible to specify a set of code-calls for the object knowledge base of a $\mathcal{MINERVA}$ agent, accessing an $\mathcal{MDLP}$ meta-interpreter, and defining the actions (corresponding to the *KABUL* commands) that change the MDLP. In other words, one could agentize a $\mathcal{MINERVA}$ agent to become an *IMPACT* agent.

8.2.4 Final Remarks

The $\mathcal{MINERVA}$ basic architecture affords us too, so we believe, with the elasticity and resilience to further support a spate of crucial ancillary functionalities, in the form of additional specialized sub-agents, via compositional, communication, and procedural mechanisms. The circum-exploration of the territories under purview has hardly started, but the means of locomotion appear to be already with us.

The use of Logic Programming for the overall endeavour is justified on the grounds of it providing a rigorous single encompassing theoretical basis for the aforesaid topics, as well as an implementation vehicle for parallel and distributed processing. Additionally, logic programming provides a formal high level flexible instrument for the rigorous specification and experimentation with computational designs, making it extremely useful for prototyping, even when other, possibly lower level, target implementation languages are envisaged.

Chapter 9

Conclusions and Future Directions

In this Chapter we single out the main conclusions and point out future directions.

Now that the end of this work is approaching, it is time for a reality check and to draw some remarks about future directions.

In the previous Chapters, we have broken a good amount of ground, previously unexplored. We believe that what has been proposed throughout this work constitutes, at different levels of polishing, solid and formal results providing solutions to existing problems, while at the same time opening several doors where new and interesting topics allow us to foresee fruitful research. Not all contributions have the same degree of importance, and we now place each in context, by commenting on what we believe to be our main achievements:

Rule Inertia: one important achievement resides, in our opinion, in the very initial motivation for this work. Realizing the importance of allowing updates of knowledge bases where the intensional and extensional knowledge are treated in a unified manner, and further showing that no existing technique was appropriate, led to the proposal that the *principle of inertia* should be applied to rules and not to the model literals, and that rules should be rejected (not carry over by inertia) by means of a notion of causal rejection, based on other rules. This led to the introduction of *Dynamic Logic Programming*, but also led to the devotion of a good research effort, by others, in the studying of other update approaches following this underlying principle. We believe that applying the principle of inertia to rules, the underlying claim and principle of this work, constitutes the adequate way to deal with logic program updates, being in our opinion one of the contributions of this work[1].

Dynamic Logic Programming: the materialization of the principles for updates, based on rule inertia and causal rejection, led to the introduction of *Dynamic Logic Programming* as a declarative framework in which to specify sequences of updates. In our opinion, DLP is probably the most important milestone of this work. Due to its very simple and intuitive declarative semantics, together with the

[1]Preliminary partial results on this subject, namely the P-Justified Updates Semantics, appeared in the authors' M.Sc. Dissertation [130].

properties it enjoys, among which we highlight the embedding of logic programs under the stable models semantics [91, 92] and revision programs [157], which no other proposal jointly obeys, place DLP as the prime candidate to become the reference for characterizing such rich logic program updates - we surely hope so. Important is also the existing transformational semantics which provides a straightforward mechanism for implementation, allowing to take advantage of recent improvements in systems for Non-monotonic Reasoning with Logic Programs such as the DLV-system [69] or SMODELS [176].

Multi-dimensional Dynamic Logic Programming: the introduction of $\mathcal{MDLP}$ to allow for logic programs arranged as nodes of an acyclic digraph, although a simple direct extension of DLP, imparts added expressiveness, thereby amplifying the coverage of its application domains far outside the domain of updates. The flexibility afforded by a *DAG* accrues to the scope and variety of the new possibilities, some presented here, some being currently developed by others. The new characteristics of multiplicity and composition of $\mathcal{MDLP}$ impart an innovative "societal" viewpoint to *Logic Programming.* Its simple semantical characterization together with its amenability to implementation add to $\mathcal{MDLP}$'s possible success story.

KABUL: languages of updates are, we believe, an important concept to allow for a joint representation of states and updates. The underlying motivation that led Alferes et al. to introduce *LUPS*, particularly in what concerns the choice of a reasonable set of commands to support the language, even though it may not be the minimal necessary, is appropriate to deal with the problem at hand. Having said this, we believe that the introduction of *KABUL*, as an extension of *LUPS* by building upon its original set of commands to allow for the specification of the KB self update behaviour and its update, together with the object knowledge base, is an important step towards the support of the specification of *Evolving Knowledge Bases.* True that some syntactical simplifications are possible, this certainly being one of our next-to-achieve goals, but we must mention that, when dealing with application examples, we found out that specifications were quite simple to encode in KABUL, in the sense that statements were easy to write, even though often quite long.

KABUL$^{m/+}$: the extension of KABUL to allow for MDLP based knowledge bases was the natural next piece of the puzzle. It allows the specification, with a precise semantical characterization, of rather elaborate *Evolving Knowledge Bases* with features such as the ability to:

- combine knowledge from different sources;
- specify external updates to the knowledge of each individual source;
- relate the sources of knowledge according to elaborate precedence relations;
- update such precedence relations;
- specify and update the evolution of such precedence relations;
- specify and update the internal behaviour of the knowledge base;
- access and reason about external observations;
- specify multiple entities (sub-agents), within an evolving knowledge base, each independently carrying out part of the internal behaviour;

- specify and update precedence relations among such sub-agents;

When establishing this most general framework, we have tried, most of all, to set forth a language which would allow for specifications of *Evolving Knowledge Bases* as general as possible. This is for example why we opted for allowing the specification of arbitrary evolutions of the MDLP DAG with prevalence modes specified by means of arbitrary functions. Even though we suspect that some of the features provided will have only a limited use in practice, and all the introduced machinery may appear too complex for such limited use, we must mention that the scenarios we have explored using this extended KABUL language, of which we have only presented one in full, were quite easy and natural to encode, with the available syntax, and the obtained results were the intuitively expected. To conclude on this topic, we believe that the definitions supplying the semantics for the language, although often with a hard-to-read appearance, provide for a language in which the specification of *Evolving Knowledge Bases* is natural and simple.

The applicability of tools such as those presented here is a crucial issue. We have attempted to illustrate all the major concepts with examples rooted in several distinct domains. It is important to stress that all the embedding Theorems presented throughout, enable for every example presented in some Chapter to carry over to subsequent ones.

To sum up, we believe that the concept of *Evolving Knowledge Bases*, as a KB that not only contains object level knowledge but also an encoding of its own evolution, and where both can be subject of updates, is an interesting and promising concept to further study and pursue. Next we elaborate on such future directions:

Well Founded Semantics: Three-valued semantics have been extensively well studied and their usefulness for representing and reasoning with incomplete knowledge established. It is therefore important to define a well founded version for the semantics of MDLP. In [130, 141–143], the notion of justified updates was also established for the three valued case. This, together with the existing well founded semantics for generalized logic programs of [49], provides a starting point for setting forth its MDLP counterpart. A well founded semantics may allow for top-down query evaluation with polynomial complexity, also opening up the possibility of using tabling techniques to further increase the overall efficiency. It would reduce the computational complexity of KABUL, by reducing the complexity of the partial evaluation step, and would allow for a well founded version of the semantics of executable commands. Also, when such unique well founded set of executable commands is specified, we no longer need the selection function. Achieving a polynomial implementable semantics of KABUL is certainly one of the most important subjects of further research.

Postulates for Updates: The basic postulates for updates in classical propositional logic, set forth in [116], do not apply when considering updates of non-monotonic theories. This was shown with the basic examples that served as the initial motivation for this work, and further explored in [77]. It is in order to establish a set of postulates to be obeyed by any reasonable semantics for such non-monotonic theory updates, and against which such semantics can be tested and compared.

Contradiction Removal: Also of importance is the subject of contradiction removal which we have previously mentioned when we addressed the several possible ways contradiction may arise in a DLP setting. One other direction for future research is the definition of paraconsistent semantics for DLP to subsequently deal with, and eventually remove, such contradictions (c.f. [51] for a recent survey article on the subject of paraconsistent semantics for logic programs). Also of interest would be the study of updates in richer LP settings such as Annotated Logic Programs [118] or Probabilistic Logic Programs [175], or even Antitonic Logic Programs [52].

Syntax Simplifications: In order to have an expressive language in which rather complex update statements are representable in a uniform way, we often loose simplicity when writing some rather simple updates. This is true, for example, for updates that just specify the assertion of some rule when a certain sequence of conditions holds, where a statement with deep nesting is required for such. One promising way to solve this issue is to adapt existing frameworks, specialized in the representation of such temporal composition of events, to KABUL. We have already mentioned one such language, the Composite Temporal Event Language of Motakis and Zaniolo [171].

Minimalist Update Language: The insight achieved with the development of KABUL by building upon the syntax of LUPS, provides the necessary maturity to focus our research effort on the other approach to update languages, consisting of identifying a rather more minimalist language, with the same representation power, and build libraries of macros to allow for the use of other intuitive constructs. This is subject of our current research, of which the first results can be found in [2].

Integration: There has been an extensive work on revision of non-monotonic theories. While revision deals with evolving representations of static worlds, updates deal with evolving worlds. One future direction for research is to study the combination of revision and updates so as to integrate them into a single unified framework. This would allow to distinguish newly incoming information as being of an update nature from that of a revision nature, i.e. information concerning one particular state for which we already have some incomplete information. But such integration work is not limited to revision. Indeed, several recent developments in non-monotonic extensions to logic programming must be integrated with MDLP, such as inductive logic programming, rule preferences, priorities, abduction, etc. Moreover, the issue is not just that of conceptual integration but that of conceptual cross-fertilization too. How can one employ learning in the service of updating? How does one remove contradictions from updates? How can rule preferences [39] be combined with the type of preferences enacted by updates, and the preferences themselves be subjected to updating? Indeed, how can other logic programming based computational reasoning abilities such as assuming by default, abducing, revising beliefs, etc., be integrated into a multi-dimensional updating framework involving a multiplicity of agents?

Application: The applicability of these theories in real application areas such as distributed knowledge bases, software development, multi-strategy learning, abductive planning, model-based diagnosis, agent architecture, legal knowledge bases, and others, are currently being investigated. But we believe that many more areas can take advantage of the update mechanisms here presented. Within the context of agent systems, even not following the architectural line here proposed, $\mathcal{MDLP}$ can easily be adapted as the core knowledge representation mechanism of other existing agent architectures.

Implementation: An efficient implementation of the full KABUL language is also in order. We are currently working towards the implementation of a three-valued approximation of KABUL, in a distributed environment, plus distributed tabling.

We began this work by praising the virtue and the promise of *Computational Logic*, most adeptly in the form of *Logic Programming*, for sketching the issues of, and the solutions for, an integrated *Evolving Knowledge Base* architecture with a precisely defined declarative semantics. As we near the end of this protracted exposition, we are confident to have brought the point home. To wit, our architectural scaffolding rests on a sound and wide basis, whose core are the multi-dimensionally configured, updatable knowledge bases.

Were it not for the impressive development in *Logic Programming* semantics in the past 12 years or so, and its extensions to non-monotonic and other forms of reasoning, we would not have today the impressive, sound, and efficient system implementations of such semantics (be it the stable or well-founded varieties or their hybrid combination), which have been opening up a whole new gamut of application areas as well as a spate of sophisticated reasoning abilities over them. This was made possible only through successive and prolonged efforts at theoretical generalization and synthesis, and by way of the combined integration of theory, procedure development, and practical implementation. The ongoing work on *Evolving Knowledge Bases* reflected here is yet another outcome of this joint enterprise.

Bibliography

[1] J. J. Alferes. An implementation of Multi-dimensional Dynamic Logic Programming, 2000. Available at `http://centria.di.fct.unl.pt/~jja/updates/`.

[2] J. J. Alferes, A. Brogi, J. A. Leite, and L. M. Pereira. Evolving logic programs. In S. Flesca, S. Greco, N. Leone, and G. Ianni, editors, *Proceedings of the 8th European Conference on Logics in Artificial Intelligence (JELIA'02)*, volume 2424 of *LNAI*, pages 50–61. Springer-Verlag, 2002.

[3] J. J. Alferes, C. V. Damásio, and L. M. Pereira. A logic programming system for nonmonotonic reasoning. *Journal of Automated Reasoning*, 14(1):93–147, February 1995.

[4] J. J. Alferes, P. Dell'Acqua, E. Lamma, J. A. Leite, L. M. Pereira, and F. Riguzzi. A logic based approach to multi-agent systems. Invited paper in The Association for Logic Programming Newsletter, 14(3): 13 pages, 2001.

[5] J. J. Alferes, J. A. Leite, L. M. Pereira, H. Przymusinska, and T. C. Przymusinski. Dynamic logic programming. In A. Cohn, L. Schubert, and S. Shapiro, editors, *Proceedings of the 6th International Conference on Principles of Knowledge Representation and Reasoning (KR-98)*, pages 98–111, San Francisco, 1998. Morgan Kaufmann Publishers.

[6] J. J. Alferes, J. A. Leite, L. M. Pereira, H. Przymusinska, and T. C. Przymusinski. Dynamic logic programming. In J. L. Freire, M. Falaschi, and M. Vialres-Ferro, editors, *Proceedings of the 1998 Joint Conference on Declarative Programming (AGP-98)*, pages 393–408, La Coruña, Spain, 1998.

[7] J. J. Alferes, J. A. Leite, L. M. Pereira, H. Przymusinska, and T. C. Przymusinski. Updates of logic programs by logic programs. In Z. Ras M. Klopotek, M. Michalewicz, editor, *Proceedings of the Seventh International Symposium on Intelligent Information Systems (IIS'98)(Former WIS Series)*, pages 160–177, Malbork, Poland, June 1998. Wydawnictwo IPI PAN.

[8] J. J. Alferes, J. A. Leite, L. M. Pereira, H. Przymusinska, and T. C. Przymusinski. Dynamic updates of non-monotonic knowledge bases. *The Journal of Logic Programming*, 45(1–3):43–70, September/October 2000.

[9] J. J. Alferes, J. A. Leite, L. M. Pereira, and P. Quaresma. Planning as abductive updating. In D. Kitchin, editor, *Proceedings of the AISB'00 Symposium on AI Planning and Intelligent Agents*, pages 1–8. AISB, 2000.

[10] J. J. Alferes and L. M. Pereira. Contradiction: When avoidance equals removal, part I. In R. Dyckhoff, editor, *Proceedings of the 4th International Workshop*

on Extensions of Logic Programming, volume 798 of *LNAI*, pages 11–23, Berlin, March 1994. Springer.

[11] J. J. Alferes and L. M. Pereira. *Reasoning with logic programming*, volume 1111 of *Lecture Notes in Artificial Intelligence and Lecture Notes in Computer Science*. Springer-Verlag Inc., New York, NY, USA, 1996.

[12] J. J. Alferes and L. M. Pereira. Update-programs can update programs. In J. Dix, L. M. Pereira, and T. Przymusinski, editors, *Selected Papers from NMELP'96*, volume 1216 of *LNAI*, pages 110–131. Springer-Verlag, 1997.

[13] J. J. Alferes and L. M. Pereira. Updates plus preferences. In M. O. Aciego, I. P. Guzmán, G. Brewka, and L. M. Pereira, editors, *Proceedings of the European Workshop on Logics in Artificial Intelligence (JELIA-00)*, volume 1919 of *LNAI*. Springer, 2000.

[14] J. J. Alferes, L. M. Pereira, and E. Orlowska, editors. *Logics in artificial intelligence: European Workshop, JELIA '96, Evora, Portugal, September 30-October 3, 1996, proceedings*, volume 1126 of *Lecture Notes in Artificial Intelligence and Lecture Notes in Computer Science*, New York, NY, USA, 1996. Springer-Verlag Inc.

[15] J. J. Alferes, L. M. Pereira, H. Przymusinska, and T. Przymusinski. LUPS : A language for updating logic programs. In M. Gelfond, N. Leone, and G. Pfeifer, editors, *Proceedings of the 5th International Conference on Logic Programming and Nonmonotonic Reasoning (LPNMR-99)*, volume 1730 of *LNAI*, pages 162–176, Berlin, 1999. Springer.

[16] J. J. Alferes, L. M. Pereira, H. Przymusinska, and T. Przymusinski. LUPS: A language for updating logic programs. *Artificial Intelligence*, 132(1 & 2), 2002.

[17] J. J. Alferes, L. M. Pereira, H. Przymusinska, T. C. Przymusinski, and P. Quaresma. An exercise with dynamic logic programming. In L. Garcia and M. Chiara Meo, editors, *Procs. of the APPIA-GULP-PRODE'00 Joint Conference on Declarative Programming AGP'00, La Habana, Cuba*, 2000.

[18] J. J. Alferes, L. M. Pereira, H. Przymusinska, T. C. Przymusinski, and P. Quaresma. Dynamic knowledge representation and its applications. In T. Eiter, M. Truszczynski, and W. Faber, editors, *Procs. of the 9th International Conference on Artificial Intelligence - Methodology, Systems, Applications (AIMSA'00)*, volume 1904 of *LNAI*, pages 1–10, Berlin, 2001. Springer.

[19] J. J. Alferes, L. M. Pereira, and T. Przymusinski. 'Classical' negation in non-monotonic reasoning and logic programming. *Journal of Automated Reasoning*, 20(1 & 2):107–142, 1998.

[20] J. J. Alferes, L. M. Pereira, T. Przymusinski, H. Przymusinska, and P. Quaresma. Preliminary exploration on actions as updates. In M. C. Meo and M. V. Ferro, editors, *Proceedings of the 1999 Joint Conference on Declarative Programming (AGP-99)*, 1999.

[21] J. J. Alferes, L. M. Pereira, and T. C. Przymusinski. Strong and explicit negation in nonmonotonic reasoning and logic programming. In J. J. Alferes, L. M. Pereira, and E. Orlowska, editors, *Proceedings of the European JELIA Workshop (JELIA-96): Logics in Artificial Intelligence*, volume 1126 of *LNAI*, pages 143–163, Berlin, 1996. Springer.

[22] G. Antoniou. *Nonmonotonic Reasoning.* The MIT Press, Cambridge, Massachusetts, 1997.

[23] K. Apt, editor. *Proceedings of the Joint International Conference and Symposium on Logic Programming (JICSLP-92)*, Cambridge, 1992. MIT Press.

[24] K. R. Apt, Howard A. Blair, and A. Walker. Towards a theory of declarative knowledge. In J. Minker, editor, *Foundations of deductive databases and logic programs*, pages 89–148. Morgan Kaufmann, Los Altos, US, 1988.

[25] K. R. Apt and R. N. Bol. Logic programming and negation: A survey. *The Journal of Logic Programming*, 19 & 20:9–72, May 1994.

[26] J. W. Backus, F. L. Bauer, J. Green, C. Katz, J. McCarthy, P. Naur, A. J. Perlis, H. Rutishauser, K. Samelson, B. Vauquois, J. H. Wegstein, A. van Wijngaarden, and M. Woodger. Revised report on the algorithmic language ALGOL 60. *The Computer Journal*, 5(4):349–367, January 1963.

[27] C. Baral and M. Gelfond. Logic programming and knowledge representation. *Journal of Logic-Programming*, 19–20, 1994.

[28] C. Baral and M. Gelfond. Reasoning about effects of concurrent actions. *Journal of Logic Programming*, 31(1–3):85–117, April–June 1997.

[29] C. Baral, J. Lobo, and G. Trajcevski. Formal characterizations of active databases: Part II. In F. Bry, R. Ramakrishnan, and K. Ramamohanaroa, editors, *Deductive and Object-Oriented Databases, 5th International Conference, DOOD'97, Montreux, Switzerland, December 8-12, 1997, Proceedings*, LNCS, pages 247–264. Springer, 1997.

[30] J. A. Barnden, S. Helmreich, E. Iverson, and G. C. Stein. An integrated implementation of simulative, uncertain and metaphorical reasoning about mental states. In Pietro Torasso Jon Doyle, E. Sandewall, editor, *Proceedings of the 4th International Conference on Principles of Knowledge Representation and Reasoning*, pages 27–38, Bonn, FRG, May 1994. Morgan Kaufmann.

[31] H. Barringer, M. Fisher, D. Gabbay, G. Gough, and R. Owens. METATEM: A framework for programming in temporal logic. In *REX Workshop on Stepwise Refinement of Distributed Systems: Models, Formalisms, Correctness (LNCS Volume 430)*, pages 94–129. Springer-Verlag: Heidelberg, Germany, June 1989.

[32] A. Benveniste, P Le Guernic, and C. Jacquemot. Synchronous programming with events and relations: the signal language and its semantics. *Science of Computer Programming*, 16:103–149, 1991.

[33] A. Bochman. A foundational theory of belief and belief change. *Artificial Intelligence*, 108(1–2):309–352, 1999.

[34] A. J. Bonner and M. Kifer. Transaction logic programming. In David S. Warren, editor, *Proceedings of the Tenth International Conference on Logic Programming*, pages 257–279, Budapest, Hungary, 1993. The MIT Press.

[35] S. Brass and J. Dix. A disjunctive semantics based on unfolding and bottom-up evaluation. In Bernd Wolfinger, editor, *Innovationen bei Rechen- und Kommunikationssystemen,* (IFIP '94-Congress, Workshop FG2: Disjunctive Logic Programming and Disjunctive Databases), pages 83–91, Berlin, 1994. Springer.

[36] S. Brass and J. Dix. Characterizations of the Disjunctive Stable Semantics by Partial Evaluation. *Journal of Logic Programming*, 32(3):207–228, 1997.

[37] S. Brass and J. Dix. Characterizations of the Disjunctive Well-founded Semantics: Confluent Calculi and Iterated GCWA. *Journal of Automated Reasoning*, 20(1):143–165, 1998.

[38] G. Brewka. Well-founded semantics for extended logic programs with dynamic preferences. *Journal of Artificial Intelligence Research*, 4, 1996.

[39] G. Brewka and T. Eiter. Preferred answer sets for extended logic programs. *Artificial Intelligence*, 109, 1999. A short version appeared in A. Cohn and L. Schubert (eds.), *KR'98*, Morgan Kaufmann.

[40] Gerhard Brewka. *Nonmonotonic Reasoning - Logical Foundations of Commonsense*, volume 12 of *Cambridge Tracts in Theoretical Computer Science*. Cambridge University Press, October 1990.

[41] A. Brogi, S. Contiero, and F. Turini. Programming by combining general logic programs. *Journal of Logic and Computation*, 9(1):7–24, Febuary 1999.

[42] L. Brownston, R. Farrell, E. Kant, and N. Martin. *Programming Expert Systems in OPS5: An Introduction to Rule-based Programming.* Addison-Wesley, 1985.

[43] M. Bruynooghe, editor. *Proceedings of the International Symposium on Logic Programming*, Cambridge, MA, USA, 1994. MIT Press.

[44] F. Buccafurri, W. Faber, and N. Leone. Disjunctive logic programs with inheritance. In D. De Schreye, editor, *Proceedings of the 1999 International Conference on Logic Programming (ICLP-99)*, pages 79–93, Cambridge, November 1999. MIT Press.

[45] P. Caspi, D. Pilaud, N. Halbwachs, and J. A. Plaice. LUSTRE: A declarative language for programming synchronous systems. In *Conference Record of the Fourteenth Annual ACM Symposium on Principles of Programming Languages*, pages 178–188, Munich, West Germany, January 21–23, 1987. ACM SIGACT-SIGPLAN, ACM Press.

[46] A. Ciampolini, E. Lamma, P. Mello, F. Toni, and P. Torroni. Co-operation and competition in alias: a logic framework for agents that negotiate. *Annals of Mathematics and Artificial Intelligence, special issue on Computational Logic in Multi-Agent Systems*, 2002. to appear.

[47] K. Clark. Negation as failure. In H. Gallaire and J. Minker, editors, *Logic and Data Bases*, pages 293–322. Plenum Press, 1978.

[48] A. Colmerauer, H. Kanoui, P. Roussel, and R. Pasero. Un systéme de communication homme–machine en français. Technical report, Groupe de Recherche en Intelligence Artificielle, Université d'Aix–Marseille II, 1973.

[49] C. V. Damásio. *Paraconsistent Extended Logic Programming with Constraints.* PhD thesis, Universidade Nova de Lisboa, 1996.

[50] C. V. Damásio and L. M. Pereira. Default negation in the heads: why not? In R. Dyckhoff, H. Herre, and P. Schroeder-Heister, editors, *Int. Ws. Extensions of Logic Programming (ELP-96)*, volume 1050 of *LNAI*, pages 103–117. Springer Verlag, November 1996.

[51] C. V. Damásio and L. M. Pereira. A survey on paraconsistent semantics for extended logic programas. In D. M. Gabbay and Ph. Smets, editors, *Handbook of Defeasible Reasoning and Uncertainty Management Systems*, volume 2, pages 241–320. Kluwer Academic Publishers, 1998.

[52] C. V. Damásio and L. M. Pereira. Antitonic logic programs. In T. Eiter, M. Truszczynski, and W. Faber, editors, *Proceedings of the 6th International Conference on Logic Programming and Nonmonotonic Reasoning (LPNMR-01)*, volume 2173 of *LNAI*, pages 379–392, Berlin, 2001. Springer.

[53] A. Damodaran. *Investment Valuation.* John Wiley & Sons, 2 edition, 2002.

[54] G. T. David. *Semantics of Multiple Inheritance with Exceptions in Hierarchically Structured Logic Theories.* PhD thesis, Faculdade de Ciências e Tecnologia, Universidade Nova de Lisboa, 1994.

[55] E. de Bono. *Lateral Thinking: Creativity Step by Step.* Harper & Row, New York, 1970.

[56] H. Decker. Drawing updates from derivations. In S. Abiteboul and P. C. Kanellakis, editors, *ICDT'90, Third International Conference on Database Theory*, volume 470 of *Lecture Notes in Computer Science*, pages 437–451, Paris, France, 12–14 December 1990. Springer.

[57] P. Dell'Acqua and L. M. Pereira. Updating agents. In S. Rochefort, F. Sadri, and F. Toni, editors, *ICLP-99 Workshop on Multi-Agent Systems in Logic*, 1999.

[58] M. d'Inverno, D. Kinny, M. Luck, and M. Wooldridge. A formal specification of dMARS. In Singh, Rao, and Wooldridge, editors, *Intelligent Agents IV: Proceedings of the Fourth International Workshop on Agent Theories, Architectures and Languages*, Lecture Notes in Artificial Intelligence, 1365, pages 155–176. sv, 1998.

[59] J. Dix. Classifying semantics of disjunctive logic programs. In K. Apt, editor, *International Joint Conference and Symposium on Logic Programming*, pages 798–812. MIT Press, 1992.

[60] J. Dix. A classification theory of semantics of normal logic programs I: Strong properties. *Fundamenta Mathematicae*, 22(3):227–255, 1995.

[61] J. Dix. A classification theory of semantics of normal logic programs II: Weak properties. *Fundamenta Mathematicae*, 22(3):257–288, 1995.

[62] J. Dix, L. del Cerro, and U. Furbach, editors. *Logics in artificial intelligence: European Workshop, JELIA'98 Dagstuhl, Germany, October 12–15, 1998: proceedings*, volume 1489 of *Lecture Notes in Computer Science and Lecture Notes in Artificial Intelligence*, New York, NY, USA, 1998. Springer-Verlag Inc.

[63] J. Dix, Ulrich Fuhrbach, and Anil Nerode, editors. *Logic programming and nonmonotonic reasoning: 4th International Conference, LPNMR '97, Dagstuhl Castle, Germany, July 1997: proceedings*, volume 1265 of *Lecture Notes in Artificial Intelligence and Lecture Notes in Computer Science*, New York, NY, USA, 1997. Springer-Verlag Inc.

[64] J. Dix, J. A. Leite, and K. Satoh, editors. *Computational Logic in Multi-Agent Systems: 3rd International Workshop, CLIMA'02, Copenhagen, Denmark, August 1, 2002, Proceedings*, number 93 in Datalogiske Skrifter (Writings on Computer Science). Roskilde University, Denmark, 2002. Appeared also in the Electronic Notes on Theoretical Computer Science 70(5), 2002.

[65] J. Dix, L. M. Pereira, and T. Przymusinski. Prolegomena to Logic Programming for Non-Monotonic Reasoning. In J. Dix, L. M. Pereira, and T. Przymusinski, editors, *Nonmonotonic Extensions of Logic Programming*, LNAI 1216, pages 1–36. Springer, Berlin, 1997.

[66] J. Dix, L. M. Pereira, and T. C. Przymusinski, editors. *Non-monotonic extensions of logic programming: ICLP '94 workshop, Santa Margherita Ligure, Italy, June 17, 1994: selected papers*, volume 927 of *Lecture Notes in Artificial Intelligence and Lecture Notes in Computer Science*, New York, NY, USA, 1995. Springer-Verlag Inc.

[67] J. Dix, L. M. Pereira, and T. C. Przymusinski, editors. *Non-monotonic extensions of logic programming: 2nd International Workshop, NMELP '96, Bad Honnef, Germany, September 5–6, 1996: selected papers*, volume 1216 of *Lecture Notes in Computer Science and Lecture Notes in Artificial Intelligence*, New York, NY, USA, 1997. Springer-Verlag Inc.

[68] J. Dix, L. M. Pereira, and T. C. Przymusinski, editors. *Logic programming and knowledge representation: Third International Workshop, LPKR'97: Port Jefferson, New York, USA, October 17, 1997: selected papers*, volume 1471 of *Lecture Notes in Computer Science and Lecture Notes in Artificial Intelligence*, New York, NY, USA, 1998. Springer-Verlag Inc.

[69] DLV. The DLV project - a disjunctive datalog system (and more), 2000. Available at `http://www.dbai.tuwien.ac.at/proj/dlv/`.

[70] P. M. Dung and P. Ruamviboonsuk. Well founded reasoning with classical negation. In A. Nerode, W. Marek, and V. S. Subrahmanian, editors, *Logic Programming and NonMonotonic Reasoning*, pages 120–132. MIT Press, 1991.

[71] R. Dyckhoff, editor. *Extensions of logic programming: 4th international workshop, ELP '93, St Andrews, UK, March 29–April 1, 1993: proceedings*, volume 798 of *Lecture Notes in Artificial Intelligence and Lecture Notes in Computer Science*, New York, NY, USA, 1994. Springer-Verlag Inc.

[72] R. Dyckhoff, H. Herre, and P. J. Schroeder-Heister, editors. *Extensions of logic programming: 5th international workshop, ELP '96, Leipzig, Germany, March 28–30, 1996: proceedings*, volume 1050 of *Lecture Notes in Artificial Intelligence and Lecture Notes in Computer Science*, New York, NY, USA, 1996. Springer-Verlag Inc.

[73] U. Eco. *Semiotics and the Philosophy of Language.* MacMillan Press, London, 1984.

[74] R. Edwards, J. Magee, and W. H. C. Bassetti. *Technical Analysis of Stock Trends.* Saint Lucie Press, 8 edition, 2001.

[75] T. Eiter, M. Fink, G. Sabbatini, and H. Tompits. A framework for declarative update specifications in logic programs. In Bernhard Nebel, editor, *Proceedings of the seventeenth International Conference on Artificial Intelligence (IJCAI-01)*, pages 649–654, San Francisco, CA, 2001. Morgan Kaufmann Publishers, Inc.

[76] T. Eiter, M. Fink, G. Sabbatini, and H. Tompits. Reasoning about evolving non-monotonic knowledge bases. In R. Nieuwenhuis and A. Voronkov, editors, *Proceedings of the 8th International Conference on Logic for Programming, Artificial Intelligence, and Reasoning (LPAR'01)*, volume 2250 of *LNAI*, pages 407–421. Springer, 2001.

[77] T. Eiter, M. Fink, G. Sabbatini, and H. Tompits. On properties of update sequences based on causal rejection. *Theory and Practice of Logic Programming*, 2002. to appear.

[78] T. Eiter and G. Gottlob. Complexity aspects of various semantics for disjunctive databases. In Catriel Beeri, editor, *Proceedings of the 12th Symposium on Principles of Database Systems*, pages 158–167, New York, NY, USA, May 1993. ACM Press.

[79] T. Eiter and G. Gottlob. Complexity results for disjunctive logic programming and application to nonmonotonic logics. In Dale Miller, editor, *Logic Programming - Proceedings of the 1993 International Symposium*, pages 266–278, Vancouver, Canada, 1993. The MIT Press.

[80] T. Eiter, G. Gottlob, and H. Mannila. Disjunctive Datalog. *ACM Transactions on Database Systems*, 22(3):364–418, September 1997.

[81] T. Eiter, N. Leone, C. Mateis, G. Pfeifer, and F. Scarcello. The KR system `dlv`: Progress report, comparisons and benchmarks. In Anthony G. Cohn, Lenhart Schubert, and Stuart C. Shapiro, editors, *KR'98: Principles of Knowledge Representation and Reasoning*, pages 406–417. Morgan Kaufmann, San Francisco, California, 1998.

[82] M. Van Emden and R. Kowalski. The semantics of predicate logic as a programming language. *Journal of ACM*, 4(23):733–742, 1976.

[83] L.-H. Eriksson, L. Hallnas, and P. J. Schroeder-Heister, editors. *Extensions of logic programming: second international workshop, Stockholm, Sweden, January 27–29, 1991, proceedings*, volume 596 of *Lecture Notes in Artificial Intelligence and Lecture Notes in Computer Science*, New York, NY, USA, 1992. Springer-Verlag Inc.

[84] M. Fisher. Concurrent METATEM — A language for modelling reactive systems. In Arndt Bode, Mike Reeve, and Gottfried Wolf, editors, *Proceedings of PARLE '93 – Parallel Architectures and Languages Europe*, Lecture Notes in Computer Science, pages 185–196, Munich, Germany, June 14–17, 1993. Springer-Verlag.

[85] M. Fitting. A Kripke-Kleene semantics for logic programs. *Journal of Logic Programming*, 2(4):295–312, 1985.

[86] P. A. Flach and A. C. Kakas, editors. *Abduction and Induction: Essays on their relation and integration.* Kluwer Academic Publishers, April 2000.

[87] P. Gärdenfors, editor. *Belief Revision*, number 29 in Cambridge Tracts in Theoretical Computer Science. Cambridge University Press, 1992.

[88] P. Gärdenfors. Belief revision and knowledge representation. In Yoav Shoham, editor, *Proceedings of the Sixth Conference on Theoretical Aspects of Rationality and Knowledge*, pages 117–118, San Francisco, March 17–20 1996. Morgan Kaufmann Publishers.

[89] A. Van Gelder, K. A. Ross, and J. S. Schlipf. The well-founded semantics for general logic programs. *Journal of the ACM*, 38(3):620–650, 1991.

[90] M. Gelfond, N. Leone, and G. Pfeifer, editors. *Logic programming and non-monotonic reasoning: 5th international conference, LPNMR '99, El Paso, Texas, USA, December 2–4, 1999: proceedings*, volume 1730 of *Lecture Notes in Computer Science and Lecture Notes in Artificial Intelligence*, New York, NY, USA, 1999. Springer-Verlag Inc.

[91] M. Gelfond and V. Lifschitz. The stable model semantics for logic programming. In R. Kowalski and K. A. Bowen, editors, *5th International Conference on Logic Programming*, pages 1070–1080. MIT Press, 1988.

[92] M. Gelfond and V. Lifschitz. Logic programs with classical negation. In Warren and Szeredi, editors, *7th International Conference on Logic Programming*, pages 579–597. MIT Press, 1990.

[93] M. Gelfond and V. Lifschitz. Classical Negation in Logic Programs and Disjunctive Databases. *New Generation Computing*, 9:365–385, 1991.

[94] M. Gelfond and V. Lifschitz. Representing actions in extendd logic programming. In *Proceedings of international joint conference and symposium on logic programming*, Boston, MA, 1992. MIT Press.

[95] M. Gelfond and V. Lifschitz. Representing actions and change by logic programs. *Journal of Logic Programming*, 17:301–322, 1993.

[96] M. Gelfond and V. Lifschitz. Action languages. *Linkoping Electronic Articles in Computer and Information Science*, 3(16), 1998.

[97] M. Gelfond, V. Lifschitz, and A. Rabinov. What are the limitations of the situation calculus? In *Automated Reasoning: Essays in Honor of Woody Bledsoe*, pages 167–179. Kluwer Academic Publishers, Dordrecht, 1986.

[98] D. Gentner, B. Falkenhainer, and J. Skorstad. Metaphor: the good, the bad and the ugly. *Theoretical Issues in Natural Language Processing*, 3:155–159, 1987.

[99] M. L. Ginsberg, editor. *Readings in Nonmonotonic Reasoning.* Morgan Kaufmann, Los Altos, California, 1987.

[100] M. L. Ginsberg. *Nonmonotonic Reasoning.* Morgan Kaufmann, 1988.

[101] E. Giunchiglia and V. Lifschitz. An action language based on causal explanation: Preliminary report. In *AAAI'98*, pages 623–630, 1998.

[102] A. Guessoum and J. W. Lloyd. Updating knowledge bases. *New Generation Computing*, 8(1):71–89, 1990.

[103] A. Guessoum and J. W. Lloyd. Updating knowledge bases II. *New Generation Computing*, 10(1):73–100, 1991.

[104] J. P. Guilford. *The Nature of Human Intelligence.* McGraw-Hill, New York, 1967.

[105] S. Hanks and D. McDermott. Default reasoning, nonmonotonic logic and the frame problem. In *National Conference on Artificial Intelligence of the American Association for AI (AAAI 86)*, pages 328–333, 1986.

[106] K. V. Hindriks, F. S. de Boer, W. van der Hoek, and J. C. Meyer. Formal semantics for an abstract agent programming language. In M. P. Singh, A. Rao, and M. J. Wooldridge, editors, *Proceedings of the 4th International Workshop on Agent Theories, Architectures, and Languages (ATAL-97*, volume 1365 of *LNAI*, pages 215–230, Berlin, July 24–26 1998. Springer.

[107] Koen V. Hindriks, Frank S. de Boer, Wiebe van der Hoek, and John-Jules Ch. Meyer. A formal embedding of AgentSpeak(L) in 3APL. In G. Antoniou and J. Slaney, editors, *Advanced Topics in Artificial Intelligence (LNAI 1502)*, pages 155–166. Springer-Verlag: Heidelberg, Germany, 1998.

[108] B. Indurkhya. *Metaphor and Cognition: an Interactionist Approach.* Kluwer Academic Publishers, Dordrecht, The Netherlands, 1992.

[109] K. Inoue. Extended logic programs with default assumptions. In Koichi Furukawa, editor, *8th International Conference on Logic Programming*, pages 490–504. MIT Press, 1991.

[110] K. Inoue and C. Sakama. On positive occurrences of negation as failure. In Pietro Torasso Jon Doyle, E. Sandewall, editor, *Proceedings of the 4th International Conference on Principles of Knowledge Representation and Reasoning*, pages 293–304, Bonn, FRG, May 1994. Morgan Kaufmann.

[111] K. Inoue and C. Sakama. Negation as failure in the head. *Journal of Logic Programming*, 35:39–78, 1998.

[112] J. Jaffar, editor. *Proceedings of the 1998 Joint International Conference and Symposium on Logic Programming (JICSLP-98)*, Cambridge, 1998. MIT Press.

[113] J. Jaffar and M. J. Maher. Constraint logic programming: A survey. *The Journal of Logic Programming*, 19 & 20:503–582, May 1994.

[114] N. R. Jennings, K. Sycara, and M. Wooldridge. A roadmap of agent research and development. *Journal of Autonomous Agents and Multi-Agent Systems*, 1(1):7–38, 1998.

[115] A. C. Kakas, R. A. Kowalski, and F. Toni. Abductive Logic Programming. *Journal of Logic and Computation*, 2(6):719–770, 1993.

[116] H. Katsuno and A. O. Mendelzon. On the difference between updating a knowledge base and revising it. In J. Allen, Richard Fikes, and E. Sandewall, editors, *Proceedings of the 2nd International Conference on Principles of Knowledge Representation and Reasoning*, pages 387–394, San Mateo, CA, USA, April 1991. Morgan Kaufmann Publishers.

[117] A. Keller and M. Winslett Wilkins. On the use of an extended relational model to handle changing incomplete information. *IEEE Trans. on Software Engineering*, 11(7):620–633, 1985.

[118] Michael Kifer and V. S. Subrahmanian. Theory of generalized annotated logic programming and its applications. *The Journal of Logic Programming*, 12(1 and 2):335–367, January 1992.

[119] R. Kowalski. Predicate logic as a programming language. In *Proceedings of IFIP'74*, pages 569–574, 1974.

[120] R. Kowalski. Algorithm = logic + control. *Communications of the ACM*, 22:424–436, 1979.

[121] R. Kowalski. Problems and promises of computational logic. In J. Lloyd, editor, *Computational Logic*, pages 1–36. Basic Research Series, Springer–Verlag, 1990.

[122] R. Kowalski and F. Sadri. Logic programs with exceptions. In Warren and Szeredi, editors, *7th International Conference on Logic Programming*. MIT Press, 1990.

[123] R. Kowalski and F. Sadri. Towards a unified agent architecture that combines rationality with reactivity. In D. Pedreschi and C Zaniolo, editors, *Proceedings of LID-96*, volume 1154 of *LNAI*, pages 137–149, 1996.

[124] K. Kunen. Negation in logic programming. *Journal of Logic Programming*, 4:289–308, 1987.

[125] G. Lakoff and M. Johnson. *Metaphors We Live By*. University of Chicago Press, Chicago, 1980.

[126] E. Lamma and P. Mello, editors. *Extensions of logic programming: third international workshop, ELP '92, Bologna, Italy, February 26–28, 1992: proceedings*, volume 660 of *Lecture Notes in Artificial Intelligence and Lecture Notes in Computer Science*, New York, NY, USA, 1993. Springer-Verlag Inc.

[127] E. Lamma, F. Riguzzi, and L. M. Pereira. Strategies in combined learning via logic programs. *Machine Learning*, 38(1/2):63–87, 2000.

[128] J. Lassez, editor. *Proceedings of the Fourth International Conference on Logic Programming (ICLP '87)*, Melbourne, Australia, 1987. MIT Press.

[129] N. Lavrac. Computational logic and machine learning: A roadmap for inductive logic programming, 2000. Available at http://www2.ags.uni-sb.de/net/Forum/.

[130] J. A. Leite. Logic program updates. Master's thesis, Dept. de Informática, Faculdade de Ciências e Tecnologia, Universidade Nova de Lisboa, November 1997.

[131] J. A. Leite. A modified semantics for LUPS. In P. Brazdil and A. Jorge, editors, *Progress in Artificial Intelligence, Proceedings of the 10th Portuguese International Conference on Artificial Intelligence (EPIA01)*, volume 2258 of *LNAI*, pages 261–275, Berlin, 2001. Springer.

[132] J. A. Leite, J. J. Alferes, and L. M. Pereira. Dynamic logic programming with multiple dimensions. In L. Garcia and M. Chiara Meo, editors, *Procs. of the APPIA-GULP-PRODE'00 Joint Conference on Declarative Programming AGP'00, La Habana, Cuba*, 2000.

[133] J. A. Leite, J. J. Alferes, and L. M. Pereira. Multi-dimensional dynamic logic programming. In F. Sadri and K. Satoh, editors, *Proceedings of the CL-2000 Workshop on Computational Logic in Multi-Agent Systems (CLIMA'00)*, pages 17–26, 2000.

[134] J. A. Leite, J. J. Alferes, and L. M. Pereira. Combining societal agents' knowledge. In L. M. Pereira and P. Quaresma, editors, *Proceedings of the 2001 Joint Conference on Declarative Programming (AGP'01)*, pages 313–327, September 2001.

[135] J. A. Leite, J. J. Alferes, and L. M. Pereira. Minerva - a dynamic logic programming agent architecture. In J. J. Meyer and M. Tambe, editors, *Pre-Procs. of the Eighth International Workshop on Agent Theories, Architectures, and Languages ATAL'01*, pages 133–145, 2001.

[136] J. A. Leite, J. J. Alferes, and L. M. Pereira. Multi-dimensional dynamic knowledge representation. In T. Eiter, M. Truszczynski, and W. Faber, editors, *Proceedings of the 6th International Conference on Logic Programming and Nonmonotonic Reasoning (LPNMR-01)*, volume 2173 of *LNAI*, pages 365–378, Berlin, 2001. Springer.

[137] J. A. Leite, J. J. Alferes, and L. M. Pereira. On the use of multi-dimensional dynamic logic programming to represent societal agents' viewpoints. In P. Brazdil and A. Jorge, editors, *Progress in Artificial Intelligence, Proceedings of the 10th Portuguese International Conference on Artificial Intelligence (EPIA01)*, volume 2258 of *LNAI*, pages 276–289, Berlin, 2001. Springer.

[138] J. A. Leite, J. J. Alferes, and L. M. Pereira. Minerva - a dynamic logic programming agent architecture. In J. J. Meyer and M. Tambe, editors, *Intelligent Agents VIII — Agent Theories, Architectures, and Languages*, volume 2333 of *LNAI*, pages 141–157. Springer-Verlag, 2002.

[139] J. A. Leite, J. J. Alferes, L. M. Pereira, H. Przymusinska, and T. C. Przymusinski. A language for multi-dimensional updates. In J. Dix, J. A. Leite, and K. Satoh, editors, *Computational Logic in Multi-Agent Systems: Proceedings of the 3rd International Workshop, CLIMA'02*, number 93 in Datalogiske Skrifter (Writings on

Computer Science), pages 19–34. Roskilde University, Denmark, 2002. Appeared also in the Electronic Notes on Theoretical Computer Science 70(5), 2002.

[140] J. A. Leite, F. C. Pereira, A. Cardoso, and L. M. Pereira. Metaphorical mapping consistency via dynamic logic programming. In G. Wiggins, editor, *Proceedings of the AISB'00 Symposium on Creative and Cultural Aspects and Applications of AI and Cognitive Science*, pages 41–50. AISB, 2000.

[141] J. A. Leite and L. M. Pereira. Generalizing updates: From models to programs. In J. Dix, L. M. Pereira, and T. C. Przymusinski, editors, *Selected Extended Papers of the ILPS'97 3th International Workshop on Logic Programming and Knowledge Representation (LPKR-97)*, volume 1471 of *LNAI*, pages 224–246, Berlin, 1997. Springer Verlag.

[142] J. A. Leite and L. M. Pereira. Generalizing updates: from models to programs. In L. M. Pereira, J. Dix, and T. Przymusinski, editors, *Proceedings of the 3th International Workshop on Logic Programming and Knowledge Representation (LPKR-97)*, pages 1–24, Port Jefferson, NY, USA, 1997.

[143] J. A. Leite and L. M. Pereira. Iterated logic program updates. In J. Jaffar, editor, *Proceedings of the 1998 Joint International Conference and Symposium on Logic Programming (JICSLP-98)*, pages 265–278, Cambridge, 1998. MIT Press.

[144] V. Lifschitz. Computing circumscription. In *International Joint Conference on Artificial Intelligence*, pages 121–127. Morgan Kaufmann, 1985.

[145] V. Lifschitz. Foundations of logic programming. In G. Brewka, editor, *Principles of Knowledge Representation*, pages 69–127. CSLI Publications, Stanford, California, 1996.

[146] V. Lifschitz and T. Woo. Answer sets in general non-monotonic reasoning (preliminary report). In B. Nebel, C. Rich, and W. Swartout, editors, *Proceedings of the 3th International Conference on Principles of Knowledge Representation and Reasoning (KR-92)*. Morgan-Kaufmann, 1992.

[147] J. Lloyd, editor. *Proceedings of the International Symposium on Logic Programming*, Cambridge, 1995. MIT Press.

[148] J. W. Lloyd. *Foundations of Logic Programming*. Springer–Verlag, Berlin, 1984.

[149] J. W. Lloyd. *Foundations of Logic Programming*. Springer–Verlag, Berlin, 2 edition, 1987.

[150] J. W. Lloyd, V. Dahl, U. Furbach, M. Kerber, K. Lau, C. Palamidessi, L. M. Pereira, Y. Sagiv, and P. J. Stuckey, editors. *Computational Logic - CL 2000, First International Conference, London, UK, 24-28 July, 2000, Proceedings*, volume 1861 of *Lecture Notes in Computer Science*. Springer, 2000.

[151] J. Lobo, R. Bhatia, and S. Naqvi. A policy description language. In *Proceedings of the 6th National Conference on Artificial Intelligence (AAAI-99); Proceedings of the 11th Conference on Innovative Applications of Artificial Intelligence*, pages 291–298, Menlo Park, Cal., July 18–22 1999. AAAI/MIT Press.

[152] C. MacNish, D. A. Pearce, and L. M. Pereira, editors. *Logics in artificial intelligence: European Workshop JELIA '94, York, UK, September 5–8, 1994: proceedings*, volume 838 of *Lecture Notes in Artificial Intelligence and Lecture Notes in Computer Science*, New York, NY, USA, 1994. Springer-Verlag Inc.

[153] M. Maher, editor. *Proceedings of the 1996 Joint International Conference and Symposium on Logic Programming*, Cambridge, 1996. MIT Press.

[154] J. Małuszyński, editor. *Proceedings of the International Symposium on Logic Programming (ILPS-97)*, Cambridge, 1997. MIT Press.

[155] V. Marek and M. Truszczyński. Autoepistemic logic. *Journal of the Association for Computing Machinery*, 38(3):588–619, 1991.

[156] V. W. Marek, A. Nerode, and M. Truszczynski, editors. *Logic programming and nonmonotonic reasoning: third international conference, LPNMR '95, Lexington, KY, USA, June 24–26, 1995: proceedings*, volume 928 of *Lecture Notes in Artificial Intelligence and Lecture Notes in Computer Science*, New York, NY, USA, 1995. Springer-Verlag Inc.

[157] V. W. Marek and M. Truszczyński. Revision specifications by means of programs. In C. MacNish, D. Pearce, and L. M. Pereira, editors, *Proceedings of the European Workshop on Logics in Artificial Intelligence (JELIA-94)*, volume 838 of *LNAI*, pages 122–136, Berlin, September 1994. Springer.

[158] K. Marriott and P. J. Stuckey. *Programming with Constraints: An Introduction.* The MIT Press, 1998.

[159] J. H. Martin. *A Computational Model of Metaphor Interpretation*, volume Volume 8 of *Perspectives in Artificial Intelligence.* Academic Press, 1990.

[160] M.Bozzano, G.Delzanno, V.Mascardi, M.Martelli, and F.Zini. Logic programming and multi-agent systems: a synergic combination for applications and semantics. In K. R. Apt, V. W. Marek, M. Truszczynski, and D. S. Warren, editors, *The Logic Programming Paradigm: A 25-Year Perspective*, Springer Series in Artificial Intelligence, pages 5–32. Springer-Verlag, Berlin, 1999.

[161] J. McCarthy. Programs with common sense. In *Proceedings of the Teddington Conference on the Mechanization of Thought Processes*, pages 75–91, London, 1959. Her Majesty's Stationary Office.

[162] J. McCarthy. Circumscription - a form of non–monotonic reasoning. *Artificial Intelligence*, 13:27–39, 1980.

[163] J. McCarthy. Applications of circumscription to formalizing common sense knowledge. *Artificial Intelligence*, 26:89–116, 1986.

[164] J. McCarthy. Artificial intelligence, logic, and formalizing common sense. In Richmond Thomason, editor, *Philosophical Logic and Artificial Intelligence*, pages 161–190. Kluwer Publishing Co., Dordrecht, Holland, 1989.

[165] D. McDermott. Non–monotonic logic II. *Journal of the ACM*, 29(1):33–57, 1982.

[166] D. McDermott and J. Doyle. Non-monotonic logic I. *Artificial Intelligence*, 13(1–2):41–72, 1980.

[167] D. Miller, editor. *Proceedings of the 1993 International Symposium on Logic Programming*, Vancouver, B.C., Canada, October 1993. MIT Press.

[168] J. Minker. *Foundations of Deductive Databases and Logic Programming.* Morgan Kaufmann, 1988.

[169] J. Minker. An Overview of Nonmonotonic Reasoning and Logic Programming. *Journal of Logic Programming, Special Issue*, 17, 1993.

[170] R. Moore. Semantics considerations on nonmonotonic logic. *Artificial Intelligence*, 25:75–94, 1985.

[171] I. Motakis and C. Zaniolo. Temporal aggregation in active database rules. In *Proceedings of the ACM SIGMOD International Conference on Management of Data*, volume 26,2 of *SIGMOD Record*, pages 440–451, New York, May 13–15 1997. ACM Press.

[172] S. Muggleton and L. De Raedt. Inductive logic programming: Theory and methods. *The Journal of Logic Programming*, 19 & 20:629–680, May 1994.

[173] A. Nerode, W. Marek, and V. S. Subrahmanian, editors. *Logic Programming and Non–monotonic Reasoning: Proceedings of the First International Workshop*, Washington D.C., USA, 1991. The MIT Press.

[174] I. Newtono. *Philosophiæ Naturalis Principia Mathematica.* Editio tertia & aucta emendata. Apud Guil & Joh. Innys, Regiæ Societatis typographos, 1726. Original quotation: *"Corpus omne perseverare in statu suo quiescendi vel movendi uniformiter in directum, nisi quatenus illud a viribus impressis cogitur statum suum mutare."*.

[175] Raymond Ng and V. S. Subrahmanian. Probabilistic logic programming. *Information and Computation*, 101(2):150–201, December 1992.

[176] I. Niemela and P. Simons. Smodels: An implementation of the stable model and well-founded semantics for normal LP. In J. Dix, U. Furbach, and A. Nerode, editors, *Proceedings of the 4th International Conference on Logic Programing and Nonmonotonic Reasoning (LPNMR-97)*, volume 1265 of *LNAI*, pages 420–429, Berlin, 1997. Springer.

[177] M. Ojeda-Aciego, I. P. Guzmán, G. Brewka, and L. M. Pereira, editors. *Logics in artificial intelligence: European workshop, JELIA 2000, Malaga, Spain, September 29-October 2, 2000: proceedings*, volume 1919 of *Lecture Notes in Computer Science and Lecture Notes in Artificial Intelligence*, New York, NY, USA, 2000. Springer-Verlag Inc.

[178] D. Pearce. Reasoning with negative information II: Hard negation, strong negation and logic programs. In D. Pearce and H. Wansing, editors, *Nonclassical Logics and Information Processing*, pages 63–79. Springer–Verlag, 1990.

[179] D. Pearce and G. Wagner. Reasoning with negative information I: Strong negation in logic programs. In L. Haaparanta, M. Kusch, and I. Niiniluoto, editors, *Language, Knowledge and Intentionality*, pages 430–453. Acta Philosophica Fennica 49, 1990.

[180] D. A. Pearce and G. Wagner, editors. *Logics in AI: European Workshop JELIA '92, Berlin, Germany, September 7–10, 1992: proceedings*, volume 633 of *Lecture Notes in Artificial Intelligence and Lecture Notes in Computer Science*, New York, NY, USA, 1992. Springer-Verlag Inc.

[181] F. C. Pereira. Modelling divergent production: A multi-domain approach. In Henri Prade, editor, *Proceedings of the 13th European Conference on Artificial Intelligence (ECAI-98)*, pages 131–134, Chichester, August 23–28 1998. John Wiley & Sons.

[182] F. C. Pereira. Construção interactiva de mapas conceptuais. Master's thesis, Dept. de Engenharia Informática, Faculdade de Ciências e Tecnologia, Universidade de Coimbra, 2000.

[183] L. M. Pereira and J. J. Alferes. Well founded semantics for logic programs with explicit negation. In B. Neumann, editor, *European Conference on Artificial Intelligence*, pages 102–106. John Wiley & Sons, 1992.

[184] L. M. Pereira and J. J. Alferes. Contradiction: When avoidance equals removal, part II. In R. Dyckhoff, editor, *Proceedings of the 4th International Workshop on Extensions of Logic Programming*, volume 798 of *LNAI*, pages 268–281, Berlin, March 1994. Springer.

[185] L. M. Pereira, J. N. Aparício, and J. J. Alferes. Counterfactual reasoning based on revising assumptions. In Ueda and Saraswat, editors, *International Logic Programming Symposium*, pages 566–577. MIT Press, 1991.

[186] L. M. Pereira, J. N. Aparício, and J. J. Alferes. Nonmonotonic reasoning with well founded semantics. In Koichi Furukawa, editor, *8th International Conference on Logic Programming*, pages 475–489. MIT Press, 1991.

[187] L. M. Pereira, C. V. Damásio, and J. J. Alferes. Diagnosis and debugging as contradiction removal. In L. M. Pereira and A. Nerode, editors, *2nd International Workshop on Logic Programming and NonMonotonic Reasoning*, pages 316–330. MIT Press, 1993.

[188] L. M. Pereira and A. Nerode, editors. *Logic Programming and Non–monotonic Reasoning: Proceedings of the Second International Workshop*, Lisboa, Portugal, 1993. The MIT Press.

[189] H. Przymusinska and T. Przymusinski. Semantic issues in deductive databases and logic programs. In R. Banerji, editor, *Formal Techniques in Artificial Intelligence, a Sourcebook*, pages 321–367. North Holland, 1990.

[190] T. Przymusinski. On the declarative semantics of stratified deductive databases. In J. Minker, editor, *Foundations of Deductive Databases and Logic Programming*, pages 193–216. Morgan Kaufmann, 1988.

[191] T. Przymusinski. Extended stable semantics for normal and disjunctive programs. In Warren and Szeredi, editors, *7th International Conference on Logic Programming*, pages 459–477. MIT Press, 1990.

[192] T. Przymusinski. Stationary semantics for disjunctive logic programs and deductive databases. In Debray and Hermenegildo, editors, *North American Conference on Logic Programming*, pages 40–57. MIT Press, 1990.

[193] T. Przymusinski. A semantics for disjunctive logic programs. In Loveland, Lobo, and Rajasekar, editors, *ILPS'91 Workshop in Disjunctive Logic Programs*, 1991.

[194] T. Przymusinski and H. Turner. Update by means of inference rules. In V. Marek, A. Nerode, and M. Truszczyński, editors, *LPNMR'95*, volume 928 of *LNAI*, pages 156–174. Springer-Verlag, 1995.

[195] T. C. Przymusinski. Extended stable semantics for normal and disjunctive programs. In P. Szerdei and D. H. D. Warren, editors, *Proceedings of the 7th International Conference on Logic Programming (ICLP '90)*, pages 459–480, Jerusalem, June 1990. MIT Press.

[196] T. C. Przymusinski. Static semantics for normal and disjunctive logic programs. *Annals of Mathematics and Artificial Intelligence*, Special Issue on Disjunctive Programs(14):323–357, 1995.

[197] T. C. Przymusinski and H. Turner. Update by means of inference rules. *Journal of Logic Programming*, 30(2):125–143, 1997.

[198] P. Quaresma and L. M. Pereira. Modelling agent interaction in logic programming. In O. Barenstein, editor, *Procs. of the INAP-98*, 1998.

[199] P. Quaresma and I. P. Rodrigues. A collaborative legal information retrieval system using dynamic logic programming. In *Proceedings of the Seventh International Conference on Artificial Intelligence and Law (ICAIL-99)*, ACM SIGART, pages 190–191, N.Y., 1999. ACM Press.

[200] R. Ramakrishnan and J. D. Ullman. A survey of deductive database systems. *Journal of Logic Programming*, 23(2):125–149, May 1995.

[201] A. S. Rao. AgentSpeak(L): BDI agents speak out in a logical computable language. In W. van der Velde and J. W. Perram, editors, *Agents Breaking Away (LNAI 1038)*, pages 42–55. Springer-Verlag: Heidelberg, Germany, 1996.

[202] A. S. Rao and N. Y. Foo. Formal theories of belief revision. In Hector J. Levesque Ronald J. Brachman and R. Reiter, editors, *Proceedings of the 1st International Conference on Principles of Knowledge Representation and Reasoning*, pages 369–380, Toronto, Canada, May 1989. Morgan Kaufmann.

[203] P. Rao, K. Sagonas, T. Swift, D. S. Warren, and J. Freire. XSB: A system for efficiently computing WFS. In J. Dix, Ulrich Furbach, and Anil Nerode, editors, *Proceedings of the 4th International Conference on Logic Programing and Nonmonotonic Reasoning*, volume 1265 of *LNAI*, pages 430–440, Berlin, July 28–31 1997. Springer.

[204] R. Reiter. On closed–world data bases. In H. Gallaire and J. Minker, editors, *Logic and DataBases*, pages 55–76. Plenum Press, 1978.

[205] R. Reiter. A logic for default reasoning. *Artificial Intelligence*, 13:68–93, 1980.

[206] R. Reiter. Nonmonotonic Reasoning. *Annual Review Comput. Science*, 2:147–187, 1987.

[207] R. Reiter. Twelve years of nonmonotonic reasoning research: Where (and what) is the beef. In William Nebel, Bernhard; Rich, Charles; Swartout, editor, *Proceedings of the 3rd International Conference on Principles of Knowledge Representation and Reasoning*, page 789, Cambridge, MA, October 1992. Morgan Kaufmann.

[208] S. Rochefort, F. Sadri, and F. Toni, editors. *Proceedings of the International Workshop on Multi-Agent Systems in Logic Programming*, Las Cruces, New Mexico, USA, 1999. Available from `http://www.cs.sfu.ca/conf/MAS99`.

[209] K. Ross and R. Topor. Inferring negative information from disjunctive databases. *Automated Reasoning*, 4:397–424, 1988.

[210] F. Rossi. Constraint logic programming, 2000. Available at `http://www2.ags.uni-sb.de/net/Forum/`.

[211] F. Sadri and F. Toni. Computational logic and multiagent systems: a roadmap. Technical report, Department of Computing, Imperial College of Science, Technology and Medicine, 1999.

[212] C. Sakama and K. Inoue. Updating extended logic programs through abduction. In M. Gelfond, N. Leone, and G. Pfeifer, editors, *Proceedings of the 5th International Conference on Logic Programming and Nonmonotonic Reasoning (LPNMR-99)*, volume 1730 of *LNAI*, pages 147–161, Berlin, 1999. Springer.

[213] E. Sandewall. Nonmonotonic inference rules for multiple inheritance with exceptions. *IEEE*, 74(10):1345–1353, October 1986.

[214] V. Saraswat and K. Ueda, editors. *Proceedings of the 1991 International Symposium on Logic Programming (ISLP'91)*, San Diego, CA, October 1991. MIT Press.

[215] E. Schapiro, editor. *Proceedings of Third International Conference on Logic Programming*, volume 225 of *LNCS*, London, 1986. Springer-Verlag.

[216] D. De Schreye, M. Hermenegildo, and L. M. Pereira. Paving the roadmaps: Enabling and integration technologies, 2000. Available from http://www.compulog.org/net/Forum/Supportdocs.html.

[217] P. Joseph Schroeder-Heister, editor. *Extensions of logic programming: international workshop, Tubingen, FRG, December 8–10, 1989: proceedings*, volume 475 of *Lecture Notes in Artificial Intelligence and Lecture Notes in Computer Science*, New York, NY, USA, 1991. Springer-Verlag Inc.

[218] SMODELS. The SMODELS system, 2000. Available at `http://www.tcs.hut.fi/Software/smodels/`.

[219] V. S. Subrahmanian, P. Bonatti, J. Dix, T. Eiter, S. Kraus, F. Ozcan, and R. Ross. *Heterogeneous Agent Systems.* MIT Press/AAAI Press, Cambridge, MA, USA, 2000.

[220] M. Turner and G. Fauconnier. Conceptual integration and formal expression. *Journal of Metaphor and Symbolic Activity*, 10(3), 1995.

[221] J. van Eijck, editor. *Logics in AI: European Workshop JELIA '90, Amsterdam, the Netherlands, September 10–14, 1990, proceedings*, volume 478 of *Lecture Notes in Artificial Intelligence and Lecture Notes in Computer Science*, New York, NY, USA, 1991. Springer-Verlag Inc.

[222] T. Veale and M. T. Keane. A connectionist model of semantic memory for metaphor interpretation. In *Proceedings of Workshop on Neural Architectures and Distributed Artificial Intelligence*, Los Angeles, CA, USA, November 1993. Centre for Neural Engineering, University of Southern California.

[223] G. Wagner. A database needs two kinds of negation. In B. Thalheim, J. Demetrovics, and H-D. Gerhardt, editors, *Mathematical Foundations of Database Systems*, pages 357–371. LNCS 495, Springer–Verlag, 1991.

[224] G. Wagner. Ex contradictione nihil sequitur. In *International Joint Conference on Artificial Intelligence.* Morgan Kaufmann, 1991.

[225] D. H. D. Warren, L. M. Pereira, and F. Pereira. PROLOG - the language and its implementation compared with LISP. In *Proc. Symp. on AI and Programming Languages SIGPLAN Notices 12 (8) SIGART Newsletter*, volume 64, pages 109–115, August 1977.

[226] D. H. D. Warren and P. Szerdei, editors. *Proceedings of the 7th International Conference on Logic Programming (ICLP '90)*, Jerusalem, 1990. MIT Press.

[227] J. Widom and S. Ceri, editors. *Active Database Systems – Triggers and Rules For Advanced Database Processing.* Morgan Kaufmann Publishers, San Francisco, 1996.

[228] M. Winslett. Reasoning about action using a possible models approach. In Reid Smith and Tom Mitchell, editors, *Proceedings of the Seventh National Conference on Artificial Intelligence*, pages 429–450, Menlo Park, California, 1988. American Association for Artificial Intelligence, AAAI Press.

[229] C. Witteveen and W. van der Hoek. A general framework for revising nonmonotonic theories. In J. Dix, Ulrich Furbach, and Anil Nerode, editors, *Proceedings of the 4th International Conference on Logic Programing and Nonmonotonic Reasoning*, volume 1265 of *LNAI*, pages 258–272, Berlin, July 28–31 1997. Springer.

[230] C. Witteveen, W. van der Hoek, and H. de Nivelle. Revision of non-monotonic theories: Some postulates and an application to logic programming. In C. MacNish, D. Pearce, and L. M. Pereira, editors, *Proceedings of the European Workshop on Logics in Artificial Intelligence*, volume 838 of *LNAI*, pages 137–151, Berlin, September 1994. Springer.

[231] XSB-Prolog. The XSB logic programming system, version 2.5, 2002. Available at `http://www.cs.sunysb.edu/~sbprolog`.

[232] Y. Zhang and N. Y. Foo. Answer sets for prioritized logic programs. In J. Małuszyński, editor, *Proceedings of the International Symposium on Logic Programming (ILPS-97)*, pages 69–84, Cambridge, October 13–16 1997. MIT Press.

[233] Y. Zhang and N. Y. Foo. Updating logic programs. In Henri Prade, editor, *Proceedings of the 13th European Conference on Artificial Intelligence (ECAI-98)*, pages 403–407, Chichester, 1998. John Wiley & Sons.

Appendix A

List of Symbols

$\mathcal{L}_{\mathcal{K}}$: propositional language generated by $\mathcal{K}$

$\mathcal{L}$: abbreviation for $\mathcal{L}_{\mathcal{K}}$

$\mathcal{K}^*$: propositional variables extended with strong negation, given $\mathcal{K}$

$\widehat{\mathcal{L}}$: extended language in which program $\biguplus_s \mathcal{P}$ is written, given $\mathcal{L}$

$\overline{\mathcal{L}}$: extended language in which program $\boxplus_s \mathcal{P}$ is written, given $\mathcal{L}$

$\mathcal{R}$: set of rules given $\mathcal{L}$

$\mathcal{E}$: language of observations

$\mathcal{S}$: set of statements given $\mathcal{L}$ and $\mathcal{E}$

$\mathcal{H}(P)$: Herbrand base of program P

$-A$: strong (or explicit) negation of A

$not\, A$: default negation of A

$\leftarrow$: rule implication symbol

$\Leftarrow$: statement implication symbol

$H(r)$: head of rule r

$B(r)$: body of rule r

M^+ : objective atoms of interpretation M

M^- : default atoms of interpretation M

$\hat{M}|\mathcal{L}$: restriction of interpretation or model $\hat{M}$ to the language $\mathcal{L}$

$least(P)$: least model of program P

$T_P(M)$: immediate consequence operator wrt. program P and interpretation M

$\preceq_T$: classical ordering among interpretations

$\vdash$: least model consequence relation

$\models$: satisfaction relation

$\models_{sm}$: satisfaction relation for the stable models semantics

$\models_{obs}$: satisfaction relation for external observations

$\models_{rule}$: satisfaction relation for rule conditions

$\frac{P}{M}$: Gelfond-Lifschitz transform of program P wrt. interpretation M

$\Gamma(I)$: $Least\left(\frac{P}{I}\right)$

$SM(P)$: stable models of P

P^{exp} : expanded extended program P

$\mathcal{P}^{exp}$: expanded extended DLP $\mathcal{P}$

P^{M} : reduct of a generalized logic program P wrt. interpretation M

$\oplus$: update operator

$\otimes$: KABUL update operator

$Rejected(M)$: rejected rules when updating P by U, given the interpretation M

$Defaults(M)$: defaults when updating P by U, given the interpretation M

$Residue(M)$: rules of P and U that are not rejected, given the interpretation M

$Reject(\mathcal{P}, s, M)$: rejected rules of (M)DLP $\mathcal{P}$ at state s wrt interpretation M

$Reject(\mathcal{P}, S, M)$: rejected rules of MDLP $\mathcal{P}$ at set of states S wrt interpretation M

$Defaults(P, M)$: defaults given a set of rules P and an interpretation M

$Rejected(M_{np}, s, \mathcal{P}')$: rejected rules for Justified Updates

$Rej(M, s, \mathcal{P})$: rejected rules for Update Answer Sets

$\rho(\mathcal{P})_s$: multi-set of (M)DLP $\mathcal{P}$ at state s

$\rho(\mathcal{P})_S$: multi-set of MDLP $\mathcal{P}$ at set of states S

$P \uplus U$: program update of P by U

$\biguplus \mathcal{P}$: dynamic program update of DLP $\mathcal{P}$

$\biguplus_s \mathcal{P}$: dynamic program update at state s of DLP $\mathcal{P}$

$\bigoplus \mathcal{P}$: DLP $\mathcal{P}$ at current state

$SM(\bigoplus \mathcal{P})$: stable models of DLP $\mathcal{P}$ at current state

$SM(\bigoplus_s \mathcal{P})$: stable models of DLP $\mathcal{P}$ at state s

$\boxplus \mathcal{P}$: multi-dimensional dynamic program update of MDLP $\mathcal{P}$

$\boxplus_s \mathcal{P}$: multi-dimensional dynamic program update at state s of MDLP $\mathcal{P}$

$\bigoplus_s \mathcal{P}$: (M)DLP $\mathcal{P}$ at state s

$\bigoplus_S \mathcal{P}$: MDLP $\mathcal{P}$ at set of states S

$\bigoplus \mathcal{P}$: MDLP $\mathcal{P}$ at at set of all states

$SM(\bigoplus_s \mathcal{P})$: stable models of MDLP $\mathcal{P}$ at state s

$SM(\bigoplus_S \mathcal{P})$: stable models of MDLP $\mathcal{P}$ at set of states S

$SM(\bigoplus \mathcal{P})$: stable models of MDLP $\mathcal{P}$ at at set of all states

D^+ : transitive closure of DAG D

D_v : relevancy DAG of D wrt vertex v

D_V : relevancy DAG of D wrt set of vertices V

$\leq_D$: relation of graph D

$\equiv$: equivalence between DLPs

$\stackrel{\oplus}{\equiv}$: update equivalence between DLPs

$\stackrel{k}{\equiv}$: k-update equivalence relation between knowledge states

$N(r)$: name of rule r

$\bowtie$: conflict relation for rules

$\stackrel{np}{\bowtie}$: conflict relation for Justified Updates

$\bar{\bowtie}$: conflict relation for alternative characterization of Justified Updates

$\dot{\bowtie}$: conflict command relation

$\rho(P^<)$: multiset of all rules in the inheritance program $P^<$

$G_I(P^<)$: reduct of inheritance program $P^<$ wrt interpretation I

$G_{\mathcal{P}}$: AND/OR-graph associated with $\mathcal{P}$

$G_{\mathcal{P}}^M$: reduced AND/OR-graph of $\mathcal{P}$ wrt. M

$\mathbf{H}(S)$: head of statement S

$\mathbf{D}(S)$: destination of statement S

$\mathbf{C}(S)$: command conditions of statement S

$\mathbf{L}(S)$: literal conditions of statement S

$\mathbf{R}(S)$: rule conditions of statement S

$\mathbf{E}(S)$: external observation conditions of statement S

$\mathbf{P}(S)$: private conditions of statement S

$Dest\,(C)$: destination of command C

$Arg\,(C)$: argument of command C

$Sel(.)$: selection function

U^r : reduced set of statements of U

U^* : logic program corresponding to the reduced set of statements U^r

$Args_R\,(U^*)$: rule arguments of U^*

$Args_S\,(U^*)$: statement arguments of U^*

$Args_H\,(U^*)$: hierarchy arguments of U^*

$Args_M\,(U^*)$: prevalence mode arguments of U^*

$BasicComm_R\,(U^*)$: basic rule commands, given U^*

$BasicComm_S\,(U^*)$: basic statement commands, given U^*

$BasicComm_H\,(U^*)$: basic hierarchy commands, given U^*

$BasicComm_M\,(U^*)$: basic prevalence mode commands, given U^*

$BasicComm\,(U^*)$: basic commands, given U^*

$PerComm\,(U^*)$: persistent commands, given U^*

$AssertComm\,(U^*)$: assert commands, given U^*

$RetractComm\,(U^*)$: retract commands, given U^*

$\mathcal{C}\,(U^*)$: commands, given U^*

$\mathcal{L}_{\mathcal{C}(U^*)}$: command language, given U^*

$Basic\,(C)$: basic command corresponding to command C

$Rejected\,(W, <, \Delta)$: rejected rules in $KABUL$

$\Omega\,(U^*)$: subsumption rules, given U^*

$Coh\,(U^*)$: coherence rules, given U^*

$Default\,(U^*, \Delta)$: default rules, given U^* and Δ

$Common\,(\mathcal{W}^*, \Delta)$: common rules in $KABUL$, given $\mathcal{W}^*$ and Δ

TF_s : transition frame at state s

I_Δ : command interpretation generated by the set of commands Δ

$\perp_{s+1}$: contradictory update atom

Γ_R : next state object level logic program operator

Γ_S : next state self update operator

Γ_H : next state hierarchy DAG operator

Γ_M : next state evolution mode operator

Γ_{PE}^+ : next state added prevalence edges operator

Γ_{PE}^- : next state removed prevalence edges operator

$\Delta^{R@\alpha}$: rule commands with destination α in Δ

Δ^H : hierarchy commands in Δ

Δ^M : prevalence mode commands in Δ

$\Delta^{S@\beta}$: statement commands with destination β in Δ

$\Delta^{H@\alpha}$: sub-agent hierarchy commands with destination α in Δ

$\Delta^{M@\alpha}$: sub-agent prevalence mode commands with destination α in Δ

EO : external observations

$\mathcal{A}$: agents

$\mathcal{SA}$: sub-agents

$\mathcal{T}$: time states

$\mathcal{H}$: agent hierarchy DAG

$\mathcal{F}$: prevalence mode functions

$\mathcal{M}$: agent prevalence modes

$\mathcal{IU}$: internal updates

$\mathcal{SH}$: sub-agent hierarchy DAGs

$\mathcal{SM}$: sub-agent prevalence modes

$\mathcal{EU}$: external updates